OXFORD MEDICAL PUBLICATIONS

# Critical appraisal
# of epidemiological studies
# and clinical trials

# Critical Appraisal of Epidemiological Studies and Clinical Trials

THIRD EDITION

J. Mark Elwood

B.C. Cancer Agency, Vancouver,
British Columbia, Canada

*Oxford   New York   Melbourne*

# OXFORD
UNIVERSITY PRESS

2007

# OXFORD

UNIVERSITY PRESS

Great Clarendon Street, Oxford OX2 6DP

Oxford University Press is a department of the University of Oxford.
It furthers the University's objective of excellence in research, scholarship,
and education by publishing worldwide in

Oxford  New York

Athens  Auckland  Bangkok  Bogotá  Buenos Aires  Cape Town
Chennai  Dar es Salaam  Delhi  Florence  Hong Kong  Istanbul  Karachi
Kolkata  Kuala Lumpur  Madrid  Melbourne  Mexico City  Mumbai  Nairobi
Paris  São Paulo  Shanghai  Singapore  Taipei  Tokyo  Toronto  Warsaw
with associated companies in  Berlin  Ibadan

Oxford is a registered trade mark of Oxford University Press
in the UK and in certain other countries

Published in the United States
by Oxford University Press Inc., New York

British Library Cataloguing in Publication Data

Data available

Library of Congress Cataloging-in-Publication Data

Elwood, J. Mark.
    Criticial appraisal of epidemiological studies and clinical trails/J. Mark
Elwood. --3rd ed.
        p. ; cm.
    Includes bibliographical references and index.
  1. Epidemiology--Research--Methodology. 2. Clinical trails. 3. Epidemiology--
Research--Evaluation. 4. Clinical trials--Evaluation. I. Title.
    [DNLM: 1. Epidemiologic Methods. 2. Clinical Trails. 3. Epidemiologic
Studies.  WA 950 E52ca 2007]
    RA652.4.E483 2007
    614.4028--dc22

                                                                            2006035976

Typeset in Minion
by Cepha Imaging Pvt. Ltd., Bangalore, India
Printed in Great Britain
on acid-free paper by
Biddles Ltd., King's Lynn

ISBN 978-0-19-921825-7 (hb)
ISBN 978-0-19-852955-2 (pb)

10 9 8 7 6 5 4 3 2 1

To Candace,
Jeremy and Briana

# Preface and acknowledgements

This book is a revised and expanded successor to *Causal Relationships in Medicine: A Practical System for Critical Appraisal*, published by Oxford University Press in 1988, and *Critical Appraisal of Epidemiological Studies and Clinical Trials*, Second Edition, published in 1998. In 1988, the book was unusual in bridging the gap between epidemiological and clinical reasoning by applying a consistent system of critical appraisal to questions of aetiology, clinical therapy, and health care management. Since that time, systematic methods of critical appraisal have been accepted as central to rational health care, both in clinical applications or with a wider health services and community perspective. Critical appraisal is the central focus of evidence-based medicine and knowledge-based health care.

The book is designed to encourage readers to apply their existing skills and knowledge within a framework of critical appraisal that can be applied to any type of study assessing the relationship between what is experienced and what eventuates. The book takes the approach that the essential issue in questions of the aetiology of disease, the effectiveness of clinical management, and the efficacy of health services is often whether a cause and effect relationship holds between the intervention or exposure and the relevant outcome. The method presented is applicable to a wide range of health care issues, to both medical and non-medical disciplines, and to many areas outside health care.

The new edition is revised throughout, and has many new sections, including those on developments in epidemiological and clinical thinking, systematic reviews and meta-analysis, and applications to clinical and health policy issues. The core text is the first nine chapters. These are followed by six examples of the application of the scheme of critical appraisal to a range of studies. Then follows an Appendix which summarizes statistical methods and useful statistical tables. Some texts of this nature are dominated by statistics; the approach here is to treat the assessment of chance variation, i.e. statistical methods, as one aspect of critical appraisal, and to review the assessment of chance variation specifically in Chapter 7. The rest of the text can be read with no mathematics beyond simple arithmetic; the essential logic of the critical appraisal approach does not require any mathematical expertise.

The extensive list of acknowledgments to colleagues and friends given in the two earlier editions applies also to this volume. For the new volume, I have greatly appreciated the untiring care in the preparation of material and in proof reading by Melissa Glogolia and Melissa Baxter at the National Cancer Control Initiative in Melbourne, Australia, and many colleagues, especially Robert Burton and Brian McAvoy, for useful discussions and suggestions. Again I thank my family for their support and patience.

I am grateful to the publishers of the *Lancet*, the *New England Journal of Medicine*, and the *Journal of the National Cancer Institute*, and to the first authors, for permission to reproduce parts of the papers shown in Chapters 10–15.

# Contents

# Introduction

*There is occasions and causes, why and wherefore in all things.*

—William Shakespeare: Henry V, v; 1599

This book presents a system of critical appraisal to help the reader evaluate studies in the health and medical fields, and also to carry out their own studies more effectively. The method emphasizes the central importance of cause and effect relationships. Over several years many doctors, nurses, health educators, health managers, and students, as well as epidemiologists and researchers, have found it interesting and useful. The great strength of the method is that it is applicable to a wide range of issues, both to intervention trials and observational studies.

The scheme is shown in **Ex. 1.** We start with a discussion of the concept of causation (Chapter 1), and then discuss the types of study design which can be used to demonstrate causation (Chapter 2) and the ways in which their key results can be expressed precisely and simply (Chapter 3). We then consider how the subjects in a study should be chosen (Chapter 4). Chapters 1–4 cover the essentials of study design, and we give examples of each of the major study designs to illustrate the concepts and some practical aspects.

We then move to the central issue of the interpretation of the results of any one study. We consider in turn each of the three non-causal explanations that have to be considered before a judgement of a causal explanation can be made. These are observation bias (Chapter 5), confounding (Chapter 6), and chance variation (Chapter 7).

In Chapter 8 we move from one study to many, reviewing the methods of systematic review and meta-analysis, the process of combining data from many studies.

We then consider features which positively support causation, and how the results from one study or set of studies can be generalized more widely (Chapter 9). Putting these steps together leads to an overall method of critical appraisal, based on the evaluation of causal relationships, which can be applied to important issues within the reader's own field of interest. This section

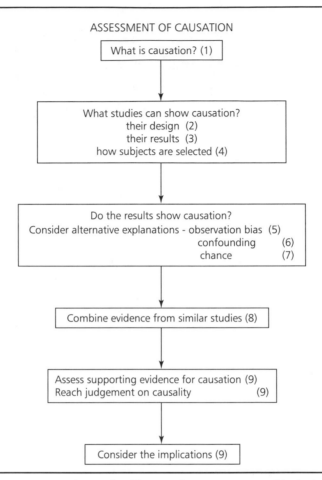

ASSESSMENT OF CAUSATION

What is causation? (1)

What studies can show causation?
their design (2)
their results (3)
how subjects are selected (4)

Do the results show causation?
Consider alternative explanations - observation bias (5)
confounding (6)
chance (7)

Combine evidence from similar studies (8)

Assess supporting evidence for causation (9)
Reach judgement on causality (9)

Consider the implications (9)

**Ex. 1.** The assessment of causation. The overall strategy presented in the book for assessing the evidence for and against causality in a particular issue. Numbers indicate the relevant chapter

concludes by reviewing the applications of critical appraisal to evidence-based medicine, knowledge-based health care, and health practice and policy.

Chapters 10–15 give six examples of the application of the scheme to studies of different designs and topics: a randomized trial of medical treatment, a randomized trial of a preventive measure, a prospective and a retrospective cohort study, a small matched case–control study, and a large case–control study. Sections of the original papers are reproduced in these chapters, although the reader will obtain the best value from them by first reading the whole of the original paper before working through the appraisal given here.

Most of this book can be understood without complex mathematics. Statistical issues are dealt with in Chapter 7 and in part of Chapter 8. The statistical methods of most value are summarized for reference in the Appendix. Statistical questions form only one aspect of the evaluation of evidence. Readers who wish to ignore the mathematical parts of this book should feel free to do so.

We use the term 'Exhibit' to refer to illustrations, to avoid the arbitrary distinction between tables and figures. In Chapters 10–15, this also distinguishes the exhibits in this book from the tables and figures in the original papers.

Chapter 1

# The importance of causal relationships in medicine and health care

*Intellectual progress is by no one trait so adequately characterized as by the development of the idea of causation.*

—Herbert Spencer: The data of ethics, IV; 1879

The study of causal relationships is essential to medicine and health care (**Ex. 1.1**). In treating a patient, the decision to offer a treatment is based on the assumption that that treatment will *cause* an improvement in the patient's condition. The study of the causes and prevention of a disease involves determining which factors *cause* the disease to occur. In health service management, the decision to provide a certain type of service or facility assumes that it will *cause* an improvement in the health of the individuals or the community that it serves. On my desk today there are new studies on whether the prenatal environment leads to diabetes, assessments of new treatments for heart disease, malaria, and bladder cancer, and a discussion on whether clinical leadership improves the performance of health services. These articles essentially ask questions of causality. Does a specific treatment cause an improvement in the patient's condition? Do particular factors cause diseases to occur? Do different systems of health management cause improvements for the users of the service? Most critical issues in health care and most controversial issues depend on the assessment of whether a cause and effect relationship exists.

In this book, we will explore the methods available to us to test whether relationships are in fact causal, and therefore to decide whether the assumptions behind decisions relating to therapy, aetiology, and health service management are true or false.

This *critical appraisal* process is central to the related topics of *meta-analysis* and *evidence-based medicine*. The evaluation of what is done and what is not done in health care, in terms of its basis in scientific evidence, depends on correct judgements being made about causal relationships.

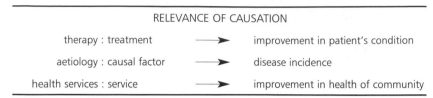

RELEVANCE OF CAUSATION

therapy : treatment    ⟶    improvement in patient's condition

aetiology : causal factor    ⟶    disease incidence

health services : service    ⟶    improvement in health of community

**Ex. 1.1.** The relevance of causal relationships in health care. Decisions on therapy, aetiology, or health services provision all make assumptions of cause and effect relationships

We will concentrate on the critical appraisal of epidemiological studies and clinical trials. We will present a practical system for critical appraisal, which can be applied to any of the main types of study that assess relationships between an *intervention or exposure* and an *outcome*. The central issue is whether any association seen between the intervention or exposure and the outcome indicates a cause and effect relationship; if so appropriate action can follow. If a cause and effect relationship does not exist, the association must be due to other mechanisms; this conclusion has different practical consequences.

## Definition of causation, and types of causation

To discuss causal relationships, we must have a definition of causation, and this definition will determine how causation can be demonstrated or disproved. The concept of causation often brings to mind only the extreme and limiting situation, which is the situation where a certain event *always and invariably* follows another event. This is a familiar notion because it is regularly observed in the physical sciences. For example, Boyle's law states that at a given temperature, the volume of a fixed mass of a gas is inversely proportional to its pressure. Thus a change in pressure results invariably and automatically in a corresponding change in volume (**Ex. 1.2**). The effect is instantaneous, can be replicated easily, and can be expressed as a simple mathematical relationship. Therefore there is little difficulty in accepting the notion that a change in pressure *causes* a change in volume. Similarly, there is little difficulty in the concept that applying heat to a metal bar *causes* it to expand; again there is an invariable and almost immediate relationship between the 'outcome', i.e. the change of length of the bar, and the 'exposure', i.e. the heat applied to the bar.

This type of causation has a number of special properties. The chief among them is that the causal agent is *sufficient*, in other words the operation of the

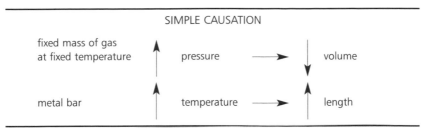

**Ex. 1.2.** Simple causal relationships. Causal relationships in the physical sciences are often simple, as in Boyle's law relating pressure and volume of a gas, or the effect of heat on a metal bar. The causal agent is sufficient, the time relationship is short, and replication is easy

one defined causal agent invariably produces the outcome. Secondly, the time relationship between the action of the causal agent and the effect produced is very short. Thirdly, because the situation can be modelled in an experiment, it can be replicated with ease under controlled conditions.

Situations that are relevant to human health and disease are rarely as simple. In human health and disease not all causal agents are sufficient. For example, the disease tuberculosis is caused by infection of the human body by the tubercle bacillus (**Ex. 1.3**). However, infection by the tubercle bacillus does not invariably lead to clinical tuberculosis. Only a small proportion of those who are infected by the bacillus develop clinical disease, and a number of other factors influence whether the disease develops, such as poor nutrition (**Ex. 1.4**). Thus a combination of tubercle bacillus infection and poor nutrition, with perhaps other factors, is required for clinical disease. We must consider both the tubercle bacillus and poor nutrition as causal factors; indeed improved nutrition was the main cause of the reduction in tuberculosis in the first half of the twentieth century.

The tubercle bacillus in this situation is a 'necessary' cause of the disease. We can now define two categories of causal factors. A *sufficient* causal factor, acting on its own, will always produce the outcome. A *necessary* causal factor is one without which the outcome cannot occur; it has acted in all instances of the

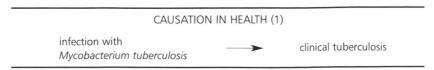

**Ex. 1.3.** Simple causal relationship? An apparently simple causal relationship in medicine. But while the causal agent is necessary, it is not sufficient and the time relationship is uncertain

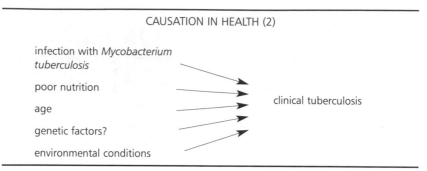

CAUSATION IN HEALTH (2)

infection with *Mycobacterium tuberculosis*

poor nutrition

age

genetic factors?

environmental conditions

clinical tuberculosis

**Ex. 1.4.** Simple causal relationship? A somewhat more complete diagram of the causes of clinical tuberculosis

outcome (**Ex. 1.5**). In the Boyle's law situation, a change in pressure was both necessary and sufficient for a change in volume, given that the other circumstances were fixed. In the metal bar example, heat was a sufficient but not a necessary cause; there are other ways of lengthening a metal bar.

Most situations in health and disease do not fulfil the criteria for either necessary or sufficient causation. If an otherwise healthy man is admitted to hospital with multiple fractures, having been hit by a bus just outside the hospital, we would conclude that there was a causal relationship between being hit by the bus and having multiple fractures. But the relationship implies neither that the cause is sufficient nor that it is necessary. Not all people hit by buses have multiple fractures. Not all patients with multiple fractures have been hit by buses.

A frequent error of logic is to define causation in a way that describes only the limiting case of the necessary and sufficient cause. Thus the fact that Uncle Joe is alive and well at age 95, having smoked 20 cigarettes a day since age 10, does not

TYPES OF CAUSAL RELATIONSHIPS

necessary — the outcome occurs only if the causal factor has operated.
sufficient — the operation of the causal factor always results in the outcome.
both     — the causal factor and the outcome have a fixed relationship; neither occurs without the other.
neither   — the operation of the causal factor increases the frequency of the outcome, but the outcome does not always result, and the outcome can occur without the operation of the causal factor.

**Ex. 1.5.** The different types of causal relationships. The last category is by far the most important

---

DEFINITION OF CAUSE

cause: a factor is a cause of an event if its operation increases the frequency of the event

---

**Ex. 1.6.** The general definition of cause. Necessary and sufficient causation are merely extremes within this definition

show that smoking is not harmful; it shows only that smoking is not a sufficient cause of death or disability before age 95. This one observation can disprove a hypothesis of sufficient causation. But to assume, on this evidence, that no type of causation exists between smoking and disease is like concluding that the existence of elderly veterans of a war means that war does not kill people.

We must use a concept of causation that is relevant to health issues, and define a causal association in a way that is applicable to real situations. The definition of cause we will use is: *a factor is a cause of an event if its operation increases the frequency of the event* (**Ex. 1.6**).

The opposite of a causal factor is, of course, a preventive factor, whose operation decreases the frequency of the outcome event. The concept of causality, and the evidence required to assess it, applies equally to preventive issues.

Returning to the man with multiple fractures, what led us to the conclusion that these were caused by having been hit by a bus? The main evidence is the immediate time relationship. Consider another situation. A woman has persistent headaches and gives a history of a head injury some months previously. Can we assume a causal relationship in this case? We cannot easily make such a judgement, because the time relation is not so clear and so many other events may have occurred. Suppose, however, we study a number of patients who have persistent headaches, and we find that most of them give a history of a head injury. We should then be justified in suspecting that the apparent connection between the two events indicates a cause and effect relationship. However, we need to be cautious about our method of recording a history of previous injury. Some people who have had an injury may not be able to remember it, and similarly many of the injuries reported might be expected as part of normal life. To go much further we need to ask whether the *frequency* with which such events have been experienced by subjects with persistent headaches is different from 'what we would expect'. To know 'what we would expect', we need to determine, by comparable methods, the frequency of such injuries in similar people who do not have persistent headaches.

So, where the time relation is not clear, and the concepts of necessary and sufficient cause do not hold, we need a *quantitative* assessment of the relationship, based on observations not on one individual but on a number of individuals. Hence the definition of causation is quantitative.

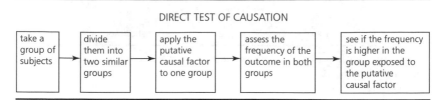

DIRECT TEST OF CAUSATION

take a group of subjects → divide them into two similar groups → apply the putative causal factor to one group → assess the frequency of the outcome in both groups → see if the frequency is higher in the group exposed to the putative causal factor

**Ex. 1.7.** One way to test causation. When applied to therapy for patients, this is the randomized clinical trial. It is also the basic controlled experiment of biology and other sciences

## A direct test of causation: the randomized trial

A direct test of the quantitative definition of causation is given if we have two groups of individuals, who are very similar in all relevant characteristics, and apply to one group the putative causative factor. 'Relevant' characteristics are those factors, other than the one under study, which affect the frequency of the outcome event. If a causal relationship exists, the frequency of the defined outcome will be higher in the group exposed to the causal factor. A study design that uses this approach is the *randomized trial*, i.e. the assignment of the treatment for each subject is made by a random or chance procedure (**Ex. 1.7**).

Randomized trials were used first in agricultural science, where, for example, fertilizers were applied to plots of soil and identical untreated plots were used for comparison; subsequently, crop yields were measured. The causal relationship between fertilizer application and crop yield was seen in the difference in crop yield between treated and untreated plots. The application of this technique to medicine dates from the late 1940s; a trial of therapy for tuberculosis (**Ex. 1.8**) is often regarded as the first such study [1], although some other early clinical trials will be mentioned in Chapter 2. The method has been used most extensively in trials of methods of treatment, where the methods compared are generally similar, for example the choice between giving one drug and giving a different drug. The ways in which randomization contributes to the study design will be discussed in later chapters; at present it is useful to note the two main features. Because the groups receiving each of the treatments being compared are selected by a chance assignment, they are likely to be similar to each other in regard to any factors (other than the treatment) which influence the outcome; therefore differences in the outcome can be attributed to the treatment. Because the different groups are being treated and assessed at the same time, it is possible to design the study so that neither the subjects nor the investigators are aware of which treatment has been given, and this *double-blind* method will allow the observations of outcome to be made in the same way for all subjects. Since that first trial, many thousand randomized trials have been carried out.

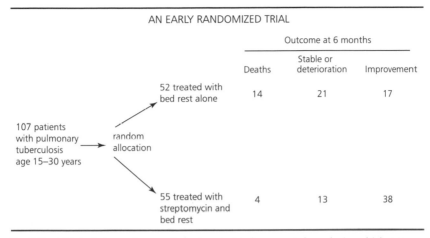

AN EARLY RANDOMIZED TRIAL

| | | Outcome at 6 months | | |
| --- | --- | --- | --- | --- |
| | | Deaths | Stable or deterioration | Improvement |
| | 52 treated with bed rest alone | 14 | 21 | 17 |
| 107 patients with pulmonary tuberculosis age 15–30 years → random allocation | | | | |
| | 55 treated with streptomycin and bed rest | 4 | 13 | 38 |

**Ex. 1.8.** A trial of chemotherapy for advanced pulmonary tuberculosis, which was organized by the British Medical Research Council and which began in 1946. Often regarded as the first randomized clinical trial. From: Medical Research Council [1]

As an aside, the tuberculosis trial arose because there was only a small amount of streptomycin in the UK immediately after the Second World War, and most of it was used for patients with advanced tuberculosis, for which the benefits were clear even without a trial, as in the absence of treatment nearly all patients would die [2]. The distinguishing mark of this trial was its use of true randomization, using random sampling numbers and sealed envelopes. The trial involved six centres, and subsequently a combined analysis of this and later trials was published, which is one of the first meta-analyses (meta-analysis will be covered in Chapter 8). There was no informed consent procedure as it was felt that if more therapy were available it would be used as the treatment of choice without specific consent, and that the consent situation for trials should not differ from routine practice.

There is no argument with the statement that the 'double-blind randomized prospective trial' is the ideal way to test a causal relationship applying to human subjects. However the procedure is not simple to carry out, not so much for scientific reasons as for practical and ethical ones. For example, to compare two types of treatment whose aim is to reduce the mortality from a chronic disease such as cancer, a large number of patients who all have a similar type of disease will have to be randomized, receive treatment, and be followed up for many years. Such a trial is obviously an expensive undertaking and will require many logistical problems to be overcome. Its results apply to the therapies used during the trial, which may be made obsolete by new therapies by the time the results of the trial are available. The absolute limitation of the prospective randomized trial is that it can be used only to assess interventions that are likely to be benefi-cial. It is clearly unethical to randomize individuals to receive a potentially harmful exposure, such as being exposed to smoking, industrial pollutants, or other toxins. Even when the comparisons are to be made between exposures that we would hope are beneficial, for example different treatments, there may well be sufficient disparity of professional opinion that many individual physicians may not judge it ethical to enter patients under their care into randomized trials.

One response to this situation is to define causation as that which can be demonstrated in a randomized trial, and to discount all other situations. This is an unrealistic stance. On this definition, we could not assume a causal rela-tionship between the multiple fractures and the bus accident. This viewpoint that a particular scientific method determines the definition of causation is the root of the commonly made assertion that epidemiological or observa-tional studies can show 'only associations'. This is not true. In the mid-1970s, several case–control studies (an epidemiological study design which will be explained in Chapter 2) suggested that women using hormonal therapy for menopausal symptoms had a substantially increased risk of cancer of the uterus. As hormonal therapy had been used for many years, the issue was very controversial and many experts strongly criticized these studies. Some of the criticism was that these were not double-blind randomized prospective trials. In a letter in response to a *Lancet* editorial which took this approach, it was pointed out that to ignore evidence other than that derived from randomized trials 'is to dismiss most of our working understanding of biology, including, for example, our presumptions about the cause of that other common intrauterine tumour, pregnancy' [3].

The argument presented in this book is that the decision as to whether a certain relationship is causal must in all cases be a balanced professional judgement. We will argue that even prospective randomized trials do not 'prove' causation, because even these trials do not give certainty; there are many practical and methodological limitations of their results. It will be argued that causation can be adequately demonstrated by other scientific methods, and that the acceptance of causation on the basis of results of such methods is essential to health care practice and planning. Only a small frac-tion of therapeutic decisions in health care can be supported by the results of randomized trials. Very few managerial or policy decisions can be so supported. Few conclusions as to the causes and natural history of disease can be supported by such evidence. For most of our knowledge of human health in terms of ther-apy, aetiology, and health care planning, we must use observational studies because of the ethical and logistical impossibility of mounting randomized trials in more than a tiny proportion of circumstances. Therefore we must be skilful in assessing such evidence and judging whether it supports a causal relationship.

## Methods of counting events: incidence and prevalence

We have seen that causation needs to be defined in terms of probabilities, and so we need to use quantitative methods. This next section reviews the terminology used in counting events in epidemiology, which may well be familiar ground to many readers.

The simplest measure of frequency is *prevalence*: the frequency of a characteristic, or the proportion of a group which has the characteristic, at one point in time. It is a simple proportion, has no units, and is measured at one point in time. In **Ex. 1.9**, there is a population of 100 000 in a community and a survey shows that at one point in time there are 800 cases of a disease present: the prevalence rate (or ratio) is 800 per 100 000. The following are real examples of prevalence rates. In a survey of 1547 people aged over 65 years in London, 563 (36 per cent) had cataract in one or both eyes, the prevalence rose from 16 per cent in men aged 65–69 to 76 per cent in women aged 85–100 [4]. This is a prevalence measure as it applies to the frequency of a condition at one point in time.

| INCIDENCE, PREVALENCE, AND DURATION | | |
|---|---|---|
| | *Time point* | *Time period* |
| | 31 Dec 2001 | 1 Jan 2001 – 31 Dec 2002 (2 years) |
| Population (average or at one time point) | 100 000 | 100 000 |
| Number of cases at one time point | 800 = prevalence prevalence rate = 800 per 100 000 | |
| Number of new cases diagnosed over a time period | | 400 = incidence incidence rate = 200/100 000 per year |
| Number of deaths over a time period | | 40 = mortality mortality rate = 20/100 000 per year |
| Average duration of disease | | $P = I \times D$ so $D = P/I = 800/200$ = 4 years |

**Ex. 1.9.** The relationship between prevalence, incidence, and duration of disease, assuming a steady state and a substantial population size

Similarly, we could say that 23 per cent of students in a university are smokers, 25 per cent are obese, and 8 per cent have red hair. In a series of autopsies, pathologists might find that the prevalence of arteriosclerosis was 60 per cent (this in particular seems to be very frequently mislabelled as incidence in pathology texts and conversation). A slightly more difficult one is that the frequency of Down syndrome in live births is about 1.5 per 1000; this is a prevalence rate, as it is the proportion of term births which show the syndrome, and may be referred to specifically as a 'prevalence rate at birth'.

An *incidence rate* is the frequency of incidents, events such as deaths or new diagnoses of disease, over a defined time period; it has units of time$^{-1}$. For example, an annual mortality rate is the number of deaths occurring in 1 year divided by the population at risk. The annual incidence of a disease is the number of new cases occurring in a year, while the prevalence at a particular date is the number of cases existing at that date. Incidence rates are numbers of cases divided by the population size. In Ex. 1.9, 400 new cases of the disease are diagnosed over 2 years, and so the incidence rate is 200 per 100 000 per year. In Australia in 2000 there was an average population of 623 134 women aged 50–54, and there were 1562 newly diagnosed cases of breast cancer, giving an incidence rate in this age group of 250.7 per 100 000 per year. In New Zealand in 1990, there were 5914 deaths from circulatory system causes in a total population of 3 379 200 people. Therefore the mortality rate for the whole population from this cause was 175 per 100 000 per year. In a study of workers at an atomic weapons establishment, 22 552 workers were identified and the average follow-up was 18.6 years, so that the total person-years of follow-up was 22 552 × 18.6 = 419 467 person-years. There were 3115 deaths during this period, giving an average death rate over the whole time period of 7.43 deaths per 1000 person-years [5]. Therefore measurement of the incidence rate requires counting events over a period of time. The term is frequently misused in place of prevalence.

In all these examples of incidence rate, the number of events (incidents) is precisely recorded, but the denominator is an approximation, representing the average or typical number of individuals at risk, or number of person-time units at risk in a whole study. This is routinely done in analysis of vital statistics and other large bodies of data. Obviously, this type of approximation is not good enough in small sets of data. More precise analysis involves life-table methods, in which the number of individuals actually at risk at any point in time is calculated precisely, and incidence rate is based on these calculations. These methods are described in Chapter 7 (p. 264).

The *population at risk* is the appropriate denominator for many rates, although in practice the total population is often used. The population at risk may be defined quite precisely in detailed studies. For example, although men can get breast cancer, in general breast cancer rates are related to the female population, and in more detailed studies the population at risk of newly incidence breast cancer may be defined more accurately by excluding women who have already developed the disease. In studying an infectious disease, the population at risk may exclude immunized subjects; in a food poisoning outbreak, the population at risk from each type of food can be defined as those who consumed that food.

*Cumulative incidence* is the proportion of a group of subjects which experiences an event from the start to the end of a specified time period, i.e. the cumulative frequency of the event. Being a measure based on incidents it requires counting events over a period of time, but as it related to one point in time, it is a simple proportion with no units. In a study of retinopathy (damage to the retina of the eye) in subjects with diabetes, the cumulative incidence by 1 year in 3743 subjects with no retinopathy at the baseline survey and an average age of 63 was 5.3 per cent, rising to 38.1 per cent by five years [6]. The outcome from major chronic diseases in patients is often expressed as a fatality rate up to a certain point in time; for example, the cumulative incidence of death for patients diagnosed with breast cancer in Norway between 1968 and 1975 reached 40 per cent at the end of 5 years after diagnosis, and, correspondingly, the survival at that point (the 5-year survival rate) was 60 per cent. In a major study of treatment of myocardial infarction, the outcome measured was cumulative mortality over 35 days since the infarction, which was about 7 per cent; i.e. by the end of 35 days, 7 per cent of the original group had died and 93 per cent were still alive [7].

If an infectious disease, or a single-source epidemic such as food poisoning, passes through a community, at the end of the epidemic we can calculate the proportion of all people who were infected as a cumulative incidence rate over the whole time period; we might find that 20 per cent of the population was affected. This is the cumulative incidence, and is also referred to as the *attack rate*. This rate is often calculated in terms of the population at risk; for example, the attack rate of measles may be calculated specifically for those who are susceptible, excluding others who are not because of immunization.

## Relationship between prevalence and incidence

Where a disease is in a stable situation in a large population (a situation of 'dynamic equilibrium'), the number of people who have a disease at one point in time (the prevalence) will depend on the incidence rate (the rate at which people develop the disease) multiplied by the average duration of the disease, ending in recovery or death. In fact, prevalence rate $(P)$ equals average incidence rate ($I$) multiplied by average duration ($D$), or $P = I \times D$. Thus, if there are 200 new cases of disease each year in a community, as shown in Ex. 1.9, and the disease lasts 4 years on average, the prevalence at one point in time will be 800 cases. The steady state assumption also means that, to keep the prevalence constant, 200 cases each year must finish; as 40 deaths each year are shown in Ex. 1.9, this implies that 40 of the 200 cases (20 per cent) are fatal, and the other people affected are either cured or die from other causes.

## Self-test questions (answers on p. 491)

**Q1.1** Give a definition of a cause or causal factor.

**Q1.2** What type of causation is shown in each of the following?
  (a) A person falls 50 feet off a roof onto concrete and sustains a fractured leg.
  (b) Exposure to the poliomyelitis virus and clinical polio.
  (c) A man smokes heavily from age 14 and develops lung cancer at age 52.
  (d) The association of extra chromosome 21 material with Down syndrome.
  (e) A change in health service purchasing policy and a reduction in health care costs.

**Q1.3** What rate, and what units, are given by:
  (a) Out of 40 children in a class, 8 wear glasses.
  (b) In a community of 50 000 people, there have been 100 road accidents in the last 2 years.
  (c) Of 100 patients who have a certain surgical operation, 14 die in hospital.
  (d) In an autopsy series, microscopic evidence of breast malignancy is found in 10 of 40 examinations.

**Q1.4** Of 1000 obese subjects, 160 already have hypertension. Over 3 years, 120 more are diagnosed with hypertension.
  (a) What is the initial, and the final, prevalence of hypertension?
  (b) What is the cumulative incidence over 3 years in the population at risk?
  (c) What is the average annual incidence rate?

**Q1.5** Consider the following data on HIV seroconversion (from negative to positive) in a high-risk group of 1000 subjects. Assume that HIV positivity is permanent, and there are no entries to or losses from the group of subjects. On 1 January 2001 there are 180 positives, on 1 January 2002 there are 200 positives, and on 1 January 2003 there are 250 positives. Calculate:

(a) the population at risk on 1 January 2001

(b) the prevalence rate at 1 January 2002

(c) the cumulative incidence over 2 years from 1 January 2001

(d) the incidence rate in 2002.

## References

1. Medical Research Council. Streptomycin treatment of pulmonary tuberculosis. *BMJ* 1948; **ii**: 769–782.
2. Yoshioka A. Use of randomisation in the Medical Research Council's clinical trial of streptomycin in pulmonary tuberculosis in the 1940s. *BMJ* 1998; **317**: 1220–1223.
3. Mack TM, Pike MC. Hormone replacement therapy and endometrial carcinoma. *Lancet* 1977; **i**(8026): 1358.
4. Reidy A, Minassian DC, Joseph J, *et al*. Prevalence of serious eye disease and visual impairment in a north London population: population based, cross sectional study. *BMJ* 1998; **316**: 1643–1646.
5. Beral V, Fraser P, Carpenter L, Booth M, Brown A, Rose G. Mortality of employees of the Atomic Weapons Establishment, 1951–82. *BMJ* 1988; **297**: 757–770.
6. Younis N, Broadbent DM, Vora JP, Harding SP. Incidence of sight-threatening retinopathy in patients with type 2 diabetes in the Liverpool Diabetic Eye Study: a cohort study. *Lancet* 2003; **361**: 195–200.
7. ISIS-4 (Fourth International Study of Infarct Survival Collaborative Group). ISIS-4: a randomised factorial trial assessing early oral captopril, oral mononitrate, and intravenous magnesium sulphate in 58 050 patients with suspected acute myocardial infarction. *Lancet* 1995; **345**: 669–685.

# Chapter 2

# Study designs which can demonstrate and test causation

*All true and fruitful natural philosophy hath a double scale or ladder, ascendant and descendent, ascending from experiments to the inventions of causes, and descending from causes to the invention of new experiments.*

—Francis Bacon: The advancement of learning, II; 1605

In the first part of this chapter, we will describe the key study designs used in clinical and epidemiological studies of causation. The designs are defined by two features: whether the study subjects are selected by their exposure or by their outcome, and the time dimensions of the study. In the second part we will describe the key strengths and weaknesses of each type of study, with many examples.

## Part 1. Types of study
## The relationship of study design to the definition of causation

The definition of a causal factor given in Chapter 1 was 'a factor whose operation increases the frequency of an event'. This implies that (i) people who are affected by the causal agent will have a higher frequency of the defined outcome, and (ii) individuals with the defined outcome will have a greater frequency of past exposure to the causal agent.

Thus there are two general types of comparative study. To test statement (i), we compare a group of people exposed to the putative causative factor with a group who are not exposed—a *cohort* study. The randomized trial introduced in Chapter 1 is a special type of cohort study, where the two groups are defined after randomization. To test statement (ii), we compare a group of people who have already experienced the outcome with a group of people without the outcome—a *case–control* study.

These studies are set up to test causal hypotheses. If the hypothesis is that the causal agent is either necessary or sufficient, or both, the results are simple to interpret. One definitive instance of mesothelioma (a type of cancer) occurring without any exposure to asbestos demonstrates that asbestos is not a necessary causal factor for mesothelioma. A single demonstration of a normal baby born to a mother who had taken thalidomide (a drug) shows that thalidomide is not a sufficient cause of birth defects. While these statements are true in logic, in real situations a single demonstration would not be enough, as the reliability of the observations would be questioned. While it is logically easy to *disprove* necessary or sufficient causation, it is impossible to *confirm* it; it is only possible to conclude on the basis of all reliably ascertained situations that the cause appears to be necessary or sufficient.

We need not pay much further attention to the unusual situations of necessary or sufficient causation. From now on we shall concentrate on the common situation: causation that is neither necessary nor sufficient. This causation gives a *quantitative relationship* between the causative factor and the outcome, and therefore the evidence for it must be expressed in quantitative terms.

## A classification of comparative studies: classification by the groups of people compared

### Cohort and intervention studies

The definition of causation leads us naturally to two basic types of study. The definition of these studies rests on the essential comparison being made. In *cohort* and *intervention* studies, groups of individuals are defined in terms of their exposure to the putative causative factor. The outcome in the 'exposed' group is compared with the outcome in the 'unexposed' group (**Ex. 2.1**). To find out if oral contraceptives cause, or protect against, heart disease, a research team could identify a group of women starting to use oral contraceptives and a group of non-users, and follow them over time to record the frequency of heart disease in each group. This is a cohort study (as it compares 'exposed' with 'unexposed' groups).

The cohort study just described is an *observational* study: the researchers observe the natural events; they do not influence which women use oral contraceptives. In *intervention* studies, the investigators control the assignment of individuals to the intervention, and so intervention studies are a special type of prospective cohort study. Thus, in the example given in Chapter 1, the clinical outcome in a group of tuberculosis patients treated with an antibiotic was compared with the outcome in a group treated without the drug.

COHORT STUDY

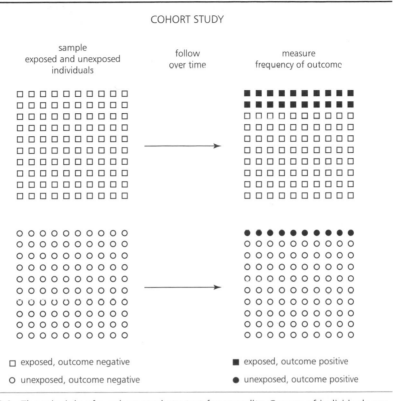

| | sample exposed and unexposed individuals | follow over time | measure frequency of outcome |

☐ exposed, outcome negative          ■ exposed, outcome positive

○ unexposed, outcome negative       ● unexposed, outcome positive

**Ex. 2.1.** The principle of a cohort study to test for causality. Groups of individuals are chosen, 'exposed' and 'unexposed' to the putative causal factor. The frequency of the outcome is measured in each group. The results would be expressed as:

| | Outcome | | Total subjects |
|---|---|---|---|
| | yes | no | |
| Exposed group | 20 | 80 | 100 |
| Unexposed group | 10 | 90 | 100 |

The term 'cohort' merely means a group of people with some common characteristic; for example, a 'birth cohort' is a group of people born in the same year or time period. Some studies merely describe the experience of such a group, and so can be called cohort studies. Thus to assess the incidence of eye disease (retinopathy) in subjects with diabetes, Younis *et al.* [1] conducted a prospective cohort study over 5 years of over 3700 patients with diabetes in England who had no retinopathy at the start of the study. As the objective was to measure the frequency of eye disease, no comparison group was needed.

However, our interest is in comparative studies, comparing people with different exposures, who may be regarded either as subsets of a single cohort or as members of different cohorts.

## Case–control studies

In *case–control* studies, groups of individuals are defined in terms of whether they have or have not already experienced the outcome under consideration, and the exposure is then measured (**Ex. 2.2**). For example, children with asthma (the 'cases') might be compared with unaffected children of the same age (the 'controls') in terms of aspects of their home environment.

In one of the earliest case–control studies of non-infectious disease, Dr Percy Stocks and Ms Mary Karn carried out a study in London in 1930 comparing patients with a range of types of cancer with subjects of the same age and sex without cancer, selected by the doctors of the cancer patients [2]. Many factors, such as keeping a dog or cat, having constipation, and pipe smoking, were assessed, but the conclusion emphasized by the authors was that the cancer patients ate vegetables less frequently than did the controls, suggesting a protective effect. This association was statistically significant, and the authors concluded that it 'seemed to be inexplicable from random causes' and suggested that further comparative studies, or an intervention study, could be undertaken to clarify it further. There is now substantial evidence that the intake of fresh vegetables and fruit, perhaps acting through vitamin C or other antioxidants, is protective against several types of cancer.

## Surveys

From the sampling perspective, surveys are carried out on subjects chosen as all members or a representative sample of a population, but the sampling is not based on any defined exposure or outcome. Thus a national census, studies of all hospital admissions, or reviews of all patients in a practice or all members of a school or workforce are all surveys. As will be seen, different types of comparison may then be made within the surveyed group.

# Classification by time relationships

## Prospective and retrospective studies

The studies are also defined in terms of their relationship to time (**Ex. 2.3**). A study in which subjects are entered and data are collected at a point in time, and then the subjects are followed and further events recorded as they happen, is a *prospective* study. The study suggested earlier, to identify a group of women starting to use oral contraceptives and a group of non-users, and follow them

CASE–CONTROL STUDY

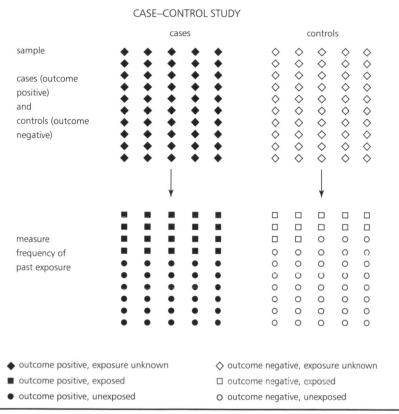

**Ex. 2.2.** The principle of a case–control design. A group of individuals who have experienced the outcome under assessment, and a group who have not, are assessed and the frequency of exposure measured in each group. The results would be expressed as:

|  | Cases | Controls |
|---|---|---|
|  | Outcome positive | Outcome negative |
| Exposed | 20 | 12 |
| Unexposed | 30 | 38 |
| Total subjects | 50 | 50 |

over time to record the frequency of heart disease in each group, is prospective; examples of such studies will be given in Chapter 4.

A *retrospective* study includes observations relating to the time at which data are collected, and also previous time. Case–control studies are always retrospective, because the outcome has already happened. To explore the

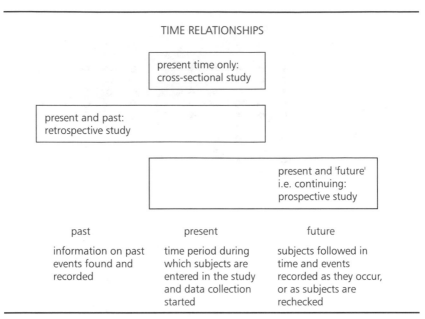

**Ex. 2.3.** The time relationships of studies

relationship between heart disease and oral contraceptive use by a retrospective case–control design, researchers would select a group of women with heart disease (cases) and a group of generally similar women without heart disease (controls), and measure for each group the frequency of exposure to oral contraceptives in the time period prior to the diagnosis of heart disease. If oral contraceptive use increases the risk of heart disease, the frequency of past use will be higher in the cases than in the controls.

## Retrospective cohort studies

A cohort study can be retrospective, in that cohorts can be defined and information collected which applies to past time. Researchers may be able to identify from medical records a group of women who were using oral contraceptives 10 years ago, and a group of women who were not. They could then go to these women, or use the medical records, to determine their subsequent history from that point to the present in terms of developing heart disease. This design can be called a *retrospective cohort study*. It is retrospective because it deals with current and past events (and so may be done fairly quickly), but it is a cohort study as the comparison made is between women who used oral contraceptives and those who did not.

In 1983 the UK Ministry of Defence commissioned a study of the health of servicemen exposed to nuclear bomb tests in Australia and the South Pacific between 1952 and 1958. In a retrospective cohort study, some 21 000 men who participated in the tests were identified and their mortality and cancer incidence from 1952 up to 1998 were compared with a comparison group of other servicemen who served in tropical and subtropical areas but were not involved in the tests. The results showed no clear increase in mortality or in any type of cancer, but there was some evidence suggesting a raised risk of some types of leukaemia [3]. Although the data were based on a follow-up of up to 45 years, the study was done in a relatively short time using the retrospective method. A major limitation is that information on other relevant exposures, including radiation exposure other than from these tests, was not available, although the choice of controls makes it likely that factors such as smoking, for example, would be similar in the two groups. Also, by relying on the Ministry of Defence records to identify both exposed and unexposed groups an estimated 15 per cent of exposed men were not identified, and it has been claimed that that omission could bias the results [4].

## Cross-sectional studies

The simplest, but weakest, type of study is one where all the information is related to one point in time and is collected at that time. Thus to assess whether high blood pressure is related to blood group O, we could survey a group of subjects and determine which of them had high blood pressure, and which were of blood group O. This is a *cross-sectional* study, as the data collected relate to a cross-section in time. Where both the putative causal factor and the outcome state are stable, so that an adequate assessment can be made (e.g. blood group), this study design may be adequate. More commonly, the exposure or outcome changes over time, and so this design is weak. For example, a cross-sectional study that compares current oral contraceptive use with current high blood pressure is a very poor method of assessing an association between oral contraceptive use and high blood pressure in women. The results will be misleading, for example, if women who develop high blood pressure stop taking oral contraceptives.

To assess the relationship between housing conditions and current health, a questionnaire was sent to a 10 per cent sample of residents in one area of England [5]. Nine per cent of the respondents reported that their housing was damp, and 49 per cent of these reported long-standing illness, compared with 37 per cent of those in dry housing. The researchers analysed these data, assessing factors such as social class, employment, and various other measures. They were aware of the limitations of the cross-sectional design, and so in their discussion they considered the possibilities that the damp housing caused the ill health, but also that people with long-standing illnesses might have more difficulty maintaining their homes, and that people who are ill may for that reason gravitate to poorer housing.

## More complex designs

The feature which defines the study is the comparison which is being made: where the groups compared are defined by their exposure, the study is a cohort study; where the groups are defined by their outcome, it is a case–control study. This principle is useful when rather more complex designs are considered.

### Case–control study within a cohort

In a cohort study, a large number of subjects may be enrolled while only a few suffer the outcome of interest. It may be useful to compare these subjects specifically with a sample of those without the outcome; this gives a case–control study within a cohort. For example, in a large prospective study in Japan between 1988 and 1990, over 65 000 subjects were surveyed and serum samples collected and stored. In 2002, an analysis was done comparing the 169 subjects who had subsequently developed colorectal cancer with 481 controls from the same cohort, using the data and samples collected earlier, and showed associations between serum fatty acid levels and cancer risk [6]. The study required analysis of a few hundred serum samples, rather than many thousand. As the case–control study is 'nested' within the larger prospective cohort study, this can be referred to as a 'nested' case–control study.

### Cohort and case–control analyses within a cross-sectional survey

Most analyses of a cross-sectional survey will examine the frequency of characteristics and associations between them in the sampled group without considerations of causality; however, in addition to such 'survey' analysis, exposure or outcome based comparisons can be made. Thus a survey may be used to identify subgroups with different exposures, who are then followed giving a prospective cohort study, or subgroups can be defined in terms of an outcome and more detailed case–control comparisons can then be made.

### Summary: types of study design

The different types of study are illustrated by work on a vitamin (folic acid) and a type of birth defect (neural tube defect) over some 20 years [7]. Descriptive epidemiological and clinical studies showed features suggesting a nutritional aetiology (such as a higher frequency in births to less affluent mothers, and time and geographical associations). A *case–control* study comparing mothers of affected babies with control mothers suggested lower levels of folic acid in the 'case' mothers [8]. Then, in an *observational prospective cohort* study, researchers measured blood levels of folic acid in about 1000 women in early pregnancy and showed that the frequency of the birth defect was higher in women with low blood levels [9]. Subsequently, in a *non-randomized intervention* study, they offered folic acid dietary supplements to some women, comparing them with others not given supplements; the frequency of the defects was reduced in those receiving supplementation, but the result was not easy to interpret as there were other differences between the two groups [10]. Finally, a *randomized intervention* study was performed, in which women were randomly assigned to receive either supplements with folic acid, or supplements without folic acid; this also showed a large reduction in the frequency of the birth defects, which is a definitive result as no other factor differed between the groups of women being compared [11]. This randomized study is described in Chapter 11.

By defining both the sampling system and the time relationships, studies can be categorized in a way that is useful in their interpretation (**Ex. 2.4**). We have now defined the most important study designs: intervention trials, observational cohort studies, case–control studies, and surveys. These main study designs have different applications, and answer different questions; the design of choice will be determined by the question to be answered, or will be dictated by practical and resource restraints. The main designs have different strengths and weaknesses, and so in assessing a study it is important to identify the design used, and then to keep these likely strengths and weaknesses in

STUDY DESIGN: SAMPLING, TIME RELATIONSHIP, AND ANALYSIS

| Sampling system | Time relationship | Type of analysis |
|---|---|---|
| COHORT: Select on exposure | prospective, retrospective, or cross-sectional | cohort |
| INTERVENTION: Assign exposure | prospective | cohort |
| CASE–CONTROL: Select on outcome | retrospective or cross-sectional | case–control |
| SURVEY: Total or sample of a defined population | cross-sectional or retrospective | survey, plus cohort or case–control analyses comparing subgroups |

**Ex. 2.4.** The different types of study design

mind when appraising it. The method of analysis depends on the sampling system used rather than on the time relationships. This is why it is essential to understand the sampling system used in a study, as only by so doing will the correct method of analysis be chosen.

That the terminology of study design can be confusing is shown by a 1996 publication which is called a 'retrospective case–control study' in the title, but a 'historical cohort study' in the abstract [12]. The confusion appears to arise because 'case–control' is sometimes used for any study that has cases and controls, which of course can be almost any design. In this study, a case series of patients with cancer of the head and neck was used to provide two cohorts: relatives of these patients, who had the exposure of a family history of the cancer, and relatives of the spouses of the original case patients, who form the unexposed cohort. The outcome was the occurrence of head and neck cancer in these two cohorts, and so the description in the abstract was correct. In another example, the incidence of malaria was monitored in villages in Ethiopia close to small dams recently constructed to assist irrigation and was found to be seven times higher than in comparison villages that were not near dams [13]. This is a prospective cohort study, yet the accompanying editorial in the *British Medical Journal* comments on the 'weakness of the case–control design'.

## Part 2. The strengths, weaknesses, and applications of the main study designs, and examples

### Intervention trials

The *purpose* of an intervention trial is to measure the effect of the intervention on certain predetermined outcomes. These trials are limited (in humans) to the evaluation of interventions that are likely to be beneficial. Their main role is in the assessment of treatment, where the randomized clinical trial is accepted as the optimal method, but they are increasingly being applied to preventive programmes and to management questions as well. Intervention trials provide a direct test of the causal hypothesis that a change in the exposure factor produces a change in the outcome.

The trials are designed so that subjects receiving the intervention are similar to those in the comparison group, with regard to both any other care they receive and other characteristics that might influence the outcome being assessed. This is best achieved by using *randomization*, i.e. by selecting people who are eligible for either the intervention under test or the comparison procedure, and then selecting those who will receive the test intervention by a random process. Usually, consent is obtained before randomization, so that each subject needs to agree to all the possible interventions offered and to the randomization process. In large trials with an option of normal care, it may be appropriate to seek consent only from those offered the new intervention, after randomization.

The randomized intervention study has *advantages* that are shared by no other type of study. Randomization is usually the best method of obtaining two or more groups of subjects whose outcome rates, in the absence of any treatment effect, are likely to be the same. A randomized design makes it easier to use techniques such as single- or double-blind methods to minimize bias in the recording of the outcome, as will be discussed in Chapter 5. Therefore, whenever a major question arises, consideration must be given to whether a randomized intervention trial can be mounted. Often the possibility is too readily dismissed. Ineffective interventions may continue to be used, or effective interventions not widely adopted, because of the inconclusive results from less rigorous study designs. This applies not only to aspects of therapy, but also to questions of prevention, public education, and the provision of services. There is a strong case for greater use of randomized intervention studies in other social areas, such as education, management, and law.

Aside from their fundamental limitation to interventions that are likely to be beneficial, the main *disadvantages* of intervention trials relate to their requirements in terms of organization, time, cost, and resources, and in the ethical questions they raise. Clinical trials of therapy to assess modest, although important, improvements in treatment need large numbers of subjects, as will be discussed in Chapter 7. Such studies require a high degree of commitment and cooperation from health professionals and their patients. Often it is more difficult to obtain cooperation from health professionals than from patients. Large-scale trials comparing different methods for the treatment of common diseases, or assessments of preventive or screening activities, often represent triumphs of organization and persistence in the face of prejudice and apathy. Time is a problem where long follow-up is required, for example to assess survival in diseases like cancer. This may mean that the therapy assessed is obsolescent by the time the results are available. The fact that the randomized trial is an excellent scientific design does not mean that all randomized controlled trials are good or that their results are correct. A survey in 1998 of 2000 randomized trials in the treatment of schizophrenia reported that the majority were of less than 6 weeks duration, included only a small number of patients, and were of poor quality [14], and many reviews in other topics have reported similar conclusions.

Clinical trials are appropriate when a new therapy looks as if it may give better results than an established therapy. A trial will be unethical if the new therapy has very little chance of being better, or if the new therapy is clearly much better, making it the treatment of choice. In the 1948 trial of treatment for tuberculosis discussed in Chapter 1, some of limited supply of streptomycin was used to treat the most severe forms of tuberculosis, miliary and meningeal tuberculosis. A comparative trial was not done, as the usual outcome was so bad that if even one patient recovered after treatment with streptomycin, this would clearly be important. On the other hand, according to the UK Medical Research Council (MRC) committee, the natural history of pulmonary tuberculosis was 'variable and unpredictable' so that 'evidence of improvement or cure following the use of a new drug in a few cases cannot be accepted as proof of the effect of that drug' [15].

There is room for much professional disagreement over the necessity for a clinical trial in a particular instance; for example, there was much debate about the need for, and the ethics of, the randomized trial of folate supplementation described above. The ethical basis of involvement of randomized trials is in the uncertainty principle. It is appropriate to offer a trial to patients if the responsible clinician is uncertain as to which of the trial treatments would be best for that particular patient, and that neither the clinician nor the patient is aware of any medical or non-medical reason why one of treatments might be inappropriate for them.

## Examples of intervention trials

The randomized clinical trial is accepted as the best method of investigation of new medical therapies; indeed, in many areas of therapeutics little attention is given to any studies other than randomized trials. One of the first such trials, of streptomycin treatment for tuberculosis in 1946–1948, was described in Chapter 1. It was a small quick trial (107 patients, and the main result was obtained in 6 months), which was possible because the effect size was large: a decrease in death rate from 27 to 7 per cent (Ex. 1.8). The *British Medical Journal* devoted its issue of 31 October 1998 to the fiftieth anniversary of this trial [16], including a reprint of the original report and several interesting papers on both past trials and issues for the future [17,18]. Sir Richard Doll gives the earliest randomized trial as the trial of immunization against whooping cough in children aged 6–18 months in the UK, which was started in 1946 but was published a few months after the report of the tuberculosis trial [17]; parents were told that half the inoculations in the study would not be active, and their consent was obtained before randomization.

The fairly late adoption of randomization in human disease trials was due to the need to gradually make this rather revolutionary method acceptable to clinicians. Randomization had been developed and used in agricultural research by R.A. Fisher and others, and had been used in trials of social programmes earlier in the century. Prior to this, some comparative trials used alternating treatments by order of entry or by day of admission, such as Fibiger's trial of serum treatment of diphtheria in Denmark in 1896–1887 [19], and several British studies in the 1930s. A large MRC trial in 1944 to assess the antibiotic patulin as a cure for the common cold used an alternate allocation system with two active and two placebo preparations [20]; the results showed no benefit. In a remarkable trial of a social programme to reduce delinquency, some 500 boys aged 5–13 were assigned either to a therapy programme or to a non-intervention control group by a coin toss, presumably without informed consent. A report after 30 years follow-up [21] showed worse outcomes in the intervention group in several respects. Lind's work on scurvy in 1747 used simple allocation between patients, as described in Chapter 4, and similar studies were proposed but not carried out by van Helmont in 1662.

While trials with short time frames and large anticipated effects can be quite small, detection of a modest, but important, improvement in outcome may require a very large trial. An example of a modern large-scale study is a trial assessing the effects of three different medications in the treatment of suspected myocardial infarction [22]. It involved some 58 000 patients in over 1000 hospitals in 32 countries, in a study that cost about £6 million sterling. The study showed no benefit of one widely used treatment (intravenous magnesium sulphate), despite the fact that benefits had been shown by many previous small studies. However, one of the other treatments was shown to reduce mortality significantly; treating 1000 patients for 1 month with the drug captopril would save about five lives at a drug cost per life saved of about £4000.

Trials in which two or more drugs are compared, all being given in similar ways, allow very comparable protocols and make double-blind designs relatively easy. This is more difficult where different types of care are being compared. For example, until the 1970s it was accepted that even uncomplicated suspected myocardial infarction required hospital treatment, but a trial comparing general practitioner care with immediate hospitalization showed no difference in mortality [23]. The trial required a skilled team to respond immediately when a general practitioner notified the hospital of a patient with suspected myocardial infarction and to visit the patient at home, and then randomized patients in whom both the options of hospital and home care appeared reasonable and the patient agreed to participate.

In the first trial of screening for breast cancer, some 62 000 women aged 40–64 in a health maintenance organization in New York were randomized into two equally sized groups; one group was offered the new screening intervention, mammography, and the other group received their normal care. Informed consent was obtained after randomization only from the group who were offered the extra intervention of mammographic screening; some 65 per cent of those women accepted the offer. No extra intervention or consent procedure was used for the comparison group, who did not necessarily know about the trial. Long-term follow-up to assess particularly the occurrence and mortality from breast cancer was instituted and is continuing. After 10–14 years of follow-up, the death rate from breast cancer in the women randomized to being offered mammographic screening was 30 per cent less than that of the comparison group [24].

The National Cancer Institute in the USA is running a complex randomized trial (the PLCO trial) to assess, in the same trial, screening techniques for prostate, lung, colorectal, and ovarian cancer, which together make up almost half of all cancers diagnosed. Over 150 000 volunteers are involved in the trial and results will accumulate over several years. Updates are available at the trial website http://www.cancer.gov/prevention/plco/.

There has been much emphasis in recent years on preserving the value of clinical trials by making sure they are done correctly and reported without bias. Standard formats for reporting results have been developed, such as the CONSORT recommended system [25], which ensure that all subjects assessed for eligibility are accounted for, whether excluded or randomized. These criteria and recommended formats are kept under review and are available from websites such as http://www.consort-statement.org. We will review this further in Chapter 4, and the CONSORT standard reporting template for a randomized trial will be shown in Ex. 4.8 (p. 96). Another emphasis has been on ensuring all trials that are performed are reported, so that all the results can be assessed to avoid publication bias. This is discussed further in Chapter 8. Investigators are encouraged to register their trial and submit the protocol when the trial is designed. Many leading medical journals will now only publish the results of trials which have been registered in advance, and which are reported according to the CONSORT criteria.

## Crossover trials

Where a treatment is designed to give short-term benefit in a continuing disease, the effects of different treatments can be tested by giving them to the same patients at different times. In a randomized crossover trial, each patient is allocated each of the treatments in random order. To ensure that the effects of one treatment have completely disappeared before the other treatment is tried, a suitable 'washout period' has to be set. The analysis is a paired analysis comparing each patient's responses, which may be quantitative or qualitative, during each treatment phase compared with the other phases. There are several specific statistical issues applying to these trials, such as assessing if the time period or order of the treatments is important, and specific methods to estimate the appropriate study size [26]. These will not be dealt with here. In suitable applications, the design is efficient as one patient provides data on all treatments, so with two treatments the number of subjects needed is about half that of a conventional two-arm trial.

As an example, a randomized crossover study was used to assess a specific treatment (lisinopril, an angiotension-converting enzyme inhibitor) compared with placebo in the prevention of migraine [27]. Participants, who were regular migraine sufferers, were observed during a 4-week run-in period during which they were given (unknown to them) the placebo drug, and then were randomized into two groups. Thirty patients received the active drug (not knowing if it was active or placebo) for 12 weeks, discontinued it for a 2-week washout period, and were then given the placebo for a second 12-week period. The other group of 30 had the placebo drug first, and the active drug later. The patients kept a daily diary of migraine attacks and other symptoms. The trial was double blind. The main results were quantitative, assessing hours and days with headache and days with migraine, and showed on a matched analysis a statistically significant 20 per cent improvement when on the active drug. The presence or absence of adverse affects was also assessed using a paired analysis.

## Individual patient (*n*-of-1) trials

In contrast with the very large studies, the efficacy of different treatments for a long-term condition in a single patient can be compared by a crossover design using randomization between different treatments given for periods of time. The '*n*-of-1' study is applicable to long-standing diseases where the objective is to improve function or decrease symptoms or disability, rather than to cure the disease. The objective is to assess the better intervention for each patient, rather than the one which is better on average; but a series of such studies can assess treatments more generally [28]. An example is a comparison of two different medications for osteoarthritis, assessing 2-week courses of each of the treatments in randomized order [29]. Other uses have been in hypertension and chronic respiratory disease. A small survey in primary care showed that patients participating in these trials appreciated their active involvement, for example through keeping symptom diaries, and had a sense of empowerment and control [30]. Mahon *et al.* [31] used a conventional two-arm randomized trial to compare conventional care with the option of selecting medication by *n*-of-1 trials. In this study, patients with chronic respiratory disease were randomized either to have an *n*-of-1 trial comparing a drug (theophylline) against placebo, continuing with the choice which gave a better outcome on the basis of the *n*-of-1 trial, or to have standard management where the theophylline was continued if the patient's respiratory disease had improved while using it. While the preliminary results showed a benefit in lower drug use at 6 months follow-up, later results showed no differences at 1 year follow-up on larger numbers of patients.

## Community-based cluster trials

Where the intervention is made on a community basis, it is appropriate to assign the intervention and make the comparisons amongst groups of people, from families to communities. Thus in an intervention study in Ethiopia, households were provided with either iron cooking pots or aluminium pots on a random basis, and the change in haemoglobin level in one child per household assessed over 12 months, with almost all children being followed; this showed that children in households supplied with iron pots had lower risks of anaemia and improved growth [32].

To evaluate the impact of improved water supplies or village health workers' activities in a developing country, comparisons between villages are appropriate. To evaluate health promotion activities, comparisons between towns, workforces, or schools may be appropriate; for example, studies of the prevention of coronary heart disease have compared workforces receiving a complex intervention programme with those not receiving it. Differences in the calculation of the necessary size of the study, and many other methodological issues, are involved when communities rather than individuals are compared [33].

Health care intervention may be done in general practices or hospitals. A trial of a new method for the diagnosis of skin lesions in primary care, with the objective of reducing unnecessary excisions, involved randomizing 223 general practices in Perth, Australia, equipping and training the 468 doctors in the intervention practices to use the new method, and comparing the ratios of benign to malignant lesions excised in the intervention and the control practices over a year [34]. The design avoided the consent processes needed if patients were to be individually randomized, and was relevant as the new system would be implemented at a practice level; but the results showed no benefit of the new method.

## Non-randomized intervention trials

Because of the logistical or ethical problems of randomization, non-randomized interventional studies may be used. However, without the strengths that randomization gives in avoiding biases, non-randomized intervention trials are more difficult to interpret. Indeed, non-randomized intervention studies may be best considered as observational cohort studies. They are especially valuable in situations where randomization would be very difficult or unacceptable.

Such intervention trials include studies of fluoridation of water supplies in which communities using fluoridated water were compared with generally similar communities continuing with unfluoridated supplies [35]. In health education, the Stanford Heart Prevention Project compared intensive methods of health education in two communities, comparing them with rather similar communities that did not receive the intervention [36,37]. A recent non-randomized study of screening has had very clear results. Neuroblastoma is a cancer affecting young children, which can be detected by a urine test in young children, and screening has been advocated, especially in Japan. In Canada, a comparison was made between a cohort of births in Quebec, where a screening programme was set up, and a comparison cohort, unscreened, in Ontario. The results showed that screening produced a great increase in the incidence rate of diagnosed neuroblastoma, but the mortality rate was not reduced. The interpretation was that screening produced a substantial number of false-positive diagnoses, and also 'silent tumours', which are tumours which were diagnosed as neuroblastoma and treated, but which if left alone would not have produced any clinical problems [38]. The results prevented further programmes from being set up, and led to the discontinuation of neuroblastoma screening in Japan.

In clinical trials of therapies, the outcome can be easily influenced by differences in the subjects selected for different treatments; the numbers of subjects are usually small, so that non-randomized trials are regarded with considerable suspicion. There are many examples of situations in which apparently similar groups of patients treated by apparently similar methods give considerably different outcomes, with no ready explanation. Several examples in surgery, such as gastric freezing, were documented in an influential book [39]. This treatment for peptic ulcer, using a gastric balloon with a coolant, was widely used in the USA in the 1960s on the basis of a logical argument that cooling reduces gastric acid secretion, and the unsystematic comparison of results after the treatment with past experience. A randomized trial then showed no benefit, and indeed somewhat worse results, when the treatment was compared with a sham treatment [40].

An unfortunate example is a study to compare the survival of patients with breast cancer attending a centre for alternative medicine in England with a comparison group selected from patients attending conventional hospitals [41]. The great difficulty in this type of study is to ensure comparability between the two groups in all other factors that relate to survival, particularly the extent (size and staging) of the breast cancer before treatment. This study showed worse survival in patients seen at the alternative medicine centre. It created much controversy, and subsequently the authors stated that they did not think the reduction in survival was due to the alternative medicine regimen, but was more likely to be due to a greater initial severity of disease in those who attended the centre. However, this explanation was not given prominence in the original paper, which was regarded by many as being seriously in error. Many correspondents felt that the problems in interpretation showed that only randomized trials should be used to assess different modes of treatment. Indeed, a randomized trial had been proposed, but agreement for such a trial could not be obtained from all parties.

A still common, but unsatisfactory, design is to compare the results of patients given a new treatment with previous patients given the previously used treatment, sometimes called *historical controls*. This is a particularly dangerous comparison, as there are many factors that may influence why a particular patient is offered or accepts the new treatment. A slightly better comparison may be to compare all patients undergoing treatment in a particular facility after the new treatment is introduced with all patients seen at the facility before it was introduced, thus avoiding the problems of individual selection and acceptance of the new treatment. However, this design is dependent on there being no change in the factors that influence patients to go to that particular facility (i.e. the referral patterns). Also, when a new intervention is introduced, the professionals who deliver it may well act differently to those who continue to use the conventional programmes. A new educational approach in schools, for example, is very likely to be first taken up and promoted by particularly interested teachers, and it may be the differences between these teachers and others which affect the educational outcome, rather than particular properties of the new programme.

In contrast, other non-randomized trials have given results that have been confirmed by a randomized study. In a non-randomized study of the prevention of congenital defects by dietary supplementation, women who came for genetic counselling in good time for their next pregnancy were offered and accepted the dietary supplement. They were compared with women who did not receive the supplement, in most cases because they did not seek professional help early enough in regard to their next pregnancy. The comparison showed a considerable reduction in birth defects in women receiving the supplement, but this could obviously be influenced by a large number of factors which would be related to whether the woman sought professional help in time for her to be offered supplementation [10]. However, a further study showed that in the area of England where this study was carried out, the recurrence rate of the defect in *all* births to at-risk women fell over time, at the same time as the proportion of all at-risk women receiving this dietary supplementation rose [42]. While still a non-randomized comparison, and open to the major problem that something else might be changing over time which affects the recurrence rate, this second comparison does avoid the individual selection effects which complicate the comparison between women being offered and not being offered the supplement. As noted earlier, these results were later confirmed by a randomized trial, which reported in 1991 [11]; it is an interesting question whether more action should have been taken after the 1981 results, rather than waiting 10 years for the later results.

## Observational cohort studies

The other types of studies involve observation rather than intervention, i.e. the researcher does not control the intervention, but merely observes its effects. A cohort study is designed to answer the question: 'What are the effects of this particular exposure?' The studies compare a group of people with the exposure under consideration with a group without the exposure, or with a different level of exposure. In a prospective cohort study, the exposure is defined and the subjects are selected before the outcome events occur. This ensures that the time relationship between exposure and outcome is appropriate; the follow-up procedures allow direct measurement of the incidence rate of the outcome(s) in each of the groups being studied.

Therefore cohort studies are the appropriate method for studying the effects of a certain exposure. Thus cohort studies were set up to follow survivors of the atomic bomb explosions in Japan in 1945 and those affected by the Chernobyl nuclear plant accident in 1986, assessing many endpoints, for example total mortality or the incidence of leukaemia. The effects of many occupational hazards have been established by studying cohorts of exposed workers, comparing their subsequent mortality or morbidity either with defined comparison groups or with the general population, which can be regarded as unexposed to the particular chemical or process.

Several studies before the Second World War showed lung scarring, and suggested a possible increase in lung cancer, in workers exposed to asbestos. Increases in several types of cancer were then shown in cohort studies, first in the UK and then in the USA [43]. These studies led to much stricter control of asbestos exposure in workplaces and in the general population, and also to legal actions that forced a major asbestos manufacturer into bankruptcy.

A major disadvantage of prospective cohort studies relates to the time required. If the outcome does not occur until after a long period the exposure, the study has to have many years of follow-up. We shall discuss in Chapter 4 the design of studies in which women using oral contraceptives were recruited either through particular clinics or through their regular doctors, and followed up over time to assess many different types of morbidity and mortality.

A retrospective cohort design will overcome this problem, but is possible only if there are adequate records for the appropriate subjects and the time period.

If the outcome does not occur frequently, the cohort study must involve large numbers of subjects to observe even a reasonable number of events. Issues of the necessary size of the study will be discussed in Chapter 7. The effective size of a study depends primarily on the number of outcome events that are observed. For example, in a prospective study of pregnancies to assess the association between a drug for maternal epilepsy and congenital malformations, data from 2332 pregnancies were obtained, but the critical figure is the number of malformed births occurring to exposed mothers, which was only six [44]. A later and larger study of this topic is discussed in the next chapter.

## Large cohort studies

The Million Women Study was set up in the UK to study the relationship between hormone replacement therapy and breast cancer incidence and mortality. Between 1996 and 2001, women coming for breast cancer screening were invited to join the study and to provide important baseline information. Follow-up was by linkage within the NHS central register to cancer registrations and deaths. As of 2003, over one million women had joined the study, with an average age of 56, and over 50 per cent had used hormone replacement therapy at some time. Over 9000 breast cancers have been reported in these women [45]. The study has enormous potential to assess other exposure factors and other disease outcomes. The study website (http://www.icnet.uk/research/studies/mws/index2.html) provides current updates and lists of publications.

The Million Women Study emphasizes relatively simple data collection at one point in time and routine follow-up through data linkage to achieve a very high sample size. This contrasts with the European Prospective Investigation into Cancer and Nutrition (EPIC), which started in 1992 and includes over 500 000 participants in 10 European countries. The participants were asked to provide extensive data including food consumption questionnaires, lifestyle data, and blood samples, resulting in the collection of nine million specimens, the largest repository of biological material in a study in the world [46]. Participants have been followed up regularly by multiple methods, and by 2004 over 20 000 cancer cases had been reported. Many of the analyses will be in the form of nested case–control studies; again a useful website gives current information (http://www.iarc.fr/epic).

Subjects may be chosen for cohort studies not because they are particularly unusual in terms of exposure, but because they can be kept under surveillance over a long period. An example of this type of study is the cohort study of the effects of smoking in British doctors started in the 1950s. Doctors were selected not because their smoking habits were particularly unusual, but because they could be followed through annual registration procedures and their rate of cooperation was expected to be high [47,48]. Using similar logic, a cohort study of American nurses was started in the late 1970s as an opportunity to assess many major health issues in women [49,50].

A cohort can be set up by doing an initial survey of a sample of subjects or of a whole community, chosen not because of any unusual characteristic of exposure but because of availability and practical considerations. Such general population follow-up studies are analysed as cohort studies comparing subjects with different exposures from within the same initial group. An important example is the Framingham Heart Study, started in the 1950s by asking for volunteers from the small town of Framingham, a short distance from Boston, Massachusetts, enrolling those who volunteered, and following them up over a long period of time [51,52].

## Cohort studies from early life

Several cohort studies have started at birth or early childhood with active follow-up. A study based on a sample of 4454 people born during a single week, 3–9 March 1946, in England, Scotland, and Wales has followed them through childhood and adolescence into adulthood; active follow-up is continuing [53,54]. A similar study in New Zealand of a group of children identified at birth in 1972–1973 in a single town has continued by inviting participants to come for a one or two day assessment of psychological and physical characteristics about every 3 years, and is now continuing to assess the children born to the original cohort members. A study of asthma from this cohort is assessed in detail in Chapter 12. An ambitious proposal for a 'conception to death' cohort study is aimed at addressing prenatal influences and events [55]. A plan for a large prospective cohort study of 500 000 individuals aged 45–69 puts emphasis on assessing biochemical and genetic parameters, using an initial questionnaire and blood sample with analyses based on different biological parameters being done later; this UK Biobank project has created considerable controversy [56].

## Case–control studies

The question asked in a case–control study is: 'What are the factors which caused this event?' Case–control studies start after the outcome event, and therefore have the opportunity to assess multiple causes relating to one event. Thus they are the prime method of assessing the causes of a new problem. A good example of the investigation of a newly recognized problem is given by studies of cancer of the vagina occurring in young women [57]. This disease had been generally described as rare, and occurring in older women, but between 1966 and 1969 seven occurrences in women aged 15–22 were reported in Boston. To investigate possible causes, these cases, plus one further patient seen in another Boston hospital, were studied, and for each 'case', four control subjects were chosen, females born within 5 days of and in the same hospital as the case women. A detailed interview schedule was drawn up, and interviews were carried out in an identical fashion on all 40 subjects. These interviews explored a wide range of possible factors, and the greatest difference between the cases and controls was in the use of diethylstilboestrol (DES) by their mothers during the pregnancy, which was documented for seven of the eight cases, but for none of the 32 controls. This suggested that it was the key causal agent, a result confirmed by further studies.

The case–control study is a natural development from the case series. If we identify people with a condition of unknown cause, we start looking for possible causes by considering the characteristics of these subjects, and we then have to consider how common those characteristics would be in an unaffected population. Beyond this, the major *advantage* of case–control studies is that they are highly efficient in terms of the numbers of subjects required. Thus, for example, in a study of the causes of breast cancer, in principle the amount of information given by studying 100 women who have developed breast cancer and 100 controls is similar to that produced by asking the same questions of a group of some 50 000 middle-aged women and following them for a year, during which 100 of them might develop breast cancer.

This advantage of numbers is because the outcome has already happened. However, that fact also results in the great *disadvantage* of case–control studies, that all information on previous events has to be collected after the outcome has happened. This produces two major problems. First, the relevant causal events may have happened a considerable time in the past, and therefore the information obtained is likely to be incomplete and inaccurate. However, the greater problem is that the case subjects, who have suffered the outcome under investigation, may tend to give different responses to the control subjects, thus introducing a bias into the information obtained on previous exposures. These problems, and methods to overcome them, will be discussed further in Chapter 4.

The advantages in the numbers of subjects and the time required for a case–control study must be compared with the disadvantages of unreliability of exposure information and possible bias in the recall of events. Often these biases are severe enough to justify a more expensive and time-consuming cohort study. Case–control studies have been of immense importance in elucidating the causes of chronic diseases, such as cancer, and the first indications of causes have often come from such studies. A good example is the association between smoking and lung cancer.

Between 1922 and 1947, the number of deaths from lung cancer in England and Wales increased by a factor of 15. While some thought this might be an artefact of diagnosis or recording, investigations suggested that the increase was real; the most favoured explanations were an effect of atmospheric pollution or of smoking tobacco, and small studies were available on each. In 1947, the MRC decided to carry out a more thorough investigation. To do this, patients with lung cancer and some other cancers in some 20 London hospitals were interviewed, along with control patients who had a range of diseases excluding cancer. The results showed that 647 of 649 men with lung cancer were smokers (99.7 per cent), but 622 out of 649 (95.8 per cent) of the control patients were also smokers. The results by detailed smoking history were more useful, and showed that the risk of lung cancer increased strongly with the amount smoked [58]. The study was then expanded, with similar results [59]. The original report of this investigation is well worth reading because of the detail given to the methodology and the consideration of biases and possible explanations of the results. For example, the issue of possible bias by the subject or the interviewer is addressed by looking at the results from a number of patients who, at the time of interview, were thought to have lung cancer, but in whom the final diagnosis was something else. The smoking habits of these patients were clearly different from those of patients who actually had lung cancer, but were similar to those of the non-cancer control patients, which would not have happened if the excess smoking recorded for lung cancer patients had been due to bias in the observations.

This was one of the first case–control studies, and acceptance of its results required several years of debate about, amongst other things, the value of the case–control approach. This study produced results in 1950; the prospective study of British doctors, published 14 years later, gave substantially the same results [47,60], as shown in **Ex. 2.5**.

## Applications of case–control studies

Although their main contribution has been to aetiological studies, case–control studies are applicable to many other questions. For example, the effect of population-based interventions can be assessed; studies of screening for cancer have been done by comparing subjects who die from the diseases in question with samples of the unaffected population [61,62]. The benefits of screening are shown by a less frequent history of screening in those who suffer the outcome which screening is designed to prevent, such as death or advanced disease; although the interpretation of these studies can be difficult [63].

---

## RISKS GIVEN BY DIFFERENT STUDIES

Relative risks of lung cancer by daily cigarette smoking from different studies

| | | | | |
|---|---|---|---|---|
| Non-smokers (referent) | 1.0 | 1.0 | 1.0 | 1.0 |
| 1–14 | 11.0 | 7.0 | 8.1 | 7.8 |
| 15–24 | 13.9 | 9.5 | 19.9 | 12.7 |
| 25+ | 27.0 | 16.3 | 32.4 | 25.1 |
| Publication date: | 1950 | 1952 | 1964 | 1976 |
| | (1) | (2) | (3) | (4) |

1. Doll and Hill (1950): 3 years' study: 1298 subjects: case–control, incidence, odds ratio [58].
2. Doll and Hill (1952): 5 years' study: 2714 subjects: case–control, incidence, odds ratio [59].
3. Doll and Hill (1964): 13 years' study: 34 445 subjects: cohort, mortality, relative risk [47].
4. Doll and Peto (1976): 25 years' study: 34 445 subjects: cohort, mortality, relative risk [60].

**Ex. 2.5.** Comparison of results. The relationship between smoking and lung cancer in men, as shown by different British reports. Relative risk, or its close approximation odds ratio, is the basic measure of association given by these studies and shows the ratio of the frequency of lung cancer at each level of smoking compared with the frequency in non-smokers (see Chapter 3)

For example, no randomized trial has yet been done to assess whether routine examination of the skin results in ultimate benefit, i.e. a reduction in mortality from the most serious skin cancer, melanoma. However a case–control study in which information was gathered from melanoma cases and comparison subjects at the time of diagnosis, and then analysed as a comparison between the skin cancer cases who went on to develop advanced disease and the control group, gives results suggestive of some benefit [64].

Case–control studies deserve to be more widely used in assessments of such population interventions, and also in assessments of different types of medical care. An interesting example of the case–control approach to a clinical topic is a study of prognostic factors in breast cancer in which long-term survivors were compared with patients who had died [65]. The method is also used in non-health areas, although often with different terminology. For example, to assess the risk of bankruptcy, studies have compared companies that went bankrupt with a sample of companies that did not, in terms of various financial parameters. These were case–control studies, and the interpretation of their results involves the same issues as apply to health-related studies [66].

Case–control studies can be quite large. In an expansion of the routine function of disease registries in Canada, information has been collected routinely from newly diagnosed cancer patients and controls chosen from the population with a similar age and sex distribution, to give a database which can be analysed for many exposure factors and different types of cancer. An analysis has been done in regard to obesity, using data on 21 000 cancer cases and 5000 population controls. It found a significant increase in cancer risk overall and increased risks for several individual cancers, and concluded that excess body mass accounted for 7.7 per cent of all cancers in Canada [67].

Unfortunately, there are many examples of badly performed case–control studies, which have led to erroneous results. There are more examples of poor quality case–control studies than there are of poor cohort studies. This is partly because the case–control design is more subtle and more difficult to apply than a cohort design, but also because case–control studies may appear deceptively easy. There has been a simplistic view that case–control studies are 'quick, simple, and cheap' compared with cohort studies, whereas in fact they may not be; to mount a well-designed case–control study of an important question is often a complex and expensive endeavour. However, because of this impression, many case–control studies have been done with inadequate resources and poor design, and not surprisingly have given erratic results. The issues are those of appropriate study design and quality control of the information collected, which will be discussed in Chapters 4 and 5, and of appropriate analysis, sample size, power, and publication bias, which will be discussed in Chapters 6 and 7.

## Case–crossover aetiological studies

The equivalent of the crossover trial in an aetiological study is to look at factors related to an episodic event, comparing them with a similar time period for the same individuals that did not result in an event. This is often called a case–crossover design. Thus in a study to assess the role of mobile phone use in motor vehicle accidents, drivers who had reported a motor vehicle accident were identified, and 74 699 of these drivers who owned a mobile phone allowed access to their phone records [68]. The study was done in Toronto before there were any legal restrictions on mobile phone use while driving. The analysis consisted of assessing from these records whether the mobile phone was being used immediately before the reported accident compared with use by the same driver in a set of control periods defined, for example, as the same time on the day before, the same time and the same day of the week before, and so on. The analysis showed an association: an increased relative risk of a motor vehicle accident if the mobile phone call was between 1 and 5 minutes prior to the accident, with the risk decreasing as the time interval between the call and the accident increased, up to 16–20 minutes. The relative risk was 4.8, and was no lower where a hands-free mobile phone was used.

## Cross-sectional surveys

The basic purpose of a survey is to measure the prevalence (frequency at one point in time) of a condition. It is therefore the appropriate method to answer questions such as: Is anaemia common in this community? What is the prevalence of hypertension in elderly people? How satisfied are patients with the health services? Surveys also allow the assessment of associations, such as whether hypertension or a poor diet is more common in one social group than another, and such comparisons can lend themselves to causal thinking. Thus Pauletto *et al.* [69] surveyed two groups of villagers in Tanzania and showed that the group who consumed a fish-based diet had lower blood pressure than the group who had a vegetarian diet. Cross-sectional surveys are limited to making observations that apply to one point in time, and therefore judgements about causation based on survey data have to be very cautious. This is because causation by its definition includes a time function, and therefore, to assess it, studies must cover a time period either prospectively or retrospectively. Our definition of a cross-sectional survey is quite narrow; if a population is surveyed to find out which subjects have a poor diet, and these subjects are then compared with those with a better diet in terms of subsequent health care utilization, we classify the first part as a survey, but the second as a prospective cohort study. Thus, a health survey was carried out in two areas of Sweden between 1963 and 1965, and subsequent linkage of the data to mortality and cancer registration data up to 1987 allowed a prospective cohort analysis of the association between obesity and cancer risk [70].

The advantages of a cross-sectional survey arise primarily because of its relative simplicity, as the complications of retrospective data collection and prospective follow-up are both avoided. Thus the methods to be used can be extensively pre-tested, applied on a large scale, and made reproducible, and at least single blind, in that the investigators need know nothing about the state of the individuals being assessed. Because of their simplicity, cooperation can be high as little is demanded of the subjects.

As the primary function of a survey is to assess prevalence, the methods obtained to draw samples from a defined population are crucial, and various randomized or systematic methods are available which have been discussed in detail in standard texts [71–73]. The use of such methods can ensure that the subjects surveyed are a representative sample of the community, and allows the repetition of the survey at other times or in other communities using identical methods and yielding comparable results. Thus surveys can monitor changes in a population in time and assess differences between population subgroups.

The main disadvantages of survey methods also arise from their simplicity. Because of their lack of a time dimension, the interpretation of their results in terms of cause and effect is very limited, and over-interpretation in this regard is a considerable danger. Their power in assessing prevalence, and therefore in assessing associations between different states, requires a reasonable prevalence of that condition in the population, otherwise they will be inefficient.

## Summary of comparisons

The major properties of the different study designs are summarized in **Ex. 2.6**. In deciding which approach to adopt to deal with a specific question, these properties can be used as a general guide, but the final decision on the appropriate method will be based on a detailed consideration of the issues to be addressed in the study, including the likely effects of bias, confounding, and chance on the interpretation of the results. These concepts will be explored in subsequent chapters.

## Self-test questions (answers on p. 492)

**Q2.1** What types of study design are illustrated by the following situations? (Consider the groups being compared, and the time relationship).

(a) The frequency of deep venous thrombosis in people who have recently had a long-distance air flight is compared with the frequency in an age-matched sample of people who have not travelled.

(b) To assess a possible protective effect of exercise, past involvement in competitive sports is assessed for women who have hypertension and for a group of women of the same age who have not.

(c) Total mortality over the last 30 years is assessed in men employed in a uranium mine at some time during that period, and compared with the general population.

(d) To assess an effect of smoking, men admitted to hospital with myocardial infarction are compared with similar unaffected men in the community.

(e) In a continuation of the same study, the risk of future repetition of the heart attack (reinfarction) is compared between those who smoked and those who did not at the time of their first heart attack.

(f) Groups of breast-fed and non-breast fed babies are identified at 6 months of age, and then surveyed at later times. To study the association with small stature, children in the lowest decile of height at

MAIN PROPERTIES OF DIFFERENT STUDY DESIGNS

| Design | Intervention trials | Cohort studies | Case–control studies | Surveys |
|---|---|---|---|---|
| Question asked | What is the effect of this intervention? | What are the effects of this exposure? | What were the causes of this event? | How common is this condition? Are conditions and exposures associated? |
| Applicability | Controlled interventions of likely benefit | Any exposure for which adequate numbers of exposed subjects can be found and studied, and outcome can be assessed | Any event for which groups of cases and appropriate controls can be found, and exposure factors can be assessed retrospectively | Any exposure, condition, or association which is reasonably common and for which assessment at one point in time is sufficient |
| | Primary method of studying new therapies | Primary method of studying unusual or new exposures | Primary method of studying unusual or new outcomes | Primary method of assessing prevalence |
| Major strengths | Allows randomization: best way to control confounding; Allows double-blind assessment: best way to control bias | Allows multiple endpoints to be assessed; Cause to effect time sequence clear; All measures of risk can be assessed; Exposure is assessed prior to outcome, avoiding bias | Usually can be done with moderate numbers of subjects; feasible even on small numbers; Retrospective method is rapid; Multiple exposure factors can be assessed | Representative samples of a population can be drawn; Methods can be standardized, reliable, and single blind; Efficient in resources needed; Cooperation may be high; Can be repeated using similar methods |
| Major weaknesses | Ethical limitations; Organizational problems; Time scale | Usually requires large numbers; Long time scale for some effects | Retrospective method limits exposure information and is open to bias; Adequate control group may be difficult to define or obtain | Lack of time dimension limits causal interpretations; Inefficient for rare exposures or conditions |

**Ex. 2.6.** Some properties of the four major study designs

age 10 years are compared with a sample of all the other children in regard to many factors.

(g) A dermatologist offers a new treatment for acne to all her teenage patients, and compares the results with those who chose to continue the traditional treatment.

**Q2.2** Do you agree with the following conclusions?

(a) A study shows higher rates of diabetes in unemployed than in employed men. This shows that becoming unemployed leads to diabetes.

(b) A survey of residents in an aged care facility shows that smoking is much less frequent in 95-year-olds than it is in 85-year-olds. This shows that many people give up smoking between these ages.

(c) In a study of breast cancer patients, 40 per cent reported stressful life events in the last 2 years compared with only 25 per cent of age-matched controls. This shows that stress increases the risk of breast cancer substantially.

(d) A survey of workers in a clothing factory shows that the frequency of repetitive strain injury is lower than the rate reported in a general population survey. This shows that repetitive strain injury is not caused by this type of work.

**Q2.3** What type of study is most useful to assess the various consequences of an environmental hazard, such as radiation exposure? What are its main disadvantages, in terms of an outcome such as cancer occurrence?

**Q2.4** What are the prime advantages and disadvantages of a case–control study in assessing the causes of a newly recognized disease?

**Q2.5** What are the main advantages of the randomized trial design?

## References

1. **Younis N, Broadbent DM, Vora JP, Harding SP.** Incidence of sight-threatening retinopathy in patients with type 2 diabetes in the Liverpool Diabetic Eye Study: a cohort study. *Lancet* 2003; **361**: 195–200.

2. **Stocks P, Karn MN.** A co-operative study of the habits, home life, dietary and family histories of 450 cancer patients and of an equal number of control patients. *Ann Eugen* 1933; **5**: 237–280.

3. **Muirhead CR, Bingham D, Haylock RGE, O'Hagan JA, Goodill AA, Berridge GL** et al. Follow up of mortality and incidence of cancer 1952–98 in men from the UK who participated in the UK's atmospheric nuclear weapon tests and experimental programmes. *Occup Environ Med* 2003; **60**(3): 165–172.

4. **Baverstock K.** The 2003 NRPB report on UK nuclear-test veterans. *Lancet* 2003; **361**(9371): 1759–1760.

5. Packer CN, Stewart-Brown S, Fowle SE. Damp housing and adult health: results from a lifestyle study in Worcester, England. *J Epidemiol Community Health* 1994; **48**: 555–559.

6. Kojima M, Wakai K, Tokudome S, *et al*. Serum levels of polyunsaturated fatty acids and risk of colorectal cancer: a prospective study. *Am J Epidemiol* 2005; **161**(5): 462–471.

7. Elwood JM, Little J, Elwood JH. *Epidemiology and Control of Neural Tube Defects*. Oxford: Oxford University Press, 1992.

8. Hibbard ED, Smithells RW. Folic acid metabolism and human embryopathy. *Lancet* 1965; **1**: 1254–1256.

9. Smithells RW, Sheppard S, Schorah CJ. Vitamin deficiencies and neural tube defects. *Arch Dis Child* 1976; **51**: 944–950.

10. Smithells RW, Sheppard S, Schorah CJ, *et al*. Apparent prevention of neural tube defects by periconceptional vitamin supplementation. *Arch Dis Child* 1981; **56**: 911–918.

11. MRC (Medical Research Council) Vitamin Study Group. Prevention of neural tube defects: results of the Medical Research Council Vitamin Study. *Lancet* 1991; **338**: 131–137.

12. Foulkes WD, Brunet J-S, Sieh W, Black MJ, Shenouda G, Narod SA. Familial risks of squamous cell carcinoma of the head and neck: retrospective case–control study. *BMJ* 1996; **313**: 716–721.

13. Ghebreyesus TA, Haile M, Witten KH, *et al*. Incidence of malaria among children living near dams in northern Ethiopia: community based incidence survey. *BMJ* 1999; **319**: 663–666.

14. Thornley B, Adams C. Content and quality of 2000 controlled trials in schizophrenia over 50 years. *BMJ* 1998; **317**: 1181–1184.

15. Silverman WA. *Where's the Evidence? Debates in Modern Medicine*. Oxford: Oxford University Press, 1998.

16. British Medical Journal. Fifty years of randomised controlled trials. *BMJ* 1998; **317**: 1167–1248.

17. Doll R. Controlled trials: the 1948 watershed. *BMJ* 1998; **317**: 1217–1220.

18. Yoshioka A. Use of randomisation in the Medical Research Council's clinical trial of streptomycin in pulmonary tuberculosis in the 1940s. *BMJ* 1998; **317**: 1220–1223.

19. Fibiger J. Om Serumbehandlung af Difteri. *Hospitalstidende* 1898; **6**: 309–325.

20. Chalmers I, Clarke M. Commentary: The 1944 patulin trial: the first properly controlled multicentre trial conducted under the aegis of the British Medical Research Council. *Int J Epidemiol* 2004; **33**(2): 253–260.

21. McCord J. A thirty year follow-up of treatment effects. *Am Psychol* 1978; **33**: 284–289.

22. ISIS-4 (Fourth International Study of Infarct Survival Collaborative Group). ISIS-4: A randomised factorial trial assessing early oral captopril, oral mononitrate, and intravenous magnesium sulphate in 58 050 patients with suspected acute myocardial infarction. *Lancet* 1995; **345**: 669–685.

23. Hill JD, Hampton JR, Mitchell JRA. A randomised trial of home-versus-hospital management for patients with suspected myocardial infarction. *Lancet* 1978; **i**: 837–841.

24. Shapiro S, Venet W, Strax P, Venet L, Roeser R. Ten- to fourteen- year effect of screening on breast cancer mortality. *J Natl Cancer Inst* 1982; **69**: 349–355.

25. Altman DG, Schulz KF, Moher D, *et al*. The revised CONSORT statement for reporting randomized trials: explanation and elaboration. *Ann Intern Med* 2001; **134**: 663–694.

26. Hills M, Armitage P. The two-period cross-over clinical trial. *Br J Clin Pharmacol* 1979; **8**: 7–20.

27. Schrader H, Stovner LJ, Helde G, Sand T, Bovim G. Prophylactic treatment of migraine with angiotensin converting enzyme inhibitor (lisinopril): randomised, placebo controlled, crossover study. *BMJ* 2001; **322**: 19–22.

28. Cook DJ. Randomized trials in single subjects: the *N* of 1 study. *Psychopharmacol Bull* 1996; **32**: 363–367.

29. March L, Irwig L, Schwarz J, Simpson J, Chock C, Brooks P. *n* of 1 trials comparing a non-steroidal anti-inflammatory drug with paracetamol in osteoarthritis. *BMJ* 1994; **309**: 1041–1046.

30. Nikles CJ, Clavarino AM, Del Mar CB. Using *n*-of-1 trials as a clinical tool to improve prescribing. *Br J Gen Pract* 2005; **55**: 175–180.

31. Mahon JL, Laupacis A, Hodder RV, *et al.* Theophylline for irreversible chronic airflow limitation: a randomized study comparing *n* of 1 trials to standard practice. *Chest* 1999; **115**: 38–48.

32. Adish AA, Esrey SA, Gyorkos TW, Jean-Baptiste J, Rojhani A. Effect of consumption of food cooked in iron pots on iron status and growth of young children: a randomised trial. *Lancet* 1999; **353**: 712–716.

33. Ukoumunne OC, Gulliford MC, Chinn S, Sterne JAC, Burney PGJ, Donner A. Methods in health service research. Evaluation of health interventions at area and organisation level. *BMJ* 1999; **319**: 376–379.

34. English DR, Burton RC, Del Mar CB, Donovan RJ, Ireland PD, Emery G. Evaluation of aid to diagnosis of pigmented skin lesions in general practice: controlled trial randomised by practice. *BMJ* 2003; **327**: 375–380.

35. Arnold FA, Dean HT, Jay P, Knutson JW. Effect of fluoridated public water supplies on dental caries prevalence. Tenth year of the Grand Rapids–Muskegon study. *Public Health Rep* 1956; **71**: 652–658.

36. Farquhar JW, Fortmann SP, Maccoby N, *et al.* The Stanford Five-City Project: design and methods. *Am J Epidemiol* 1985; **122**: 323–334.

37. Fortmann SP, Flora JA, Winkleby MA, Schooler C, Taylor CB, Farquhar JW. Community intervention trials: reflections on the Stanford Five-City Project experience. *Am J Epidemiol* 1995; **142**: 576–586.

38. Soderstrom L, Woods WG, Bernstein M, Robison LL, Tuchman M, Lemieux B. Health and economic benefits of well-designed evaluations: some lessons from evaluating neuroblastoma screening. *J Natl Cancer Inst* 2005; **97**: 1118–1124.

39. Bunker CB, Barnes JA, Mosteller F, (Eds.). *Costs, Risks and Benefits of Surgery.* New York: Oxford University Press, 1977.

40. Ruffin JM, Grizzle JE, Hightower NC, McHardy G, Shull H, Kirsner JB. A co-operative double-blind evaluation of gastric 'freezing' in the treatment of duodenal ulcer. *N Engl J Med* 1969; **281**: 16–19.

41. Bagenal FS, Easton DF, Harris E, Chilvers CE, McElwain TJ. Survival of patients with breast cancer attending Bristol Cancer Help Centre. *Lancet* 1990; **336**: 606–610.

42. Smithells RW, Sheppard S, Wild J, Schorah CJ. Prevention of neural tube defect recurrences in Yorkshire: final report (Letter). *Lancet* 1989; **ii**(8661): 498–499.

43. Selikoff IJ, Churg J, Hammond EC. Asbestos exposure, smoking and neoplasia. *JAMA* 1968; **204**: 106–112.

44. **Lindhout D, Schmidt D.** *In-utero* exposure to valproate and neural tube defects. *Lancet* 1986; **i**: 1392–1393.

45. **Million Women Study Collaborators.** Breast cancer and hormone-replacement therapy in the Million Women Study. *Lancet* 2003; **362**: 419–427.

46. **Bingham S, Riboli E.** Diet and cancer—the European Prospective Investigation into Cancer and Nutrition. *Natl Rev Cancer* 2004; **4**: 206–215.

47. **Doll R, Hill AB.** Mortality in relation to smoking: ten years' observations of British doctors. *BMJ* 1964; **i**: 1399–1410.

48. **Doll R, Gray R, Hafner B, Peto R.** Mortality in relation to smoking: 22 years' observations on female British doctors. *BMJ* 1980; **i**: 967–971.

49. **Hennekens CH, Speizer FE, Rosner B, Bain CJ, Belanger C, Peto R.** Use of permanent hair dyes and cancer among registered nurses. *Lancet* 1979; **i**: 1390–1393.

50. **Stampfer MJ, Colditz GA, Willett WC,** *et al.* Postmenopausal estrogen therapy and cardiovascular disease. Ten-year follow-up from the Nurses' Health Study. *N Engl J Med* 1991; **325**: 756–762.

51. **Dawber TR.** *The Framingham Study: The Epidemiology of Atherosclerotic Disease.* Cambridge, MA: Harvard University Press, 1980.

52. **Wilson PW.** Established risk factors and coronary artery disease: the Framingham Study. *Am J Hypertens* 1994; **7**: 7S–12S.

53. **Kuh D, Hardy R, Langenberg C, Richards M, Wadsworth ME.** Mortality in adults aged 26–54 years related to socioeconomic conditions in childhood and adulthood: post war birth cohort study. *BMJ* 2002; **325**: 1076–1080.

54. **Wadsworth MEJ.** *The Imprint of Time: Childhood, History, and Adult Life.* Oxford: Oxford University Press, 1991.

55. **Susser E, Terry MB.** A conception-to-death cohort. *Lancet* 2003; **361**: 797–798.

56. **Barbour V.** UK Biobank: a project in search of a protocol? *Lancet* 2003; **361**: 1734–1738.

57. **Herbst AL, Ulfelder H, Poskanzer DC.** Adenocarcinoma of the vagina: association of maternal stilbestrol therapy with tumor appearance in young women. *N Engl J Med* 1971; **284**: 878–881.

58. **Doll R, Hill AB.** Smoking and carcinoma of the lung. Preliminary report. *BMJ* 1950; **ii**: 739–748.

59. **Doll R, Hill AB.** A study of the aetiology of carcinoma of the lung. *BMJ* 1952; **ii**: 1271–1286.

60. **Doll R, Peto R.** Mortality in relation to smoking: 20 years' observations on male British doctors. *BMJ* 1976; **ii**: 1525–1536.

61. **MacGregor JE, Moss SM, Parkin DM, Day NE.** A case–control study of cervical cancer screening in north east Scotland. *BMJ* 1985; **290**: 1543–1546.

62. **Selby JV, Friedman GD, Quesenberry CP, Jr, Weiss NS.** Effect of fecal occult blood testing on mortality from colorectal cancer: a case–control study. *Ann Intern Med* 1993; **118**: 1–6.

63. **Weiss NS, McKnight B, Stevens NG.** Approaches to the analysis of case–control studies of the efficacy of screening for cancer. *Am J Epidemiol* 1992; **135**: 817–823.

64. **Berwick M, Begg CB, Fine JA, Roush GC, Barnhill RL.** Screening for cutaneous melanoma by skin self-examination. *J Natl Cancer Inst* 1996; **88**: 17–23.

65. **Fentiman IS, Cuzick J, Millis RR, Hayward JL.** Which patients are cured of breast cancer? *BMJ* 1984; **289**: 1108–1111.

66. **Taffler RJ.** Forecasting company failure in the UK using discriminant analysis of financial ratio data. *J R Statist Soc* 1982; **145**: 342–358.

67. **Pan SY, Johnson KC, Ugnat AM, Wen SW, Mao Y.** Association of obesity and cancer risk in Canada. *Am J Epidemiol* 2004; **159**: 259–268.

68. **Redelmeier DA, Tibshirani RJ.** Association betweeen cellular-telephone calls and motor vehicle collisions. *N Engl J Med* 1997; **336**: 453–458.

69. **Pauletto P, Puato M, Caroli MG,** *et al.* Blood pressure and atherogenic lipoprotein profiles of fish-diet and vegetarian villagers in Tanzania: the Lugalawa study. *Lancet* 1996; **348**: 784–788.

70. **Törnberg SA, Carstensen JM.** Relationship between Quetelet's index and cancer of breast and female genital tract in 47 000 women followed for 25 years. *Br J Cancer* 1994; **69**: 358–361.

71. **Cartwright A.** *Health Surveys in Practice and in Potential: A Critical Review of their Scope and Methods.* London: King Edward's Hospital Fund for London, 1983.

72. **Abramson JH.** *Survey Methods in Community Medicine: Epidemiological Research, Programme Evaluation, Clinical Trials*, 5th edn. Edinburgh: Churchill Livingstone, 1999.

73. **Aday LA, Cornelius LJ.** *Designing and Conducting Health Surveys: A Comprehensive Guide*, 3rd edn. San Francisco, CA: Jossey-Bass, 2006.

Chapter 3

# The results obtained from studies of causation

*When you can measure what you are speaking about, and express it in numbers, you know something about it; but when you cannot measure it, when you cannot express it in numbers, your knowledge is of a meagre and unsatisfactory kind: it may be the beginning of knowledge, but you have scarcely, in your thoughts, advanced to the stage of science.*

—William Thomson, Lord Kelvin: Popular lectures and addresses; 1891–1894

In the previous chapter we presented a classification of study design which separated the criteria used to select the groups of individuals to be compared from the time relationships of the study. The logic of this system will appear clear when we discuss the results obtained from these studies. The format of the results and therefore the appropriate methods of interpreting them depend on the groups being compared. The extent to which particular problems and biases occur depends largely on the time relationships.

## Cohort and intervention studies

We shall first consider the cohort design, which applies to both observational cohort studies and intervention trials. In this design we are comparing groups of individuals who are classified by their exposure to the putative causal factor. The simplest situation is with two groups, which we can regard as 'exposed' and 'non-exposed'. This will often be the real situation; for example, we might compare women using oral contraceptives with women who do not use oral contraceptives, or patients on one therapy with patients on another. In other situations, the cohorts may be more numerous and may be ordered, such as groups of individuals characterized by the amount they smoke, or groups of patients with different severities of disease. The format of the results in any cohort study is the same. The same method of analysis is used for aetiological studies looking at individuals exposed to external agents in the environment, observational studies comparing the outcome of groups of patients given different therapies, and randomized trials. It makes no difference to the analysis whether the cohort study is prospective (where subjects were identified at the start of the study and followed forward in time), or retrospective, where the subjects are identified using records and their experience up to the current time provides the outcome data.

The simplest situation is illustrated by **Ex. 3.1** which shows the results of a study in expectant mothers who had epilepsy during pregnancy, which was treated with one anti-epileptic drug, i.e. monotherapy. The comparison is between those treated with one specific drug, valproic acid, and those treated with other single agents. Mothers with epilepsy who required no drug treatment and those who received two or more drugs are excluded, as they are likely to have less or more severe epilepsy. The data come from a prospective cohort study in the UK based on enrolments of women during pregnancy from both general practitioners and specialists [1]. Since this is a study of pregnancy outcome, the follow-up period is fixed and relatively short, and the outcome of interest is the frequency of a major congenital abnormality in the offspring. Therefore the results have a simple format. For each group of mothers, exposed and unexposed, we have the number of infants delivered, and the number of these infants who has an abnormality.

The results show the two proportions, or prevalence rates at birth. If there were no difference in outcome between the two groups i.e. if the 'null hypothesis' were true, the prevalence rates in the two groups would be the same, apart from random variations. It is logical to compare either the difference in the rates, or the ratio of the rates, and these considerations lead to important and widely used epidemiological measures. **Ex. 3.2** shows the measures which can be derived.

## Relative risk and relative odds

The *relative risk* or *risk ratio* is the ratio of the rate of disease among those exposed (mothers using valproic acid) to the rate in those not exposed

| | RESULTS OF A COHORT STUDY (1) | | | |
|---|---|---|---|---|
| | Number of infants | | | |
| Exposure | Malformed | Not malformed | Total | Prevalence of malformation (%) |
| Valproic acid | 44 | 647 | 715 | 6.15 |
| No valproic acid | 47 | 1697 | 1710 | 2.75 |

**Ex. 3.1.** Results of a cohort study comparing among mothers with epilepsy, those treated with valproic acid with those receiving other drugs (each as single agents) with regard to the occurrence of major malformations in their offspring. From Morrow *et al.* [1]

---

## RESULTS OF A COHORT STUDY (2)

| Exposure | Number of infants | | | Prevalence of malformation (%) |
|---|---|---|---|---|
| | Malformed | Not malformed | Total | |
| Valproic acid | 44 | 647 | 715 | 6.15 |
| No valproic acid | 47 | 1697 | 1710 | 2.75 |
| Whole population | 91 | 2344 | 2425 | 3.75 |

(assuming sample is representative)

*RR, Relative risk* or risk ratio = 6.15/2.75 = 2.24

*OR, Odds ratio* = (44/647)/(47/1697) = 2.46

*AR, Attributable risk* or risk difference = 6.15 – 2.75 = 3.41%

$AP_{exp}$, *Attributable proportion in exposed subjects* = attributable risk / total risk in exposed = 3.41/6.15 = 55.3%

Also, $AP_{exp} = (RR–1)/RR = (2.24 – 1)/2.24 = 55.3\%$

$AP_{pop}$, *Attributable proportion in the population*:

For the whole population, risk – 3.75%
attributable proportion in the whole population = (3.75 – 2.75)/3.75 = 26.8%
(using full data to avoid rounding errors)

More generally, where *p* = the proportion of the population exposed, estimated from the study or from other sources, the attributable proportion in the population is given by

$$AP_{pop} = \frac{p(RR - 1)}{p(RR - 1) + 1}$$

Here *p* = 715/2425 = 29.4%
So $AP_{pop}$ = 26.8%

---

**Ex. 3.2.** Derivation of measures of association from the results of the cohort study shown in Ex. 3.1. Note: in this and subsequent exhibits, the calculations are shown with limited decimal places for clarity, but the calculations themselves are carried out from the basic data to avoid rounding error.

(mothers taking other drugs), and as it is a ratio it has no units. In this example the relative risk is 2.24.

We can also consider a further measure, the *odds ratio*. The odds of a baby in the exposed group being malformed are 44:647 (approximately 1 in 15), compared with odds of 47:1697 (about 1 in 36) in the unexposed group. The ratio of these is the odds ratio, which is 2.46, similar but not identical to the relative risk. The odds ratio and the relative risk are similar when the frequency of the outcome is low; they diverge as the outcome becomes more frequent.

For example, if the prevalence in the exposed group is 50 per cent (odds 1:1), and that in the unexposed group is 25 per cent (odds 1:3), the risk ratio is 2, but the odds ratio is 3. For both relative risk and odds ratio, the value of 1.0 corresponds to the situation of no association between exposure and outcome.

## Risk difference (attributable risk)

The difference between the two rates is the *risk difference*, or *attributable risk*. The latter term is less satisfactory as it implies that there is a causal relationship. The risk difference gives, in absolute terms, the frequency of the outcome which is associated with the exposure. In this example the attributable risk is 3.41 per cent. If there were no association present, the risk difference would be zero.

If we divide the attributable risk by the total risk in the exposed group, the result is the proportion of disease in those exposed to the factor which is associated with the exposure; this can be called the 'attributable proportion in exposed subjects'. Here it is $3.41/6.15 = 55$ per cent.

If, for the population under study, the proportion of subjects who are exposed is known, the proportion of total disease in the population which is associated with the causal factor can be calculated; this is the 'attributable proportion in the population'. In this example it is 27 per cent.

## The uses of risk difference and relative risk

Unlike relative risk, the risk difference, or attributable risk, describes the absolute quantity of the outcome which is associated with the exposure. Therefore it is useful in considering the practical implications of studies once a decision has been reached that the association represents causation. Thus a comparison of the attributable risks in terms of total mortality conferred by a number of environmental exposures gives an indication of how much mortality will be prevented by successful action on each one of the exposures, and such an approach has been useful in setting priorities for public health and health promotion campaigns. A similar consideration in terms of the long-term outcome of a complex disease such as diabetes, whose course may be influenced by a large number of factors, may be used to indicate what aspects of care, if dealt with successfully, will result in the greatest improvement in outcome. Therefore attributable risk is particularly useful in well-researched situations where the implications of soundly supported results are being considered. It is of less value in the preliminary stages of assessment of a possible causal relationship.

The great advantage of the relative risk estimate is the empirical finding that in many human disease situations, the relative risk of disease incidence or mortality associated with a particular exposure is fairly constant over a wide range of populations and groups of subjects, even where other factors differ. If the relative risk for a particular exposure is the same in two different populations, but because of differences in other factors the total risks of the outcome are different, then the attributable risks will be different. In comparing evidence from a number of sources concerning a particular causal relationship, it is more reasonable to expect consistency in terms of relative risk than of attributable risk. This property of consistency makes relative risk more valuable in evaluating whether a particular relationship is or is not likely to be causal. It is also rather easier to predict the effects of non-causal factors on the observed relative risk than on the observed attributable risk.

There is another important reason for concentrating on relative risk, and that is because this measure, unlike attributable risk, can be derived from any of the main study designs. As will be shown, case–control studies provide estimates of relative risk (by the odds ratio), but do not provide direct measures of attributable risk. For these reasons the relative risk is the more useful index to summarize the results of a study in order to discuss the interpretation of the association. Therefore in the rest of this book we will concentrate on the interpretation of relative risk.

## Preventive factors and application to intervention studies; number needed to treat

If the factor under consideration is protective, the rate of outcome in the exposed group will be less than in the unexposed group, and therefore the relative risk will be less than 1, and the risk difference will be negative. There is no difficulty with this apart from terminology.

Ex. 3.3 shows the result of a large-scale randomized trial in which patients with myocardial infarction (a heart attack) were treated with a new drug (captopril), and compared with a placebo group [2]. This was a very large trial with about 29 000 subjects in each group. As shown, there was a protective effect of the new drug, with a relative risk of 0.94 and a risk difference of –4.9 deaths per 1000 subjects. Rather than calling this a risk difference or, if we assume causality, an attributable risk of –4.9 deaths per 1000, a better terminology is to call it an attributable benefit of 4.9 deaths averted per 1000 subjects. Such terminology is logical, although not widely used. We can also simply refer to this absolute benefit as the 'number of deaths averted per 1000 treated', which will again be 4.9. We can also invert that figure, and express the results of the trial in terms of the 'number of subjects treated with the new drug to prevent one death', often called the 'number needed to treat' (NNT). This is a 1000/4.9, or approximately 200. This is an easily understandable and readily applicable figure [3]. Thus the result of this study (assuming we interpret

---

BENEFICIAL EFFECTS AND NUMBER NEEDED TO TREAT

*Actual results*

|  | Deaths | Survivors | Total | Death rate per 1000 |
|---|---|---|---|---|
| Treated with captopril | 2088 | 26940 | 29028 | 71.9 |
| Placebo group | 2231 | 26791 | 29022 | 76.9 |

| | | | |
|---|---|---|---|
| Relative risk | = 71.9/76.9 | = | 0.94 |
| Risk difference per 1000 | = 71.9 − 76.9 | = | − 4.9 |
| Deaths averted per 1000 treated | = 76.9 − 71.9 | = | 4.9 |
| Number treated to prevent one death | = 1000/4.9 | = | 202 |

*Hypothetical results if relative risk remains the same, but baseline mortality rate doubles*

|  | Deaths | Survivors | Total | Death rate per 1000 |
|---|---|---|---|---|
| Treated with captopril | 4176 | 24852 | 29028 | 143.9 |
| Placebo group | 4462 | 24560 | 29022 | 153.7 |

| | | | |
|---|---|---|---|
| Relative risk | = 143.9/153.7 | = | 0.94 |
| Risk difference per 1000 | = 143.9 − 153.7 | = | − 9.9 |
| Deaths averted per 1000 treated | = 153.7 − 143.9 | = | 9.9 |
| Number treated to prevent one death | = 1000/9.9 | = | 101 |

---

**Ex. 3.3.** Results of a clinical trial: number needed to treat. Results of randomized trial of a drug treatment (captopril) in patients with suspected myocardial infarction; deaths in first 35 days. From ISIS-4 study [2]. As noted in Ex. 3.2, calculations avoid rounding errors, which is why the risk difference is −4.9, not −5.0 from the simple calculation shown.

it as a causal relationship) is that treatment of these patients with this new drug resulted in a reduction in death rate, with one death averted for every 200 subjects treated. Whether this benefit is worthwhile will depend on how it is balanced by the disadvantages of the new drug, in terms of side effects, costs, and so on. (More correctly, one death is averted for every 200 offered treatment, as not all those randomized to captopril would have necessarily accepted it or taken the full dosages.)

Consider what would happen if the relative effect of the drug were the same, i.e. a relative risk of 0.94, but the death rate of both the treated and the comparison groups were higher, as would happen if the treatment were offered to patients with particularly severe disease. If the relative risk is constant and the mortality rate in the non-treated group is doubled, the number of deaths averted per 1000 treated (the attributable benefit) is doubled, and the number who are treated to prevent one death falls to about 100. The difference between 100 and 200 patients treated to avert one death could well be important in terms of the comparison with ill effects and costs. Although in this example only the data on early mortality are shown, the overall results of this major study looking at longer-term mortality were essentially similar, and from consideration of this and other literature, the authors indeed concluded that the use of the captopril therapy would save about one life per 200 treated in average-risk patients, and about one life per 100 treated in higher-risk groups.

## Perceptions given by relative and absolute risks: framing

Therefore the association shown by studies can be expressed as a ratio measurement, or a measurement on an absolute scale. Results which are actually the same can produce different impressions when presented in different ways, an effect referred to as 'framing', and the question of whether relative or absolute measurement of benefits or risks should be used can be controversial. Effects expressed as absolute benefits are usually numerically smaller than when expressed as relative risks, and often have a lesser impact [4], for example on influencing doctors to prescribe cholesterol-lowering drugs [5]. In a population survey, 80 per cent of people said that they would accept a screening test when presented with data on relative risk reduction, while only 45 per cent would accept it when given equivalent data expressed as number needed to screen [6]. Both absolute and relative measures have value. The trial just described shows a very useful property of relative risk, in that this was fairly constant over the range of underlying absolute mortality rates. The absolute benefit measure, which can be expressed as the number needed to treat to avert one outcome, is a very useful interpretation in terms of clinical and cost implications. For example, in recent trials of the monoclonal antibody trastuzumab (Herceptin), use of this drug in addition to standard chemotherapy after primary surgery in suitable patients with breast cancer (adjuvant treatment) gave a relative risk of 0.67, i.e. a one-third reduction in the average death rate [7]. This is quite dramatic, but these are early results. At 3 years follow-up, the absolute mortality was reduced from 8.3 per cent to 5.7 per cent, which is a risk difference of 2.6 per cent, corresponding to a number needed to treat of 38 (1/0.026). Thus treating 38 eligible women with the new drug would result in one less death. Given that the cost of a course of the drug may be around US $50 000, the cost of averting one death would be about US $2 million. Understandably, these important new results are causing considerable discussion in terms of appropriate drug costs. Longer follow-up in the trial may change the results; if the relative risk persists, the absolute mortality reduction will increase and the number needed to treat will fall. Indeed, the estimated 4-year follow-up results show this; the mortality is reduced from 13.4 per cent to 8.6 per cent, giving a risk difference of 4.8 per cent and a number needed to treat of 21.

## Person-time as the denominator of rates

In the data for pregnancies in Ex. 3.2, the outcome measure is the proportion of malformed births. In cohort studies of other outcomes, the follow-up time is not fixed and may not be the same for each subject. Consider a cohort study in which men are classified by their level of exercise, and subsequently the occurrence of deaths from heart disease is recorded. Each subject contributes information from the time he enters the study until his death, until the end of the follow-up period, or until some specified time at which the data collection ends. Some subjects may leave the study before any of these endpoints; they are 'censored', or become 'lost to follow-up', but still contribute to the study up to the time at which their outcome status was last known. To assess the incidence rate, the number of heart disease deaths is divided by the total follow-up period, i.e. the sum of the follow-up times for all individuals, expressed as person-time (person-years, man-months, etc.).

One of the classic studies showing a relationship between physical exercise and coronary heart disease mortality was the prospective cohort study of longshoremen (dock workers) in San Francisco [8]. Between 1951 and 1961, men who were assessed at a health screening clinic and were aged 35–74 were entered into the study; men first assessed at a younger age entered the study when they turned 35. The follow-up continued until death, attaining the age of 75, the end of the follow-up period in 1972, or the date of loss to follow-up. Less than 1 per cent were lost to follow-up. Thus the follow-up varied from very short, if an early death occurred, to 22 years. In total, 6351 men entered the study, contributing 92 645 man-years of experience; there were 598 deaths from coronary heart disease, giving a crude death rate of 598/92 645 = 64.5 deaths per 10 000 man-years. The total incidence rate in this example is the average for the whole follow-up period. If the rate of outcome varies greatly over the follow-up period, this simple average will not be adequate and more complex methods of analysis are necessary. As the issues of interpretation can be adequately dealt with using simple data, such methods are not discussed here but are presented in Chapter 7 as survival and life-table methods (p. 264).

## More than one causal agent

Ex. 3.4 shows death rates from cardiovascular disease in cohorts of women defined by two exposures, smoking and contraceptive usage, from a large prospective cohort study [9]. Women exposed to neither oral contraceptives nor smoking had a cardiovascular death rate of 3.0 per 100 000 woman-years. Those who smoked but did not use oral contraceptives had a death rate of 8.9/100 000, while those who used oral contraceptives but did not smoke had a death rate of 13.8/100 000. In this joint exposure situation, it is appropriate to regard the women who were exposed to neither factor as the baseline or 'referent' group, and to consider attributable risks and relative risks as compared with this group. What rate would we expect in women who both used oral contraceptives and smoked?

There are two simple methods by which we could derive such a rate. The first is to assume that women who are exposed to both agents have the baseline risk of the unexposed group, plus the attributable risk associated with smoking, plus the attributable risk due to oral contraceptive use, and so end up with a cardiovascular mortality rate of $3.0 + 5.9 + 10.8 = 19.7$ deaths per 100 000 woman-years. We are assuming that the two effects work in an *additive* fashion. Therefore the excess risks produced by each exposure add together, and add to the baseline risk, which is due to the effects of other factors, to give the total risk. The relative risk for the group exposed to both factors, compared with the unexposed group, is $19.7/3.0 = 6.6$. We can derive the same figure using relative risk estimates by combining what is called the *excess relative risk,* which is the relative risk minus 1. Therefore the additive calculation is the excess relative risk from smoking ($3.0 - 1 = 2.0$), added to the excess relative risk from oral contraceptive use ($4.6 - 1 = 3.6$) plus the baseline relative risk ($1.0$), which sums to give 6.6 as the relative risk for subjects with both exposures compared with those with neither.

Another simple argument is that if smoking increases an individual's risk by a factor of 3.0, and oral contraceptive use increases it by a factor of 4.6, the joint effect of smoking and oral contraceptive use may increase the risk by a factor of $3.0 \times 4.6 = 13.8$. If we multiply this relative risk of 13.8 by the baseline absolute risk of 3.0 deaths per 100 000 woman-years, we obtain an expected death rate of 41.4 deaths per 100 000 woman-years. We are assuming here

| COHORT STUDY WITH TWO CAUSAL FACTORS | | | |
|---|---|---|---|
| Exposure | Mortality from circulatory system diseases, per 100 000 woman-years | Relative risk | Attributable risk/$10^5$ woman-years |
| Non-smoker, no OC use | 3.0 | 1.0 | 0 (referent) |
| Smoker, no OC use | 8.9 | 3.0 | 5.9 |
| Non-smoker, OC user | 13.8 | 4.6 | 10.8 |
| Smoker, OC user | ? | ? | ? |

**Ex. 3.4.** Two causal factors. Results of a prospective cohort study comparing women classified by smoking habit and oral contraceptive (OC) use in terms of deaths from circulatory system diseases. For effects of joint exposure, see text. From Royal College of General Practitioners [9]

a *multiplicative* model, i.e. the effect of two exposures is the multiple of the effects of each. In few studies of human disease have we enough information on biological mechanisms to predict confidently which of these models, or indeed which of a large range of other models, fit the real situation. We have to observe what happens in practice. In this oral contraceptive study the cardio-vascular death rate per 100 000 woman-years in women who both smoked and were exposed to oral contraceptives was in fact 39.5 per 100 000 woman-years. This is close to the expected result on a multiplicative model, and so this is the more appropriate model for these data.

However, we should be cautious, as the numbers of deaths in each group shown in Ex. 3.4 are small (2, 3, 5, and 19 in the four groups) and more infor-mation would be needed to be confident that the multiplicative model is a better fit to the data than the additive model. This example is based on a early report of this cohort study with follow-up from the start of the study in 1968 to 1976. A later report from this study, based on follow-up to 1993, showed that the increased mortality from circulatory diseases is largely restricted to current and recent users of oral contraceptives [10], and a further report from another cohort study of the topic showed that the increase in deaths from ischaemic heart disease associated with oral contraceptive use was confined to heavy smokers [11].

## Case–control studies

The other major design is the case–control study, comparing a group of indi-viduals who have experienced the outcome under study with a group who have not. The exposure of each subject in the study to the factor under consideration is ascertained retrospectively. The results appear as a 2 × 2 table as shown in **Ex. 3.5**. In the case–control design, a sample of all available cases is taken $(a + c)$, and a sample of unaffected subjects (controls) is drawn independently $(b + d)$. As these two groups are sampled separately, rates of disease in the exposed or unexposed groups cannot be calculated, nor can relative risk be measured directly. However, the *odds ratio* can be obtained, and so it is the primary measure of association in case–control studies.

Note the simple algebra of the calculation of odds ratio; the number $a$ of exposed cases is multiplied by the number opposite it on the diagonal of the table, and this result is then divided by the two other numbers multiplied together; because of this simple arithmetic, the odds ratio is sometimes referred to as the *cross-products ratio*.

To understand how the odds ratio in a case–control study is derived, it is useful to consider an unusual example in which we can compare the results with the situation in the whole population from which the study participants

CASE-CONTROL STUDY RESULTS

|  | Cases | Controls |
|---|---|---|
| Exposed | a | b |
| Unexposed | c | d |
|  | a + c | b + d |

Odds ratio = (a/b)/(c/d)
        = ad/bc the 'cross-products' ratio

**Ex. 3.5.** Simplest form of results for a case-control study. The odds ratio, or relative odds, is the key measure of association. Because of the sampling used, the total number of exposed subjects is *not a + b*, and the risk in exposed subjects is *not a/(a + b)*; see text for explanation

CASE-CONTROL STUDY RESULTS

|  | Cases numbers | Controls numbers |
|---|---|---|
| Exposed (one or more previous stillbirths) | 141 | 133 |
| Unexposed (no previous stillbirths) | 1250 | 4867 |
|  | 1391 | 5000 |

(a) Odds ratio = $(141 \times 4867)/(133 \times 1250) = 4.13$

(b) Relative risk undetermined but will be similar to relative odds as other information shows that anencephalus is uncommon (about 1–2 per 1000 births).

Attributable risk undermined.

Attributable proportion in exposed subjects $= \dfrac{4.13 - 1}{4.13} = 75.8\%$

Attributable proportion in population; if controls are representative of all unaffected births, then prevalence of exposure $p = 133/5000 = 0.0266$ and attributable proportion in the population =

$$\frac{p(RR - 1)}{p(RR - 1) + 1} = \frac{0.0266 \times 3.13}{(0.0266 \times 3.13) + 1} = 7.7\%$$

**Ex. 3.6.** Format of results from a case-control study assessing the relationship between a history of a previous stillbirth and the occurrence of anencephalus. Mothers of all notified babies with anencephalus in a defined population form the case series ($n = 1391$); an arbitrary number of 5000 mothers of liveborn babies were chosen as controls. From Elwood *et al.* [12]

were selected. **Ex. 3.6** shows the results of a case–control study in which 1391 births with anencephalus, a severe and fatal abnormality, were compared with 5000 live births; the exposure was the mother's past history of stillbirth [12]. The odds ratio is 4.13, showing a strong association. Ignore the results under (b) at present.

To see how these results were derived, **Ex. 3.7** shows the source population, i.e. all births in certain cities in Canada over a 20-year period. There were 1391 births with anencephalus, all of which were included in the case–control study; and 1 193 600 live births, of which only 5000 were selected to form the control series. From Ex. 3.7, all the measures of risk can be calculated as shown. Note that the relative odds and the relative risk are virtually the same; this is because the frequency of the disease is low, and so the numbers of unaffected and of total subjects are not very different.

Now, return to Ex. 3.6 and see what measures can be calculated. The odds ratio estimate is valid, differing from that in the whole population only by sampling variation; knowing that the outcome being studied is uncommon allows us to use the odds ratio as an estimate of relative risk. What cannot be calculated from Ex. 3.6 is the actual rate of disease in either the exposed or unexposed groups, or the attributable risk. If Ex. 3.6 is misinterpreted by a failure to consider that the data come from a case–control study, it might be thought that the risk of this defect in births to mothers who had had a previous stillbirth was $141/(141 + 133) = 51$ per cent, an order of magnitude greater than the true value (4.4 per 1000) given in Ex. 3.7.

## Attributable proportion in case–control studies

In Ex. 3.2 it was shown that there is a simple formula linking the attributable proportion in exposed subjects to the relative risk, with the attributable proportion being equal to $(RR - 1)/RR$; thus this can be estimated in a

---

A RELATIONSHIP IN A POPULATION

| | Anencephalus births | Unaffected births | Total births | Prevalence of anencephalus per 1000 births |
|---|---|---|---|---|
| Previous stillbirth | 141 | 31 750 | 31 891 | 4.42 |
| No previous stillbirth | 1250 | 1 161 850 | 1 163 100 | 1.07 |
| | 1391 | 1 193 600 | 1 194 991 | 1.16 |

relative odds = $(141/31\ 750)/(1250/1\ 161\ 850) = 4.13$
relative risk = $(141/31\ 891)/(1250/1\ 163\ 100) = 4.11$
attributable risk = $4.42 - 1.07 = 3.35$ per 1000 births
attributable proportion in exposed subjects = $3.35/4.42 = 75.8\%$
attributable proportion in population = $(1.16 - 1.07)/1.16 = 7.8\%$

---

**Ex. 3.7.** Relationships in a population. The relationships between anencephalus and previous stillbirths in all pregnancies in the population in which the case-control study shown in Ex. 3.6 was conducted. From Elwood *et al.* [12]

case–control study, as shown in Ex. 3.6. The attributable proportion in the population can be calculated if there is an estimate of the proportion of the total population which is exposed to the causative factor (Ex. 3.6). In some circumstances the control group in a case–control study can be considered as a representative sample of the total population, and this proportion is given by the proportion of controls exposed. However, often this is not so; for example, if the controls have been matched to the cases on certain characteristics, they will not be representative of the population and an independent source of evidence will be necessary to give the proportion of the population which is exposed.

## Use of the odds ratio

As has been already shown, the odds ratio is a very good estimate of relative risk in most situations, the exception being where the outcome is very frequent. Cohort designs for outcomes which are frequent will be efficient, as a reasonable number of subjects will have to be followed to obtain an adequate number who experience the outcome under study. The great disadvantage of cohort studies is in attempting to study outcomes which are uncommon, so that many hundreds or thousands of individuals have to be followed before a reasonable number of them experience the outcome. It is in this situation that case–control studies are most useful. Therefore in most situations for which case–control studies are advantageous, the difference between relative odds and relative risk will be trivial, and certainly much less important than other potential sources of error in the study. Therefore in most literature odds ratios produced from case–control studies are referred to as relative risks.

## Odds ratio from case–control studies; a more formal derivation

(For the more curious reader; others may wish to skip to the next section.)

The difference between the results from a case–control study and those from the entire source population arise because the sampling fractions are different for cases and controls. In the study shown in Ex. 3.6 and Ex. 3.7, the sampling fraction for the cases was 1.0, and that for the controls was $5000/1\,193\,600 = 0.00419$. Usually the sampling fractions are unknown in a case–control study, but they will often be of this nature, in that the sampling fraction of the cases will be 1.0 or very high, and the sampling fraction of the controls will be very low.

**Ex. 3.8** summarizes the algebra of case–control studies, showing that in the odds ratio calculations the sampling fractions cancel out, and therefore the odds ratio is a direct estimate of the odds ratio in the source population, even if the sampling fractions are unknown. This simple algebra emphasizes a crucial

---

ODDS RATIO IN A CASE-CONTROL STUDY

|  | Cases | Controls |
|---|---|---|
| Exposed | $a = fA$ | $b = gB$ |
| Unexposed | $c = fC$ | $d = gD$ |
|  | $a + c = f(A + C)$ | $b + d = g(B + D)$ |

odds ratio in population $= (A/B)/(C/D) = AD/BC$
odds ratio in study $= (a/b)/(c/d)$
$= (fA/gB)/(fC/gD)$
$= AD/BC$

---

**Ex. 3.8.** Algebraic justification for the calculation of odds ratio from a case-control study.
Capital letters = numbers of individuals in the population ($A$, $B$, $C$, $D$).
Lower case letters = numbers of individuals in the study ($a$, $b$, $c$, $d$).
$f$ = sampling fraction for cases = $(a + c)/(A + C)$
$g$ = sampling fraction for controls = $(b + d)/(B + D)$
The essential design characteristic of case-control studies is that the fractions $f$ and $g$ are the same for both exposed and unexposed subjects

point in the design of case–control studies: the sampling system used for cases must be 'without bias' with respect to exposure, i.e. the same sampling fraction $f$ must apply to both exposed and unexposed cases. If that is so, the ratio of the numbers of exposed to unexposed cases in the study will be the same as the ratio in the population. The same logic applies to the controls, which must also be sampled without bias with regard to exposure status, so that the (different) sampling fraction $g$ applies to both exposed and unexposed controls.

## Different sampling schemes in case–control studies: why a case can also be a control

The traditional, and intuitively clear at first glance, process of selecting controls in a case–control study is to select them as a representative sample of the *unaffected* subjects from a particular population. In **Ex. 3.9** we present a hypothetical set of data concerning an exposure in pregnancy and a malformation, which is based loosely on the data presented in Ex. 3.1, but quite deliberately shows a much greater prevalence of the malformation at birth. Therefore in this hypothetical example, the exposure is associated with a relative risk of 4.23, but an odds ratio of 5.65. The substantial difference between these two measures is because the frequency of the malformation overall is quite high.

Now suppose we set up a case–control study in this situation. One design of case–control study would take a representative sample of *malformed* infants as cases, and a representative sample of the *not malformed* infants as controls. Let us assume we sample all the malformed infants (260) and an arbitrary sample

---

SAMPLING OF CONTROLS IN A CASE-CONTROL STUDY

A: Total population

| Exposure | Malformed | Not malformed | Total | Prevalence of malformation (%) |
|---|---|---|---|---|
| Exposed | 120 | 273 | 393 | 30.5 |
| Unexposed | 140 | 1799 | 1939 | 7.2 |
| Total population | 260 | 2072 | 2332 | 11.1 |

Odds ratio = 5.65
Relative risk (prevalence ratio) = 4.23

B: Case control design, sampling controls from non-affected only

| Exposure | Malformed | Controls = not malformed |
|---|---|---|
| Exposed | 120 | 53 |
| Unexposed | 140 | 347 |
| Total population | 260 | 400 |

Sample estimate of odds ratio $= (140 \times 347)/(53 \times 140) = 5.61$

C: Case control design, sampling controls from all pregnancies

| Exposure | Malformed | Controls = not total pregnancies |
|---|---|---|
| Exposed | 120 | 67 |
| Unexposed | 140 | 333 |
| Total population | 260 | 400 |

Sample estimate of relative risk $= (120 \times 333)/(67 \times 140) = 4.26$

---

**Ex. 3.9.** Different sampling schemes for controls in a case–control study. Subtable A shows the whole population data; both odds ratio and relative risk can be calculated. Subtable B shows controls drawn as a random sample of unaffected pregnancies; the results yield the odds ratio. Subtable C shows controls drawn as a random sample of all pregnancies; the results yield relative risk.

of 400 of the unaffected infants (there is nothing magical about having an equal number, or a fixed ratio of controls to cases, and the actual size chosen will depend on practical issues such as cost). The numbers in subtable B are calculated by integer numbers given by a random sample of 400 controls. This sample yields an *odds ratio* of 5.61, which is a good estimate of the actual odds ratio of 5.65 in the population, but is clearly different from the relative risk.

A second type of case–control design would again sample all the 260 malformed infants as cases, but take a representative sample of *all infants* as controls. Therefore the distribution of the controls would reflect the exposure frequency in the whole population, not just the unaffected babies. The cross-products ratio from this design yields a sample estimate of *relative risk* directly, as the control sample represents the total population rather than only the 'non-case' population. As can be seen, a good estimate of the relative risk is obtained, which is clearly different from the odds ratio. This is '*incidence density*' sampling.

The practical ways in which these studies would be carried out clarify another seemingly complex issue. In the first design, comparing cases with non-cases, malformed infants would be entered into the study as cases as they are recognized; and a sample of non-malformed infants would be chosen, for instance by selecting a number of such infants from the same hospitals each week and interviewing their mothers, as non-diseased controls.

The second design is equally simple. Again, malformed infants would be classified as cases as they occur, but the comparison sample here would be a representative, perhaps random, sample of all births occurring in the birth population which yields the cases. In this sampling design, an affected 'case' infant is also eligible for selection as a control; if that case infant appears in the representative sample of controls, it should be used as a control. Thus the same individual can appear as both a case and a control. Although this seems obscure, it is simply analogous to the calculation of any measure of occurrence rate, such as prevalence or incidence rate. In these rates (as noted in Chapter 1), the number of affected individuals is the numerator, and it is divided by the total number of individuals at risk which of course includes those who are affected. Therefore affected individuals appear in both the numerator and the denominator of a calculated frequency rate. Thus in a case–control study designed to produce an estimate of the ratio of such rates, i.e. a relative risk, the same individual can appear as a case and a control.

As was shown earlier, if the odds ratio is calculated, affected and unaffected infants appear as the numerator or the denominator respectively, and there is no figure which includes both. The case–control design which produces estimates of the odds ratio keeps the cases and controls separate, and an individual cannot appear in both affected and unaffected samples.

Many case–control studies of major diseases are of the type which directly yields an estimate of the relative risk. A typical design for a case–control study of a chronic disease such as cancer is to enter individuals as cases as soon as they are diagnosed with the disease, and to obtain a control at that time from the entire population from which that case is sampled. Therefore the control series provides a sample based on the population at risk at the time when the case became an incident case. The cross-products ratio, as in subtable B of Ex. 3.9, gives an estimate of the relative risk. In this design, an individual can be sampled as a control, and then shortly afterwards could become a case and be eligible to be sampled as a case. This is quite appropriate theoretically.

## Surveys

In principle, survey designs yield the same type of results as cohort studies; in cross-sectional surveys, all information on both exposures and outcomes is in terms of prevalence. The terms relative risk, relative odds, and so on can be used, remembering that in this situation these apply to ratios of prevalence rates rather than ratios of incidence rates as in a prospective cohort design. The use of relative odds is also more limited because frequently in a survey the prevalences of conditions being studied are quite substantial, and therefore the relative odds may be substantially different from the relative risk. Thus in the survey comparing Tanzanian villagers with different diets, the prevalence of borderline or frank hypertension was 38.7 per cent in those with a vegetarian diet, and 12.5 per cent in fish-eaters, giving a prevalence rate ratio of 3.1; the odds ratio is 4.4 [13].

**Ex. 3.10** shows the results of a cross-sectional survey of the prevalence of smoking in a sample of schoolchildren in England, and explores the association, at that point in time, between the parents' current smoking habit with that of the children [14]. Where one or both parents smoked, the prevalence of 'ever smoking' in the children was 57.0 per cent; where neither parent smoked, it was 51.5 per cent. The relative risk, the prevalence ratio, is 57.0/51.5 = 1.11. The odds ratio can be calculated, as shown, but tends not to be used as it is different from the relative risk as the prevalence of the outcome is high. The attributable risk, and proportions, are calculated as shown and expressed in terms of prevalence.

## General applicability of these analytical approaches

We have now presented a format of results for a cohort study and for a case–control study. The cohort format applies to any study in which the comparison is between two or more groups defined by differences in the exposure. Thus, for example, Sloan *et al.* [15] compared the assault and murder rates in Vancouver, Canada, and Seattle, USA, two generally similar cities which have different laws affecting access to firearms. This is a descriptive study, but as the comparison is between the 'exposure' to different legislative systems, the results can be expressed in the format of a cohort study and show the great excess of assault and murder related to firearms in Seattle compared with Vancouver, in contrast with similar rates of assault and murder involving other weapons (**Ex. 3.11**). Relative risks are calculated, and the other measures shown in Ex. 3.2 can be derived.

Other surveys may equate to the case–control design, where the essential comparison is between groups with and without the outcome of interest, in which case the format of results applicable to case–control designs is applied.

---

### RESULTS OF A CROSS-SECTIONAL SURVEY

Smoking in young children

| Parent's smoking | Ever smoked | Never smoked | Total | Prevalence, ever smoked (%) |
|---|---|---|---|---|
| One or both smoke | 3203 | 2418 | 5621 | 57.0 |
| Neither smokes | 1601 | 1508 | 3109 | 51.5 |
| Total | 4804 | 3926 | 8730 | 55.0 |

Prevalence ratio (relative risk) = 57.0/51.5 = 1.11
Odds ratio = (3203/2418)/(1601/1508) = 1.25

The odds ratio is not a very useful measure, as the prevalence ratio can be calculated as easily, and it is substantially different from the prevalence ratio as the outcome is common.

Attributable risk or prevalence difference = 57.0 − 51.5 = 5.5%

Attributable proportion in exposed $= \dfrac{5.5}{57.0} = 9.6\% = \dfrac{(RR-1)}{RR}$

Attributable proportion in population $= \dfrac{55.0 - 51.5}{55.0} = 6.4\%$

$$= \dfrac{p(RR-1)}{p(RR-1)+1}$$

where $p = 5621/8730 = 0.64$

**Ex. 3.10.** Results of a cross-sectional survey in which questionnaires were given to 8–9-year-old subjects in industrial areas of northern England; these results show the smoking history of the subjects, compared with their report on their parents' smoking. Note: for the attributable proportion calculation, rounding errors can be considerable. Thus $RR = (3203/5621)/(1601/3109) = 1.1066$; $(RR − 1)/RR = 0.1066/1.1066 = 9.6\%$ although $(1.11 − 1)/1.11 = 9.9\%$. From Charlton [14]

---

### EXPOSURE-BASED COMPARISON OF DESCRIPTIVE DATA

| Crime | Annual rate per 100 000 population | | Relative risk |
|---|---|---|---|
| | Seattle, USA | Vancouver, Canada | |
| Aggravated assault using: | | | |
| Firearms | 87.9 | 11.4 | 7.7 |
| Knives | 78.1 | 78.9 | 1.0 |
| Other means | 320.6 | 330.2 | 1.0 |
| All aggravated assault | 486.5 | 420.5 | 1.2 |
| Murder (homicide) using: | | | |
| Firearms | 4.8 | 1.0 | 5.1 |
| Knives | 3.1 | 3.5 | 0.9 |
| Other means | 3.4 | 2.5 | 1.3 |
| All homicide | 11.3 | 6.9 | 1.6 |

**Ex. 3.11.** Descriptive study with results in a cohort format. These annual rates of assault and murder in Vancouver (Canada) and Seattle (USA) represent the outcome; the city of residence, and its legal system, is the exposure. From Sloan *et al.* [15]

## Self-test questions (answers on p. 494)

**Q3.1** The trial of tuberculosis treatment shown in Chapter 1 showed four deaths from 55 patients treated by streptomycin, compared with 14 deaths from 52 controls. Calculate:

    (a) The mortality rates in each group. What type of rates are these?

    (b) The relative risk.

    (c) The odds ratio.

    (c) The attributable risk.

    (d) The attributable benefit.

    (e) The 'number needed to treat' for one death prevented.

**Q3.2** In a cohort study of diet and heart disease in men, the study population is considered in two groups. In the high fat diet group there were 12 500 man-years of observation and 48 deaths; in the lower fat group there were 22 000 man-years of observation and 64 deaths.

Calculate:

    (a) The mortality rates in each group.

    (b) The relative risk.

    (c) The attributable risk of the high fat diet.

    (d) What proportion of disease in the high fat diet group is attributable to the high fat diet?

    (e) What proportion of disease in the whole population group is attributable to the high fat diet?

**Q3.3** If the incidence rate of asthma is 400 per 10 000 person-years in those who smoke, 100 in those who are exposed to air pollution, and 50 in those with neither exposure, what is the expected incidence in those with both exposures, assuming:

    (a) an additive model

    (b) a multiplicative model.

**Q3.4** In a case–control study of arthritis of the knee, there are 500 cases, and 180 have a history of a previous knee injury; of 800 controls free from knee arthritis, 120 had a history of injury. Calculate:

    (a) The relative risk.

    (b) The odds ratio.

    (c) The attributable proportion in those with a previous injury.

**Q3.5** If, in Q3.4, the cases were all newly diagnosed cases in a given community and the controls were a random sample of that community, each selected at the time a case occurred, what difference would that make to the answers to Q3.4 (a) and (b)?

**Q3.6** If we assume that the effects seen in Ex. 3.11 represent an effect of the difference in gun laws, and if Canadian gun laws could be introduced to Seattle:

    (a) What proportion of murders in Seattle, using firearms, would be prevented?

    (b) How many people would be affected by the change for each firearm-linked murder prevented?

    (c) What proportion of all murders in Seattle would be prevented?

# References

1. **Morrow J, Russell A, Guthrie E,** *et al.* Malformation risks of antiepileptic drugs in pregnancy: a prospective study from the UK Epilepsy and Pregnancy Register. *J Neurol Neurosurg Psychiatry* 2006; **77**(2): 193–198.

2. **ISIS-4** (Fourth International Study of Infarct Survival Collaborative Group). ISIS-4: A randomised factorial trial assessing early oral captopril, oral mononitrate, and intravenous magnesium sulphate in 58 050 patients with suspected acute myocardial infarction. *Lancet* 1995; **345**: 669–685.

3. **Cook RJ, Sackett DL.** The number needed to treat: a clinically useful measure of treatment effect. *BMJ* 1995; **310**: 452–454.

4. **Edwards A, Elwyn G, Covey J, Matthews E, Pill R.** Presenting risk information: a review of the effects of "framing" and other manipulations on patient outcomes. *J Health Commun* 2001; **6**: 61–82.

5. **Bucher HC, Weinbacher M, Gyr K.** Influence of method of reporting study results on decision of physicians to prescribe drugs to lower cholesterol concentration. *BMJ* 1994; **309**: 761–764.

6. **Sarfati D, Howden-Chapman P, Woodward A, Salmond C.** Does the frame affect the picture? A study into how attitudes to screening for cancer are affected by the way benefits are expressed. *J Med Screen* 1998; **5**: 137–140.

7. **Romond EH, Perez EA, Bryant J,** *et al.* Trastuzumab plus adjuvant chemotherapy for operable HER2-positive breast cancer. *N Engl J Med* 2005; **353**: 1673–1684.

8. **Paffenbarger RS, Hale WE.** Work activity and coronary heart mortality. *N Engl J Med* 1975; **292**: 545–550.

9. **Royal College of General Practitioners' Oral Contraception Study.** Mortality among oral-contraceptive users. Royal College of General Practitioners' Oral Contraception Study. *Lancet* **1977**; **ii**: 727–731.

10. **Beral V, Hermon C, Kay C, Hannaford P, Darby S, Reeves G.** Mortality associated with oral contraceptive use: 25 year follow up of cohort of 46 000 women from Royal College of General Practitioners' oral contraception study. *BMJ* 1999; **318**: 96–100.

11. **Vessey M, Painter R, Yeates D.** Mortality in relation to oral contraceptive use and cigarette smoking. *Lancet* 2003; **362**: 185–191.

12. **Elwood JM, Raman S, Mousseau G.** Reproductive history in the mothers of anencephalics. *J Chronic Dis* 1978; **31**: 473–481.

13. **Pauletto P, Puato M, Caroli MG,** *et al.* Blood pressure and atherogenic lipoprotein profiles of fish-diet and vegetarian villagers in Tanzania: the Lugalawa study. *Lancet* 1996; **348**: 784–788.

14. **Charlton A.** Children's coughs related to parental smoking. *BMJ* 1984; **288**: 1647–1649.

15. **Sloan JH, Kellermann AL, Reay DT,** *et al.* Handgun regulations, crime, assaults, and homocide. *N Engl J Med* 1988; **319**: 1256–1262.

# Chapter 4

# Selection of subjects for study

On the 20th of May, 1747, I took twelve patients in the scurvy, on board the Salisbury at sea. Their cases were as similar as I could have them. They all in general had putrid gums, the spots and lassitude, with weakness of their knees. They lay together in one place ... and had one diet common to all... Two of these were ordered each a quart of cyder a-day. Two others took twenty-five gutts of elixir vitriol three times a day ... Two others took two spoonfuls of vinegar three times a day ... Two of the worst patients ... were put under a course of sea water ... Two others had each two oranges and one lemon given them every day ... The two remaining patients, took the bigness of a nutmeg three times a-day, of an electuary recommended by an hospital surgeon ... The consequence was, that the most sudden and visible good effects were perceived from the use of the oranges and lemons.

—James Lind: A treatise of the scurvy; 1753

This chapter deals with how subjects are selected for inclusion in analytical and intervention studies. To interpret a study, we must assess the problems that may have been overcome, or introduced, by the methods used to select subjects for the study. Again, we shall be dealing with the simplest possible situation, where two groups of subjects are being compared. In observational cohort studies, we have to select subjects who are or have been exposed to the putative causal factor and a suitable comparison group who are unexposed or less exposed. In the case–control design, we have to select subjects in whom the outcome has occurred (cases) to compare with subjects in whom the outcome has not occurred (controls). In intervention studies, we select subjects who are suitable and willing to have either the intervention being assessed or the alternative with which it is compared, which may be no intervention. Part 1 of this chapter will cover the general principles, and Part 2 will show the application of these principles to each type of study.

## Part 1. Principles of subject selection

### Target, source, eligible, entrant, and participant populations

As the derivation of subjects in a study is sometimes quite complex, we shall use five terms to describe the selection process in most studies (**Ex. 4.1**).

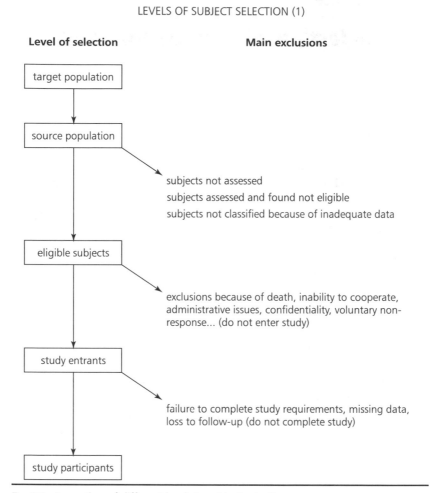

**Ex. 4.1.** Formation of different levels in subject selection

The information in any study is derived from the individuals who complete the study and contribute information to it, and we refer to these subjects as *participants*. They may be the same as the study *entrants*—those who enter the study—but some people may enter the study but not complete it. The study entrants are derived from the *eligible* population—those individuals who have been defined as eligible for entry into the study. Some members of the eligible population will not become study entrants. This may be because they are not invited although eligible, or they are unable to participate because of death, illness, administrative, or confidentiality issues, or they do not wish to participate. Such subjects do not enter the study. Eligible subjects may also fail to become study participants because although they enter the study, they do not complete its requirements and undergo the procedures or provide the data that are necessary. The correct handling of subjects who enter but who do not complete the study is an important issue, particularly in intervention trials, and will be discussed specifically in that context. Some individuals may complete part of a study (e.g. they may complete a clinical examination, but not provide a blood sample), and so they will be participants for some analyses, but only study entrants for others.

The eligible population is in turn a subset of the *source* population. The source population is determined by practical considerations, and might consist of patients in a hospital or in an individual doctor's practice, members of a particular community, a workforce, or some other group. For some studies the source population can be strictly defined and enumerated, and the proportion eligible can be calculated; in other studies the source population cannot be measured exactly, although it still needs definition. Within the source population there will be four groups of subjects: those who are eligible, those who are adequately assessed and found not to be eligible, those who cannot be classified because of inadequate information, and those who are not assessed because of lack of resources, unavailability, or other reasons.

To have practical value the study results must be applicable to subjects other than those in the original source population; for example, a study of medical treatment needs to give information that will be relevant to future patients. We shall call the population to which we aim to apply the results the *target* population, or rather target populations; unlike the other entities in the scheme, the target population is not fixed, and its definition can be modified by information from outside the study results.

In terms of subject selection, these five levels give five successively smaller subsets of subjects, each derived from the one preceding it (**Ex. 4.2**). In terms of the application of the study results, they are five successively larger populations, for each of which a further generalization of the results derived from the participants is needed.

As an example, consider a clinical trial assessing different treatments in the management of acute myocardial infarction, carried out, as most such trials are, in a major teaching hospital. The study *participants* are those patients who enter the study, are randomized, and provide outcome data; their outcome information is used in the results. Some subjects may be study *entrants*, but for some reason their outcome information is not available, and so they are not full participants as they do not contribute to the key analysis. The *eligible* population consists of all patients with an appropriate diagnosis seen at the participating hospital, within preset limits of age and perhaps other factors, who do not

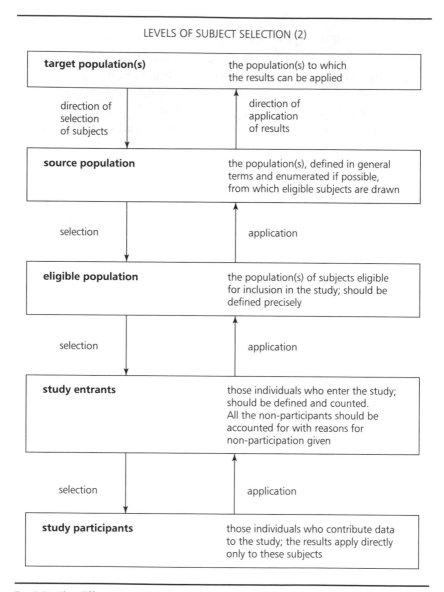

**Ex. 4.2.** The different groups of subjects to be considered in interpreting studies

have the various clinical contraindications that will be defined in the trial protocol. The study will be of little value unless we can assume that the results
based on the study participants will apply to this eligible population. If many
subjects enter but do not complete the trial, many others do not give their
consent to enter the trial, and many are excluded for reasons other than those

stipulated in the trial protocol, there will be substantial differences between the eligible and participant populations. Then we have to question whether the results apply to the eligible population.

A low participation rate raises questions of interpretation. For example, Slanetz et al. [1] assessed the opinions of doctors on whether mammograms would be better read immediately by one radiologist, or sent away for reading by two radiologists. Of 278 doctors responding to a questionnaire, 90 per cent favoured off-site double reading. This seems a conclusive result, but is based on a survey of 1000 doctors, and a response rate of 28 per cent. The results are valid only if the views of those who returned the questionnaires (the participants) are similar to those of the whole group sent questionnaires (the eligible population); as the opinions of those who did not respond are unknown, this cannot be ascertained.

For the trial of treatment for myocardial infarction, the *source* population consists of the patients admitted to the teaching hospital, or to the particular clinical unit, over a certain period of time. In principle all such patients should be assessed to see if they are eligible for the study. The *target* population is much wider, and will include patients seen in other geographical areas, perhaps even other countries, and certainly include patients seen at a future time. The definition of the target population will reflect the eligibility criteria, but also the characteristics of the source population, with regard to how individuals become part of the source population. The particular issues will be specific to the subject matter. For example, if the trial concerns therapy for myocardial infarction given immediately on admission to the clinical unit, results based on a unit which has a very rapid referral procedure from the community might not be applicable to another institution which admits only patients who have survived a considerable time since the infarct.

The choice of the source population will affect the interpretation of the results. For example, studies assessing whether children who had convulsions related to fever (febrile convulsions) also had an increased risk of further convulsions showed results ranging from 60 per cent subsequent risk down to 2–5 per cent [2]. The studies showing high risks were based on hospitals or speciality clinics, relating to children referred to them, whereas the studies with low subsequent risks were based on children identified through community-based or primary care sources. The hospital studies relate to children with more severe initial disease, which probably explains the higher subsequent rate of convulsions recorded; differences in subsequent ascertainment and follow-up methods could also be important. Similarly, the remission rate in patients with leukaemia varied from 44 to 85 per cent, depending on the eligibility criteria applied [3].

The procedure for selection of subjects who participate in the study can affect not only how widely the results of the study can be applied, but also whether the results of the study are in fact valid. To go further, it is helpful to distinguish two important aspects of study validity.

## The distinction between internal and external validity

All these studies involve a comparison between, at the simplest level, two groups of subjects. Thus, in the cohort study or intervention trial we compare subjects who have been exposed to the putative causative factor with subjects who have not been exposed. The *internal validity* of a study is a measure of how confident we can be that a difference in outcome between these two groups can be attributed to the effects of the exposure or intervention. The alternative explanations, which will each be discussed in detail in subsequent chapters, are that the observed difference in outcome between the groups being compared is due to *bias* in the way the observations are made, to differences between the groups in terms of other relevant factors (*confounding*), or to *chance* variation. As an example of a study with high internal validity, consider an experiment to test the cancer-causing potential of a chemical. This can be done by taking a large number of laboratory rats, bred from the same genetic strains and kept under identical conditions of diet, environment, and handling, and from these randomly selecting some animals to receive the chemical in their food, while the other animals receive a similar amount of an inert substance. The outcome would be determined by post-mortem examination of all animals at the end of their natural lifespan to determine the prevalence of cancers, with these examinations being done by a pathologist who is unaware of which animals have been given the chemical. In such a study the possibility of the observations of cancer occurrence being biased can be dismissed, the likelihood of there being some systematic difference between the animals who received the chemical and those who did not is small, and if adequate numbers are used the possibility of chance variation will be small. Therefore it is relatively easy to interpret differences in cancer occurrence between the exposed and unexposed animals as reflecting a cause and effect relationship; this ease of interpretation is due to the high *internal validity* of the study.

In contrast, consider a study attempting to look at the relationship between regular exercise and heart disease, in which a group of men who report that they take regular exercise is compared with a group of men who do not take regular exercise, with the outcome of the study being determined by the diagnoses of heart disease made by the subjects' doctors over the following few years. A difference in the recorded frequency of heart disease between these groups could be due to differences in ascertainment, for example if there were differences in the frequency with which subjects visit their doctors, or differences in the doctors' diagnostic criteria, or differences in their record keeping. A difference in outcome could also occur because of other differences between the two groups of men that could affect their frequency of heart disease, such as variations in cigarette smoking or diet. If the two groups of men being compared were small, the likelihood of the difference seen having arisen through chance variation might be considerable. We would say that such a study has low internal validity.

The *external validity* of a study refers to the ability to apply the results of the study to a wider population. Despite the very high internal validity of the rat experiment described above, we would hesitate to use the results to conclude that the chemical causes cancer in humans, because the species, the dosages given, the route of administration, and various other factors differ between the experimental situation and the situation which interests us. An epidemiological study of the same topic, for example comparing workers who use the chemical in their job with workers who do similar jobs but without such exposure, could give us a result that would have much higher external validity.

It is obvious that the best studies are those that have high internal validity and also high external validity; however, such studies may be difficult or impossible. Often the design considerations which help to increase the internal validity of a study may work against its external validity. Difficult choices in study design often have to be made. Going back to the example of the comparison between exercising and non-exercising men, one could argue that this study might have acceptable external validity as it is, after all, looking at the topic in free-living individuals. However, the internal validity of that study is so low that its external validity is irrelevant. It is important to realize that *external validity is useful only if the internal validity of a study is acceptable*; studies with very low internal validity have very little value. Studies that have high internal validity always have some value, even if the external validity is low. Therefore we can conclude that in designing and interpreting studies we need to pay attention to both internal validity and external validity, but internal validity is the more important.

In considering a study, each step in the chain from target population to study participants should be examined. We should ask whether the losses seen at each point produce differences between the groups of individuals being compared which may compromise the internal validity of the study, or produce a limited or atypical group of study participants which may compromise the external validity of the results.

## Selection bias and its effects

Selection bias can be regarded as any potentially misleading effect caused by the way subjects are selected to participate in a study. The selection processes can potentially affect both the internal validity and the external validity of a study, and can result in changing the hypothesis being assessed (**Ex. 4.3**).

## Effects on internal validity

First, selection effects can influence the *internal validity* of the study. This will occur only if the selection process has different effects on the different groups being compared. Suppose we compare the frequency of smoking in men and women by sending a questionnaire to all residents in a community. The response rate could well be higher for women than for men (which we will know if the gender distribution of the source population is known), and it may be lower for smokers than for non-smokers (we may not know that without further information). The survey will then underestimate the prevalence of smoking, and this underestimation will be greater in women. Thus the internal validity of the study in assessing differences in smoking between men and women is compromised.

Subjects who participate readily in a study often differ from those who are less enthusiastic. In an early demonstration of this, in a survey of psychosocial issues in the 1950s major psychosomatic problems were found in three out of 20 families who showed good cooperation with the survey, but in 11 out of 17 families who were less cooperative [4]. Selection factors affect internal validity only if they have *different* effects on the groups of subjects being compared within the study; this is the important distinction from the effect on external validity discussed next. As we have seen, internal validity is the more important concept, and so the primary objective in designing appropriate selection procedures is to preserve internal validity.

---

SELECTION BIAS

Selection bias can have three types of effects on a study.
It may:

affect the internal validity

affect the external validity

modify the hypothesis being tested

---

**Ex. 4.3.** Three effects of selection bias on a study

## Effects on external validity

Secondly, selection issues can affect the *external validity* of the study. If a trial of two treatments for myocardial infarction is restricted to patients who are male, aged under 55, and have a particular pattern of infarction, the results can be directly applied to a target population which shares these features, but extension beyond needs to be justified by other evidence. Thus the selection criteria control the nature of the target population, and so limit its external validity. As these selection restrictions apply to both the groups being compared, they should not impair the internal validity. External validity may also be influenced by the participation rate, i.e. the proportion of eligible subjects who participate in the study, as a low participation rate makes it more likely that the participants are not representative of the eligible population.

Examples of studies with limited external validity which have already been given include the survey of doctors about mammography, which suffered from a very low response rate, and the studies of subsequent convulsion frequency in children who have had febrile convulsions; here, each individual study may have been internally valid, but their results depend greatly on the sources from which the subjects included were chosen.

## Effects on the hypothesis being tested

The effects of selection bias may mean that the study as performed tests a different hypothesis to that originally envisaged. Consider a case–control study of the causes of 'rheumatoid arthritis'. The selection procedure used to identify cases may mean that the study actually assesses possible causative factors for 'rheumatoid arthritis that is sufficiently severe to lead to hospital treatment', which may be a hypothesis considerably different from that originally envisaged.

This issue is closely related to that of misclassification. External validity will be highest where the cases in the case–control study, or the exposed group in a cohort study, can be regarded as representative of all cases or of all exposed individuals in the source population. However, frequently the attempt to maintain high external validity introduces the risk of inaccuracies in the definition of these study groups, so that they include non-cases or non-exposed individuals. For example, in the case–control study of rheumatoid arthritis there are choices between the two extremes of entering all individuals in a defined community (the source population) who have any type of diagnosis of rheumatoid arthritis, or of entering only those who have rheumatoid arthritis defined by specific criteria and supported by specific laboratory and radiological investigations. The latter procedure will lead to less misclassification, but if a full investigation is performed only on patients with severe disease, the participants will be less likely to be representative of all individuals with rheumatoid arthritis. The balance between these two options will depend on the particular circumstances of the investigation.

For example, several case–control studies in the 1970s (e.g. [5]) compared women with endometrial (uterus) cancer with control groups selected on various criteria, and showed a much higher frequency of the use of oestrogens, prescribed mainly for the control of menopausal symptoms, in the endometrial cancer cases. However, a subsequent case–control study showed no association; the controls for that study were chosen as women who had been investigated for endometrial cancer, but found not to have it. The argument made for the comparison was that using such a control group would ensure that no controls had unrecognized endometrial cancer, i.e. misclassification was avoided. However, the comparison being made was between women with endometrial cancer and other women investigated because of similar symptoms, such as bleeding. If oestrogens cause both endometrial cancer and other conditions that lead to bleeding, the lack of association reported in that comparison would be expected, and would not assess whether the risk of cancer was increased. A further study compared women with endometrial cancer with three other groups: women having investigation for gynaecological symptoms, other gynaecological patients, and a community-based group. Oestrogen use was highest in the women with cancer and the first of these comparison groups, showing that it caused both endometrial cancer and other non-cancer conditions leading to similar investigations [6]. One of the first of these studies is discussed in detail in Chapter 14.

There have been several investigations of the relationship between psychological parameters, previous life events, and breast cancer by studying women attending breast clinics for diagnosis. This has the advantage of allowing interviews or questionnaires to be applied prior to diagnosis, avoiding the response bias that might arise after the diagnosis. Factors that are more common in women who are subsequently diagnosed with breast cancer than in women without cancer have then been interpreted as causal factors for breast cancer. However, the comparison being made is not between women with breast cancer and women representative of the general population, but between women with breast cancer and women with other breast problems which bring them to a diagnostic clinic. A positive association with breast cancer could arise because the factor prevents other breast conditions that would lead to attendance at that clinic; one such factor is oral contraceptive use, which decreases the risk of some benign breast conditions.

# Methods of reducing selection biases

Selection effects are of two kinds: first, effects of incomplete *participation*; secondly, effects produced by the selection *criteria*. The investigator should have knowledge and control over the selection criteria; only partial control of participation is possible.

## Reporting, and optimizing, participation and response

The *participation rate* indicates how the participants in a study may differ from the eligible population. The participation rate is defined as the number of study participants divided by the number of eligible subjects. It is particularly useful to compare the participation rates of the different groups of subjects in the study, as differences may affect the internal validity of the study.

The *response rate* is one component of the participation rate. The response rate is the number of study participants divided by the number of eligible subjects who were identified, contacted, and asked to participate; it is a measure of the completeness of voluntary response by the subjects. As such, it is useful and indicates one important part of the selection process. As it does not account for losses by mortality, failure to locate, exclusion by doctors, and so on, it should not be used as the only or main estimate of participation, although it frequently is in publications, perhaps because it is often impressively high. The participation rate is, of course, always lower than, or at the maximum equal to, the response rate.

Ideally, all studies should report on the participation and response rates, but this is not always done. In a survey of the published information on participation in 355 epidemiological studies published in 10 major journals in 2003, information on participation was given in only 32 per cent of cohort studies, 44 per cent of case–control studies, and 59 per cent of surveys. The information given was sparse; for example, participation and subject response rates could both be calculated in only 16 per cent of reported case–control studies [7]. Participation rates declined over the period 1970 to 2003.

Obtaining high response rates in surveys and questionnaires is a major subject in its own right. A systematic review of randomized controlled trials of strategies to increase response rates to postal questionnaires based on information up to 2003 included 372 trials [8]. The review reported that many methods had been shown to increase response rates. These included monetary and non-monetary incentives, a promotional message on the envelope, a more interesting topic, pre-notification of the subjects, follow-up contact, shorter questionnaires, providing a second copy of the questionnaire at follow-up, mentioning an obligation to respond, university sponsorship, personalized questionnaires, coloured as opposed to black or blue ink, stamped returned envelopes instead of franked returned envelopes, an assurance of confidentiality, and first class mailing. The response rate was reduced when sensitive questions were included, when questionnaires began with the most general questions, and when participants were offered the opportunity to opt out of the study. Of course the various trials reviewed were all in different contexts, and not all factors would be relevant to all questionnaires.

## Selection effects with different study designs

As the maintenance of internal validity is the most important objective in study design, the stronger study designs are those in which the selection criteria apply equally and with the same effects in each of the groups being compared. The outline diagram of a randomized intervention trial (**Ex. 4.4,** type (a)) illustrates the value of this design. Only subjects who are eligible and have given their consent to the study, including consent to randomization and to each of the interventions being offered, enter the study. The selection criteria are identical to the point of randomization. The factors influencing participation act prior to randomization, and so will affect the intervention and comparison groups equally. From the point of randomization, all subjects will be included in the analysis, irrespective of whether they accept the prescribed intervention and complete the follow-up procedures or not (this issue will be described more fully when we consider the role of randomization in preventing confounding in Chapter 6). As the selection criteria apply to each of the groups in an identical fashion, selection issues will not affect internal validity. However, the external validity of this design may be quite limited, as the strict eligibility criteria and the requirement for consent prior to randomization may make the participant group a relatively small and perhaps unrepresentative sample of the eligible and source populations.

The effects of selection on internal validity become more severe as the design departs from the ideal of the randomized trial. Exhibit 4.4, types (b), (c), and (d), shows designs in which the differences in selection appear at the levels of the participant, eligible, and source populations respectively. As an illustration, consider the design of a prospective cohort study comparing women using oral contraceptives with those using other methods of contraception in terms of later disease. The ideal scientific design would be a randomized trial, but clearly this is ethically impossible. The next strongest design is one in which a suitable source population is identified and eligibility criteria are set which are identical for exposed and unexposed women; this is design (b). For example, the eligible population could be defined as all women

SELECTION LEVELS IN DIFFERENT DESIGNS

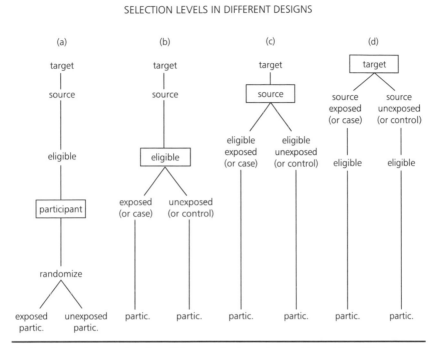

**Ex. 4.4.** Study designs showing different selection schemes. From (a) to (d), the pathways for selection of groups to be compared become more different, and so the possible influence of selection on *internal* validity increases. (a) is a randomized trial design; (b), (c), and (d) are varieties of non-randomized intervention, cohort, or case–control designs. Partic. = participants

attending a defined group of doctors who start a new contraceptive method (oral contraception or other method); an example of this design will be described subsequently. By having the same eligibility criteria for both groups, some similarity is ensured; however, the eligible groups of oral contraceptive users and non-users may differ in other factors that affect their outcome rates, and the participation rates for users and non-users may differ. The analysis of the study needs to take account of these possible differences between the groups.

If the eligibility criteria for oral contraceptive users and for the comparison subjects are not the same, greater differences will be introduced, and this becomes design (c). For example, oral contraceptive users might enter the study from the time of their first use of an oral contraceptive, but it may be convenient to enrol comparison subjects using other contraceptive methods whether they were just starting on these methods or had used them for some time. This difference in eligibility criteria could introduce further differences between the groups being compared, giving greater effects on internal validity.

Another design would be of type (d), where the source populations are different. For example, the oral contraceptive users might be identified as women who had received their contraceptive prescriptions from a certain clinic, while comparison subjects might be taken as women using other methods of contraception, identified in other ways. Therefore the source populations are different, and factors affecting this difference, such as factors influencing whether women go to a particular clinic, can then contribute to the differences between the exposed and unexposed groups.

The same types of consideration apply to case–control studies. Therefore it is helpful in assessing or designing studies to define the participant, eligible, source, and target populations, as this may illustrate where problems of validity may arise.

## Selection of subjects for comparative studies

A few clear principles apply to the selection of subjects for all comparative studies, whether intervention trials, cohort studies, or case–control studies. While the details are specific to each study design, the principles apply to all these studies.

In comparative studies, there are two groups of subjects: the group of prime interest (the cases in a case–control study, the exposed group in a cohort study, and the intervention group in a trial) and the comparison group. There are four principles relating to the selection of the group of prime interest, shown in **Ex. 4.5.**

1.  The groups should be what they are designed to be, i.e. the group of prime interest should truly be cases, or exposed, or an intervention group. If we

---

QUALITIES OF THE 'EXPOSED' GROUP IN A COHORT STUDY
AND THE 'CASE' GROUP IN A CASE–CONTROL STUDY

1.  should be truly 'exposed' or a 'case'

2.  should be newly exposed, or be a newly incident case

3.  should be representative of a defined eligible population

4.  should be available for study so that necessary information can be collected in the same way as it is for the comparison subjects

---

**Ex. 4.5.** Criteria for the groups of prime interest in a comparative study. Total fulfilment of all criteria is rarely possible.

include amongst a cohort defined as exposed some subjects who are not exposed, we will underestimate the true size of the association between exposure and outcome. Misclassification by exposure status in a cohort study, or case status in a case–control study, will bias the results of the study towards the null hypothesis. The direction of this effect is useful to note. In assessing published work, misclassification is not a serious issue in studies that show a strong association, as a reduction of the misclassification will actually strengthen the observed association. However, in interpreting studies that show no association, perhaps a true association exists and there has been sufficient misclassification to disguise it. In some circumstances quantitative estimates of the degree of misclassification can be made, and the results adjusted accordingly; this will be discussed in Chapter 5.

2. The group of prime interest should be ascertained from the beginning of the factor's operation, i.e. a case group should be selected from newly incident cases, and an exposed or intervention group from the beginning of the exposure or intervention. Consider a study to look at the frequency of muscular pain in workers doing repetitive jobs in a factory. The simplest design is to go to the factory, examine workers who are doing the particular job, and find out how many of them have evidence of muscular problems. This will almost certainly underestimate the problem, as the study includes only workers who have started the job and continued it for various periods until the time of the investigation. If, instead, we study all workers who start on the job, we might find that many of them develop muscular problems and then change their job or leave the workforce entirely.

3. The exposed or case subjects should be representative of a defined eligible population. As we have seen, this defined eligible population is the essential link between the exposed or case group in the study and the comparison group.

4. The subjects must be chosen so that the necessary other investigations can be carried out, i.e. the assessment of outcome in a cohort study, exposure in a case–control design, and related factors in either. These other investigations should be carried out in a similar manner in the control groups chosen, and with similar completeness. For example, one of the main cohort studies of the effects of smoking was the study of British doctors started in the 1950s. The decision to base the study on doctors was made largely because they would be interested in participating in the study, and as they had to re-register formally each year to maintain their license to practice, the difficulties of keeping them under follow-up were minimized.

A little consideration will show that feature 4 above relates primarily to dealing with bias in observations. Feature 3 is mainly concerned with dealing with differences between the groups in regard to other factors, i.e. confounding. Feature 2 will also relate to this, and feature 1 relates to the points we have just reviewed, that the selection of subjects may affect both the internal and external validity of the study, and may modify the hypothesis under test. Good study design requires a balance between these four features; often a strategy to improve one of these features may compromise another.

## Selection of the comparison subjects

The essential characteristics of the comparison group, whether it be the unexposed group in a cohort study or the unaffected group in a case–control study, follow logically from, and are equivalent to, the criteria for the exposed or case groups (**Ex. 4.6**).

1.  The controls must be representative of the group they are designed to be. In cohort studies, that means they should be unexposed or minimally exposed. In many case–control designs, controls are defined as free of the outcome of interest, and so should be selected to fit that definition. Alternatively, the design may call for the controls to be a sample of the whole population, as discussed in Chapter 3. As pointed out above, misclassification in this regard will have the effect of biasing the measured association towards the null value, and cannot exaggerate the true association. Therefore a small degree of misclassification may be acceptable, particularly if to avoid it would compromise other valuable parts of the research design.

2.  The control group should be chosen so that the relevant information can be collected in a manner analogous to that used for the exposed or case series.

---

QUALITIES OF THE COMPARISON GROUP IN A COHORT OR
CASE–CONTROL STUDY

1.  Should be truly 'non-exposed' or 'non-diseased'

2.  Should be available for the study so that necessary information can be obtained in the same way as it is for the exposed or case subjects

3.  Should be representative of a defined eligible population, analogous to that for the 'exposed' or 'case series'; this can be modified in that comparison subjects may be chosen specifically to be similar to the exposed or case series with regard to particular factors

---

**Ex. 4.6.** Criteria for the comparison groups in a cohort or case–control study. Total fulfilment of all criteria is rarely possible.

3. A useful general concept is that comparison subjects should be representative of the unaffected (or of all) members of the same eligible population that provided the exposed or case subjects. While this general statement is usually applicable, the choice of appropriate comparison subjects is a complex issue and the ideal characteristics cannot be fully described in a simple inclusive statement. Therefore we shall explore this issue more fully in the context of the different study designs.

## Assessment of selection issues in a completed study

We have seen how the selection of subjects for a study can influence both internal and external validity, and affect the hypothesis under test. In assessing a study, it is useful to examine the component populations, and a simple scheme is shown in **Ex. 4.7**. The general questions, applying to the whole study, are relevant to external validity and to the hypothesis; the questions concerning differences between the groups being compared are also relevant to internal validity.

---

ISSUES IN THE SELECTION OF SUBJECTS

| General questions | Comparison of the groups |
| --- | --- |
| What is the definition of the eligible population? | Are the definitions comparable? |
| How do the participants relate to the eligible population? | |
| What is the participation rate? | Compare the groups |
| What are the reasons for losses, and how frequent is each? | Compare the groups. Are differences likely to affect internal validity? Do the losses compromise external validity? |
| What is the source population? | Is it the same for each group? |
| How do the source and eligible populations relate? | Is the relationship similar for each group? Is the main result likely to apply to the source population? |
| What is the target population? | Is the main result applicable to this target population? |

**Ex. 4.7.** Selection of subjects. An outline scheme to assist in the consideration of issues of subject selection in a particular study. The questions should be considered generally, and specifically in regard to the comparability of the relevant groups: exposed and unexposed in cohort and intervention studies; affected and unaffected in case–control studies.

## Part 2. Application of the principles of selection of subjects to each type of study, and examples

### Selection of subjects in randomized intervention trials; intention to treat analysis

This design is conceptually the simplest. In the design used most commonly, exemplified by the trial of treatment for tuberculosis discussed in Chapter 1 (Ex. 1.8), a group of participants is selected on the basis of eligibility criteria and informed consent, and divided into the intervention and comparison groups by randomization. In an alternative design, eligible subjects are identified and randomization is then performed; those randomized to be offered the intervention are then approached for consent and participation, while those randomized to the comparison group receive their normal care, and may indeed be unaware that the trial is proceeding. This design is often used in large-scale interventions comparing a new intervention with routine care, as consent is required only for those who will be offered the new intervention. Thus, in a trial of breast cancer screening, some 64 000 women were randomized into two equal groups; one group was offered screening and their consent to screening was sought, while the other group continued with normal care without any need for consent [9].

We can apply the four principles of subject selection, which were shown in Ex. 4.5, to the intervention group. Ideally, those randomized to the intervention receive the intervention, and the comparison group do not. In practice, this is rarely likely to happen without some compromises. Some subjects randomized to the intervention may never receive it because they do not accept it, or clinical contraindications arise, or there are administrative difficulties, and some of those who start may not continue it for very long. Therefore there some misclassification is produced which will reduce the difference between the intervention and comparison groups. Despite this, the appropriate analysis compares the ultimate outcome in the original total groups defined by the randomization. Only this comparison maintains the advantages of the randomized design; this is the *intention to treat* analysis. If comparisons are based only on the subjects who accept the intervention, or complete it, the comparisons are open to all the difficulties of comparing non-randomized cohorts. Thus in the breast cancer trial noted earlier, death rates were compared between all women in the control group and all women in the group randomized to be offered screening, although only about two-thirds of them accepted the offer.

Similarly, the comparison group may be influenced by the intervention. This may mean that the association actually assessed is different from that originally envisaged. For example, in a trial of health education, an intervention

group may be selected by randomization and offered a new education programme, but the comparison group, which is not offered the intervention,
may make similar changes themselves. This is referred to as *contamination* or
*dilution*. The comparison actually being made is between the specific intervention and the other changes affecting the control group. In the Multiple
Risk Factor Intervention Trial (MRFIT) in the USA 12 866 men at high risk of
coronary heart disease were randomly allocated to a special intervention programme or to normal care [10]. Men allocated to the intervention programme
showed substantial reductions in blood pressure, cholesterol levels, and smoking. However, substantial, although lesser, reductions were also seen in the
group randomized to normal care. The trial results showed only a small and
non-significant reduction in mortality from heart disease in the intervention
group. This was an *'open'* trial, i.e. both the participants and their own doctors
were aware of the trial. For men in the control group, the information from
the assessments made was sent to their own doctors, although without any
recommendations for action. The changes seen in the normal care group
could have been produced by several factors: enrolment in the trial, even
although they were randomized to the normal care group; those volunteering
for the trial being already motivated to change; the impact of the new knowledge of risk factors from the examinations carried out in the trial; or the doctors of men in the normal care group making their own intervention
recommendations. Carrying out the trial in a more rigorous fashion, without
giving feedback on the results of the regular examinations to men in the normal care group, was regarded as unethical. Similarly, in trials offering screening mammography to randomized groups of women, substantial numbers of
women in the non-intervention group will also receive mammography
through their own initiative or through other programmes [11].

As the interventions are under the control of the investigators, the issue of
being newly exposed should be well defined. Sometimes prior exposure to a
similar intervention (e.g. the same drug) is expected to influence the effect of
the exposure under test, and so lack of prior exposure may be used as an eligibility criterion.

The great strength of the randomized design is with regard to representativeness, i.e. both the intervention and comparison groups are representative of a
defined eligible or participant population. The random selection procedure, if
done on adequate numbers, will result in two groups which are likely to be similar in terms of any particular factor. Further, the exposure is added independently to one group, and so should not be associated with other factors
influencing the outcome. Thus it is reasonable to assume that the frequency of
outcome seen in the comparison group would also be seen in the exposed

group if the exposure had not occurred or had no effect. This does depend on adequate numbers, so, a small randomized trial may well show differences between the groups in relevant factors, as will be discussed in Chapter 6.

Also, in a randomized design the methods of ascertaining outcome and other relevant factors can be identical in the two groups. There is the special opportunity, rarely provided in the other designs, to use single-blind and double-blind techniques, i.e. study designs where the subjects are not aware of which intervention they are receiving (*single-blind*) or where neither the subjects nor those making the observations of outcome are aware of this (*double-blind*). This is obviously easiest with drug trials, and more difficult with trials of other interventions. (In a *triple-blind* design, in addition those analysing the data only have a code indicating which intervention has been given, and do not know what the code means).

Randomized trials have a potential weakness in that the application of strict eligibility criteria and management protocols may mean that the subjects who participate in the trial are unrepresentative of the wider group of relevant subjects in the community. This raises the question of whether the results of the trial can easily be applied to a wider population. Another criticism of trials is that many are designed to address scientific issues predominantly, and there is a need for more clinical trials to address questions faced by decision-makers providing health care. Such trials have been called *pragmatic* or *practical* clinical trials [12]. They are designed to address important clinical or management issues, to include a diverse population of participants recruited from a range of health care settings, and to collect data on a wider range of health outcomes, adding patient-centred outcomes, such as symptom control and quality-of-life measurements, and economic outcomes to the more traditional clinical outcomes.

In the design of clinical trials, the number of subjects required is estimated by methods that are discussed further in Chapter 7. In many trials, particularly large and long-term trials, the results are monitored as they come in by an independent data monitoring committee which is separated from the principal investigators of the trial, and can operate in a 'triple-blind' fashion. This is to fulfil the ethical ideal of stopping the trial as early as possible so that a conclusion can be reached and the optimum treatment can be offered to all participants in the trial and to other people. This issue is also discussed further in Chapter 7. The decision of whether or not to stop a trial can be complex and is often controversial. Stopping a trial too late delays results and will mean that more participants of the trial are given the inferior treatment; but stopping a trial too early can make interpretation difficult and may lose the scientific value of the trial not only for all its participants but for people in general. For example, a randomized trial was started in 1997 to investigate whether hormone replacement therapy for menopausal symptoms was safe in women with a previously treated breast cancer. The trial had a data monitoring committee and a preset protocol for examining the results regularly. In September 2003, after a median follow-up of 2.1 years, 26 of 174 women in the hormone replacement therapy group and seven of the 171 women in the comparison group had signs of breast cancer progression, and the trial was stopped [13]. Other trials are stopped because there is clear evidence of benefit before the predetermined study size is reached. This occurred in a trial of the benefits of folic acid in preventing birth defects, which is described in Chapter 11.

In summary, in the randomized intervention design, the prime advantages are that both groups are drawn from the same eligible or participant populations, and that the randomization is likely to lead to comparability in regard to other factors, and to similarity in how the observations of outcome are made. These characteristics, features 2, 3, and 4 on the generic list in Ex. 4.5, are given prominence over feature 1, so that the analysis by comparing randomized groups may accept a degree of misclassification because of incomplete participation of those randomized, or other influences.

## The CONSORT report format for randomized trials

The CONSORT (Consolidated Standards of Reporting Trials) statement is a recommended way of describing the results of randomized trials which has been adopted by many leading medical journals [14,15]. It follows the principles set out already, and emphasizes the need to document all exclusions or departures from the protocol after randomization. The use of the format has been shown to improve reporting [16]. The CONSORT scheme is shown in **Ex. 4.8**, and is described at http://www.consort statement org, where amendments and new publications are given. As can be seen, it deals with the trial from randomization onwards, and so addresses issues of internal validity; it does not deal with questions of external validity. Another emphasis has been on ensuring that all trials that are performed are reported, so that all the results can be assessed to avoid publication bias; this is discussed further in Chapter 8. Investigators are encouraged to register their trial and submit the protocol when the trial is designed. Many leading medical journals will now only publish the results of trials which have been registered in advance, and which are reported according to the CONSORT criteria.

## Examples of randomized trials

A trial of an innovative laser treatment for facial acne illustrates the issues in the selection of subjects for a small randomized clinical trial [17]. **Exhibit 4.9** shows the conduct of the trial, following the CONSORT scheme. Eligible patients were selected from one hospital clinic or recruited by a public

CONSORT FLOWSHEET FOR RANDOMIZED TRIALS

**Ex. 4.8.** The CONSORT (Consolidated Standards of Reporting Trials) recommended flowchart to describe a randomized trial. From www.consort-statement.org [14]

advertisement, and had to be aged between 18 and 45 years and have mild to moderate facial inflammatory acne, which was assessed on a scoring system accepted by dermatologists. Because previous treatments could affect the trial, minimum time intervals were set; for example, patients had to have had no oral antibiotic treatment during the previous 4 weeks, but no treatment by isotretinoin (a vitamin A derivative), which has a much longer effect, during the previous 52 weeks. Sixty-two such patients were assessed for eligibility, of whom 15 did not meet the entry criteria and a further six chose not to partici-pate, giving 41 patients who were randomized. A three-to-one randomization

A SMALL CLINICAL RANDOMIZED TRIAL

Ex. 4.9. CONSORT flowchart for a randomized trial of laser treatment compared with sham treatment for inflammatory acne. Reprinted from The Lancet 362(9393), Seaton ED, Charakida A, Mouser PE, Grace I, Clement RM, Chu AC. Pulsed-dye laser treatment for inflammatory acne vulgaris: randomised controlled trial. 1347–1352. Copyright 2003, with permission from Elsevier. [17]

scheme was used, resulting in 31 patients allocated the new laser treatment and 10 allocated sham treatment, where the disconnected laser handpiece was moved across the face in an identical manner to that of the active treatment group. All patients wore opaque goggles to protect their eyes, which also ensured that they were unaware of which therapy they received. Four of the 31 patients allocated laser treatment discontinued it for reasons which are given in the report, and one of the 10 patients allocated sham treatment discontinued it, giving 27 and nine, respectively, who completed the study. However, follow-up examinations were done on all patients initially randomized, and so the comparison for the primary outcome, based on a clinical assessment of the acne after 12 weeks, was made using all 41 originally randomized subjects. There was a substantial improvement in acne in the laser group, with no change in the sham treatment group. Some other secondary endpoints could only be assessed on those who completed the study, which is less satisfactory, although here the number of subjects discontinuing the trial is small.

Although this randomized trial is small, information is given on the comparability of the laser and sham treatment groups with regard to demographic factors, previous treatments, and characteristics of the initial acne. The internal validity of the results is good. The subjects to whom the trial was offered are defined in a clinically relevant way in terms of an accepted severity scoring system, and so the results should be applicable to similarly defined patients elsewhere. However, there is no guarantee that the patients seen at this particular clinic are representative of any wider group, and verification of that would logically come from repetition of the study with other populations.

An example of a much more complex community-based trial is one comparing two methods of providing maternity care in Scotland [18]. The objective was to study women coming for prenatal care, exclude high-risk women, and assess for the other women whether a specialist-led care system (which was the norm at that time) produced any different results from a new system of care led by general practitioners (GPs) and midwives. As shown in **Ex. 4.10,** this required a great deal of set-up work, starting with obtaining the consent of 51 general practices to participate in the study so that women could be assessed and excluded if there were indicators of high risk, and obtaining the support of all the specialist obstetricians in the area. Of the 2642 women assessed as eligible, 475 were excluded because they were already beyond 18 weeks of pregnancy or had already seen an obstetrics specialist. A further 402 women did not consent to the study, leaving 1765 who were randomized into two approximately equal groups. A small number of women withdrew from the trial but could be included in the analysis. The analysis was based largely on clinical records, and further exclusions were because records were missing; to assess the patients' opinions of their care, a questionnaire was used which had an incomplete response so that the results for that part of the trial were based on smaller numbers. This was a complex design, but there is little doubt that the randomized trial design ensured that the women treated with each of the alternative systems of care were generally comparable, and the general design of the study ensured that the results are relevant to the community and health care system in which the study was done. The study showed that the new GP and midwife care system produced better continuity of care, fewer antenatal hospital admissions, a modest reduction in routine clinic visits, and

A LARGE COMPLEX RANDOMIZED TRIAL

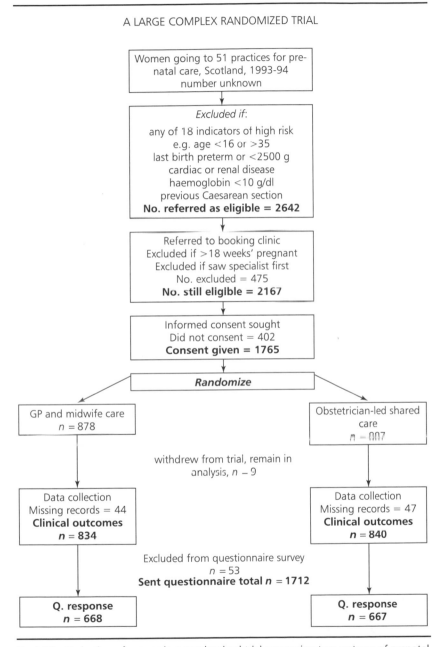

Ex. 4.10. Derivation of groups in a randomized trial comparing two systems of prenatal care for low-risk women in Scotland. Data from Tucker *et al.* [18]

a lower frequency of some of the more common complications of pregnancy. The levels of satisfaction of both groups of women with their care were very similar, and high. The authors concluded that GP and midwife care was an acceptable alternative to obstetrician-led care, which was the norm at the time.

## Selection of the subjects for a cohort study

In an observational cohort study, the groups compared are the exposed group and a comparison group. The 'exposed' group should truly be exposed, and misclassification by exposure status in a cohort study will bias the results of the study towards the null value. However, misclassification is often severe in cohort studies because an indirect indicator of exposure is used. To assess the health effects of exposure to asbestos, for example, an 'exposed' group of subjects who have worked in an environment where asbestos was used may be chosen, even though many of them may have had little or no exposure. The results will demonstrate the health effects of the average exposure of this group; a real effect may be missed if there are many individuals in the group who have not had exposure.

A related issue is that the exposure may change over time. In the study of asbestos, the initial cohorts of exposed and unexposed workers may be set, but as the study follow-up proceeds some exposed workers will cease exposure and some unexposed workers will begin exposure, introducing further misclassification. If such variations are large, special types of analysis will be necessary, such as defining each subject on the basis of total length of exposure. This method was used in a study of oral contraceptive users discussed later in this chapter.

Subjects should ideally be newly exposed to the causative agent under study. As noted above, a prevalence survey of currently employed workers will underestimate a problem that leads some workers to quit. This consideration of being newly exposed must be taken along with the definition of the exposure. In studying the frequency of cancer in workers exposed to a particular chemical through their occupation, we might assume that a substantial amount of exposure would be necessary before any detectable increase would occur, and therefore we might define exposure as a minimum of 5 years occupational exposure to the chemical. In this situation, being newly exposed means that this 5-year period has just been completed, and the study may include the total follow-up period subsequent to that time for each subject, but exclude subjects who leave the workforce or change jobs before they have 5 years exposure.

Similarly, the comparison group of subjects who are regarded as unexposed, should actually be unexposed. As pointed out above, misclassification in this regard will have the effect of biasing the measured association towards the null value, and cannot exaggerate a true association. Therefore a modest degree of misclassification may be acceptable, particularly if to avoid it would compromise other valuable parts of the research design.

The exposed and unexposed subjects must be chosen so that the appropriate investigations can be carried out, i.e. the assessment of outcome and of related factors. These investigations should be carried out in a similar manner in the control groups chosen, and with similar completeness.

## Choices with regard to the control group in cohort studies

It is helpful to concentrate on the *purpose* of the control group. In a cohort study, we measure the frequency of the outcome in exposed subjects. The function of the control group is to estimate what that rate would be in those same subjects, had they not been exposed. The frequency observed in the exposed group will depend on the effects of the exposure factor, but also on the other characteristics of that exposed group that influence the outcome. Therefore an appropriate comparison is a group of subjects who share, as far as possible, all the other factors which influence the outcome, apart from the exposure.

The best way to achieve this is by a randomized trial. However, random allocation and an intervention design are often not possible. In the randomized trial design, the control group has two properties; it is a representative sample of the original eligible population, and it is likely to be similar to the exposed group with regard to other relevant factors. Procedures for selecting controls in non-randomized studies can be logically determined by starting from one or other of these properties.

The control series can be chosen as *a representative sample of the unexposed members of the eligible population from which the exposed subjects are also drawn*—design (b) in Ex. 4.4. A useful practical guiding point is that all potential controls, if they were exposed, should be eligible for inclusion in the exposed group. This approach ensures comparability of the exposed and unexposed groups with regard to characteristics that define the eligible population.

In an observational study the subjects themselves or, in the case of therapy, their medical advisers, have chosen whether they are to be exposed or unexposed to the factor in question. This self-selection will usually mean that the exposed and unexposed groups differ with regard to other factors that influence the outcome. For example, smokers and non-smokers differ with regard to other aspects of lifestyle such as alcohol use and diet; a non-randomized comparison of patients who have been given different treatments will often be made difficult because the patient's clinical findings and current prognosis will influence the treatment given.

If we know a great deal about the factors that influence the outcome under study, we could choose a comparison group that is *deliberately made similar to the exposed group* in terms of the other factors that determine outcome. This results in a matched design, in which for each exposed subject, one or more unexposed subjects are chosen because they share the other characteristics that affect the frequency of the outcome variable. Thus in a study of the long-term outcomes of amniocentesis, Baird *et al.* [19] identified a cohort of 1296 live-born infants whose mothers had had amniocentesis during that pregnancy, and compared them in terms of later disabilities with 3704 control liveborns whose mothers were matched for sex, maternal age, area of residence, and time of birth. No differences were found except for an increase in haemolytic disease due to iso-immunization. Matching can give a powerful design, but it has several disadvantages. It is not often that we know all the factors that influence the outcome under study. For this design we not only have to know them but we have to be able to measure them, and we have to be able to find matched comparison subjects who share those characteristics with the exposed subjects. Therefore matched designs, although elegant in theory, are often difficult to employ in practice. Matching is discussed more fully in Chapter 6.

The designs we have described so far involve *internal control groups*, i.e. controls derived from the same source population as the exposed subjects (e.g. the same community, workplace, or medical practice). A rather weaker design uses an *external control group*, from a different source population. While the source populations for the exposed and unexposed groups are not the same, they must both relate to a common target population. Thus the health effects of asbestos could be examined by comparing workers who use asbestos with workers in the same industry who have generally similar jobs but do not use asbestos—an internal control group. The health effects of asbestos could also be assessed by comparing the death rates of workers using asbestos with the death rates for the whole population in that area or country—an external control group. If the effects are large, this may be an adequate design, but it is clearly a rather weak one. In a prospective cohort study of vegetarians, with some 17 years of follow-up, the overall mortality was much lower than that of the general population—a comparison with an external control group; in one of many internal comparisons, the mortality rate from all causes was reduced in those who consumed fresh fruit daily compared with the other members of the cohort [20]. The main options in the design of cohort studies are summarized in **Ex. 4.11**.

## Examples of prospective cohort studies

We will describe two studies, which, while set up some time ago, have interesting design features and may be regarded as classic studies. Both are continuing

SOME OPTIONS IN THE DESIGN OF COHORT STUDIES

| Design | Exposed group | Comparison group | Applicability |
|---|---|---|---|
| *Randomized* | | | |
| randomized trial | random selection from eligible population: intervention applied | random selection from same eligible population: intervention not applied | only for ethical interventions of likely benefit |
| *Unmatched internal controls* | | | |
| one or more outcomes, confounders not fully known | exposed subset of an eligible population | representative sample of unexposed members of same eligible population; no individual matching | preferable if multiple outcomes; confounders controlled in analysis |
| *Matched internal controls* | | | |
| specific outcome, main confounders known | exposed subset of an eligible population | unexposed subjects matched for other factors which influence outcome | only if outcome specified and main confounders known in advance |
| *External controls* | | | |
| | exposed subjects, or all members of a population with high exposure | all or sample of another population with no exposure or lower exposure | if internal controls not possible |

**Ex. 4.11.** Design of cohort studies. Some methods of selection of exposed and comparison groups in cohort and intervention studies. The list is not meant to be exhaustive

to produce new results. Consider the situation faced by investigators in the mid-1960s concerning the effects of the contraceptive pill. Here was a new pharmacological preparation being used by very large numbers of women which could have major effects on their health. To show such effects, or to demonstrate their absence, required a long-term cohort study capable of assessing multiple endpoints and of giving results that would be widely applicable. Such a study would be a large, expensive, and long-term commitment, not easily repeated; therefore the design needed to optimize both internal and external validity. Two such studies were set up in the UK.

The first study (**Ex. 4.12**) was set up in 1968 by the Royal College of General Practitioners (RCGP), using patients registered with 1400 volunteer general

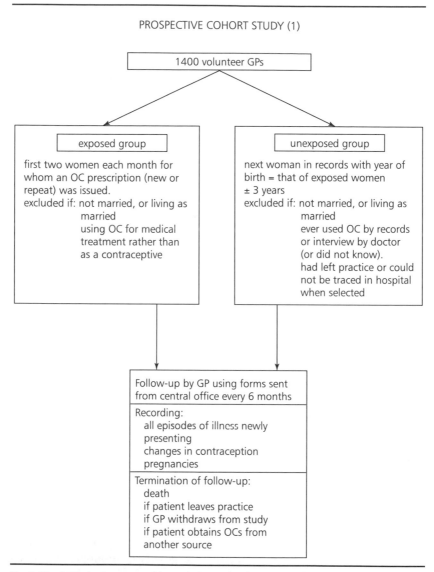

PROSPECTIVE COHORT STUDY (1)

1400 volunteer GPs

**exposed group**

first two women each month for whom an OC prescription (new or repeat) was issued.
excluded if: not married, or living as married
using OC for medical treatment rather than as a contraceptive

**unexposed group**

next woman in records with year of birth = that of exposed women ± 3 years
excluded if: not married, or living as married
ever used OC by records or interview by doctor (or did not know).
had left practice or could not be traced in hospital when selected

Follow-up by GP using forms sent from central office every 6 months

Recording:
all episodes of illness newly presenting
changes in contraception
pregnancies

Termination of follow-up:
death
if patient leaves practice
if GP withdraws from study
if patient obtains OCs from another source

**Ex. 4.12.** Design of a prospective cohort study: derivation of groups of exposed and non-exposed women in a prospective cohort study of oral contraceptive (OC) use. From Royal College of General Practitioners [21]

practitioners [21]. The general practitioners selected the first two women in each month for whom they prescribed an oral contraceptive, either for the first time or as a repeat prescription. For each, a control was selected as the next woman identified from the practice records who was aged within 3 years of the oral contraceptive user, but who had never used an oral contraceptive.

PROSPECTIVE COHORT STUDY (2)

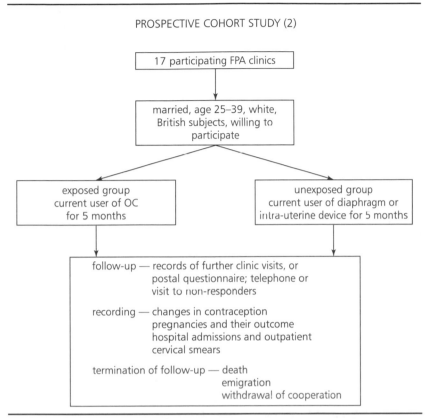

**Ex. 4.13.** Design of a prospective cohort study of oral contraceptive (OC) use: based on Family Planning Clinics. From Vessey et al. [23]

Both users and non-users had to be married or living as married, and thus were likely to be sexually active. The follow-up was based on the general practitioner's regular records, including further information on oral contraceptive use, pregnancies, and related events. Patients who had left their original practitioner, or whose practitioner withdrew from the study, or who were supplied with oral contraceptives from other sources ceased follow-up at that time. This study has continued: follow-up over 25 years has shown the same overall death rate in oral contraceptive users and non-users of oral contraceptives, but increases in deaths from cervical cancer and from cerebrovascular disease, and a decrease in ovarian cancer deaths, in current and recent users [22].

The other study was based on 17 of the largest clinics run by the Family Planning Association (FPA) [23] (**Ex. 4.13**). Eligible subjects had to be married, aged 25–39, a white British subject, and be willing to participate; these criteria were primarily to ensure adequate follow-up. Oral contraceptive users were defined by current and past use over 5 months, and the unexposed group was defined as women using a diaphragm or an intra-uterine device for at least 5 months without prior exposure to oral contraceptives. The 5-month duration criterion was to eliminate substantial numbers of women who would change their method of contraception only a few months after starting. Follow-up information was based on the FPA clinic records, but if no further appointments were recorded, a follow-up form was sent directly to the patient, supported by telephone calls or home visits where necessary. Patients were asked on recruitment to give the name of their family doctor and of two contact persons to assist in follow-up. Information about hospital visits was sought on both clinic and direct mail follow-up forms; the primary outcome measures used in analysis were mortality and morbidity recorded as inpatient or outpatient visits. Follow-up ceased at death, emigration from the UK, or at the subject's request. This study has also continued: follow-up to the year 2000 showed no effect of oral contraceptive use on total mortality, increased deaths from cervical cancer, and, in agreement with the RCGP study, a decreased death rate from ovarian cancer [24].

In both these studies, the prime considerations were to achieve high follow-up and high internal validity, after choosing source populations which gave reasonable external validity. In the FPA study, the loss to follow-up was only around 0.7 per cent per year, and was similar in the different contraceptive groups. This good follow-up was achieved by the eligibility criteria which tended to select women with a stable lifestyle, and applied to both the oral contraceptive and comparison groups. This advantage in internal validity was achieved at the cost of some external validity. The women in the FPA study are not representative of all oral contraceptive users in the UK, and exclude, for example, women of non-white origin and younger unmarried women who may have different sexual behaviours. However, any major biological associations assessed in this study might well apply to other groups. A greater limitation is that the comparison was between oral contraceptive users and women using a different method of contraception, so that any differences in a particular outcome may be due to either the oral contraceptive or the other method. However, it was useful that the comparison group comprised two major subgroups, users of a diaphragm or of an intrauterine device. Thus in one study it was shown that the frequency of cervical cancer and dysplasia was lower in women who used a diaphragm than in either of the other two groups, suggesting a protective effect of diaphragm use rather than an increased risk from the other methods. To assess whether cervical cancer was increased in oral contraceptive users, the relevant comparison was between oral contraceptive users and users of an intra-uterine device, excluding diaphragm users entirely from that analysis [25].

The external validity of the RCGP study may be somewhat greater, as the criteria are looser, and the users and non-users chosen may be representative of all users in a particular practice. However, the number of eligible women who were selected but did not choose to enter the study was not recorded. The non-users included women who were not using any method of contraception, which is probably not particularly beneficial, as differences between them and oral contraceptive users in regard to other features related to sexual activity may be substantial. However, the participating general practitioners are unlikely to be representative of all practitioners, and therefore in this study the women cannot be regarded as a representative sample of British oral contraceptive users.

Both these designs fail to fulfil one of the criteria set out in Ex. 4.5; the exposed group were not defined from the time of first exposure, but were identified as a prevalent sample of oral contraceptive users. The recruitment process would have been much more difficult if women had to be recruited at first use only, as many women would stop oral contraceptive use after only a short time and therefore contribute little to the study. As a result, neither of these studies is powerful in the assessment of short-term effects of oral contraceptive use, as women who started oral contraceptives and had ill effects immediately would be under-represented in both studies. In both studies, a degree of external validity has been sacrificed to facilitate follow-up and achieve good internal validity. The ways in which the data were collected in these studies will be reviewed in Chapter 5.

# Retrospective cohort studies

The prospective cohort studies described above are clearly very major undertakings, requiring many years of follow-up to produce results. If the essential information for a particular study can be obtained from records that already exist, the advantages of a cohort study can be exploited without the need for the long length of time required for prospective follow-up. Many such studies have been done on groups of people who can be identified as sharing an important exposure in the past, such as occupational groups. Very powerful studies can be carried out efficiently using computer-based record linkage techniques if high-quality databases are available.

## Example of a retrospective cohort study

A good example of a retrospective cohort study is a study set up to assess possible links between the use of cellular (mobile) telephones and cancer in Denmark [26] (**Ex. 4.14**). Cell phone services in Denmark started in 1982 and were provided by two operating companies. After scientific and ethical review,

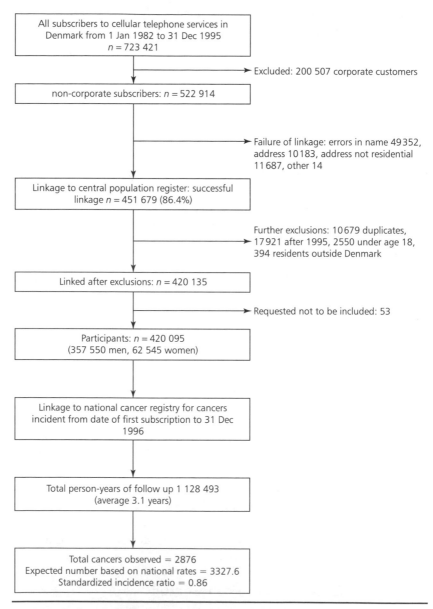

A RETROSPECTIVE COHORT STUDY

All subscribers to cellular telephone services in
Denmark from 1 Jan 1982 to 31 Dec 1995
*n* = 723 421

→ Excluded: 200 507 corporate customers

non-corporate subscribers: *n* = 522 914

→ Failure of linkage: errors in name 49 352,
address 10 183, address not residential
11 687, other 14

Linkage to central population register: successful
linkage *n* = 451 679 (86.4%)

→ Further exclusions: 10 679 duplicates,
17 921 after 1995, 2550 under age 18,
394 residents outside Denmark

Linked after exclusions: *n* = 420 135

→ Requested not to be included: 53

Participants: *n* = 420 095
(357 550 men, 62 545 women)

Linkage to national cancer registry for cancers
incident from date of first subscription to 31 Dec
1996

Total person-years of follow up 1 128 493
(average 3.1 years)

Total cancers observed = 2876
Expected number based on national rates = 3327.6
Standardized incidence ratio = 0.86

**Ex. 4.14.** Design of a retrospective cohort study: a national study of cancer occurrence
in mobile phone subscribers in Denmark. From Johansen *et al.* [26]

both companies made their records available for the study, and it was possible to link the lists of subscribers to a central population register which carried information on mortality and date of emigration, and in turn to link this to the Danish cancer registry which records information on all cancers diagnosed. This demonstrates the immense potential for research of the use of linkable population registries, which here include a unique 10-digit personal identification number that assists accurate linkage between the registers. In many other countries such links are impossible either because the registries do not exist, or because legal issues prevent the linkages being established; in fact, a similar proposed study using subscriber lists for cell phone customers in the USA had to be abandoned after a legal challenge.

Thus the investigators were able to identify all 723 421 subscribers to cell phone accounts, from which they excluded 200 507 corporate customers, leaving 522 914 non-corporate subscribers. A key assumption is that the non-corporate subscriber is the user of the cell phone, which is obviously not always true. Further exclusions were because of errors in name or address of the telephone user, addresses which were not residential, duplicates, subscriptions initially identified but which were outside the eligibility period chosen, persons under the age of 18, and residents in Greenland and the Faroe Islands. The study needed only access to the registers, and the subjects were not asked for consent and were not informed if they were included. The study was publicly announced, and the two telephone companies issued a notice that subscribers could contact them if they wished to be excluded; only 53 people actively excluded themselves in this way. The final cohort was of 420 095 cellular telephone subscribers, representing 80.3 per cent of the non-corporate subscribers initially identified. Linkage to the cancer registry then allowed the calculation of incidence rates for various cancers, which were compared with the incidence in the whole country as the comparison population. Using information from the cell phone service providers, the data could be analysed by the year of first subscription, age at first subscription, the type of telephone system, and the duration of subscription. Special attention was paid to tumours of the brain, which were analysed in detail with respect to site within the brain and pathological subtype. The results showed no indication of an increased risk of cancer in total or in any tumour type, even in subjects with the longest duration of exposure, which was the only measure of intensity of exposure in the study.

The design makes this study strong in that the participants are likely to be representative of all subjects in Denmark using cellular phones, although it has been pointed out that the exclusion of corporate subscribers could exclude subjects with the most intense usage, such as sales people. The weaknesses of the study are that there is no information on the individual extent of use or, for example, on which side of the head the cell phone was normally used, which has been assessed in case–control studies using questionnaires, and the short latency period. In this study the eligible cell phone subscriptions started between 1982 and 1995, and cancer incidence was analysed for each subscriber from the start of their subscription up to 1996. Thus the study includes those in whom the occurrence of cancer would have been shortly after their first subscription, and is limited to a maximum of 14 years between first cell phone use and cancer incidence. The mean follow-up time was only 3 years. This is too short to demonstrate a classic cancer incidence effect, although it could detect a promotion effect, and this limitation is acknowledged by the authors. A strength of the study is its precision, as the study is extremely large. For all cancers, there were 2876 cancers in men compared with 3327.6 expected, giving a relative risk of 0.86, with statistical 95 per cent confidence limits of 0.83–0.90. These are explained later in Chapter 7, but illustrate the precision of this result. On the other hand, for the tumours of greatest interest, those of the brain and nervous system, the numbers were much more modest, there being 135 observed cases compared with 142.8 expected giving a risk ratio of 0.95 with considerably wider confidence limits of 0.79–1.12; the study does not confidently exclude a 12 per cent increase in risk for these tumours.

## Selection of subjects for a case–control study

We will now look at the selection of subjects for a case–control study, which follows very similar principles to those outlined in Ex. 4.5. Here we are selecting groups on the basis of outcome—selecting a case group who have already suffered the outcome and a control group.

The cases should truly be cases. The inclusion of some individuals who do not in fact have the outcome in question within the case group will tend to dilute the case group and bias the results of the study towards the null value. However, as we have seen earlier, this ideal has to be balanced with the logistical difficulties of ascertaining a representative case group. Suppose that the diagnosis of the disease requires complex procedures. Then, to ensure that all those classified as cases do in fact have the disease may involve restricting the study to subjects who have had the opportunity to go through such diagnostic tests. This will exclude individuals who have the disease but have not been investigated so thoroughly. The restricted case series may not be representative of the disease in the wider community; it may be slanted towards individuals with more severe or more manifest disease. The dilution effect of including some non-cases within the case series has to be balanced against the possible non-representativeness of a limited case series. It may be helpful to categorize cases in terms of the certainty of their definition; thus in a case–control study of venous embolism and hormone replacement therapy, the association seen was stronger for the cases with a definite rather than a possible diagnosis [27].

Ideally, the cases should be recently diagnosed. A series of prevalent cases, such as all cases currently being seen in a clinic or existing in a community, will exclude those subjects who have developed the disease and then left the area, died, or recovered. Such subjects will be different in a number of ways from those who still have the disease and therefore are included in the sample. In studies of the outcome of disease in groups of subjects seen in hospital, a frequent error is to study only those subjects who are still under follow-up by the hospital, rather than all patients diagnosed with the disease, irrespective of whether they are being followed up or not. The patients not under follow-up include those with particularly bad outcomes, who may have died or been admitted elsewhere, and sometimes those with particularly good outcomes, who need not return for further care.

A major issue in case–control studies of disease is the choice between a case series chosen from one or more hospitals, or one derived from a community. Hospital series are acceptable if a very high proportion of those developing the disease will come into hospital for diagnosis or treatment. If that is not so, the hospital-based cases may differ substantially from those in the community. This restriction may be accepted in view of the logistic advantages of basing a study on hospital cases, but considerable care is then needed in the generalization of the results.

## Choice of the control group in case–control studies

Choosing control groups in case–control studies is more complicated than in cohort studies. In the most frequently used design, subjects in the control group are chosen to be truly without the outcome of interest at the time the study is performed. The objective of this design is that by comparing representative samples of cases and of controls who do not have the outcome, the study will provide an estimate of the odds ratio in the underlying population. Misclassification, i.e. including some who are actually cases in the control group, will have a dilution effect and bias the results of the study towards the null value. If the prevalence of the outcome under study is small (such as cancer), only a few controls are likely to have the disease and the effect of this misclassification will usually be too small to be important. Where the outcome is relatively common in the underlying source population (such as hypertension or depression), this effect could be considerable, and it may be necessary to assess potential controls to exclude disease. The benefits of doing this must be compared with the likely fall in participation rate produced by such an assessment, added to the logistic, cost, and ethical issues.

However, as noted in Chapter 3, there is an alternative design for a case–control study, in which the controls are selected not to be representative of subjects without the case condition, but designed to be representative of the eligible population at risk. In this design, the format of the results directly produces a relative risk estimate, and a case subject is also eligible for sampling as a control. On this basis, because relative risk is being estimated, there is no issue of misclassification in terms of the controls.

**Exhibit 4.15** illustrates some of the designs that are often used for case–control studies. A primary choice is between selecting cases and controls from the community, or from a health care facility or similar 'institutional' source. One strong design uses a case series that is a total or representative sample of all affected subjects drawn from a specified source population, and a control group that is chosen as a representative sample of unaffected members of that same source population. The source population may be a community or a health care source.

## SOME OPTIONS IN CASE–CONTROL STUDIES

| Design | Case group | Control group | Applicability |
|---|---|---|---|
| *Unmatched community-based* | all or representative sample of all affected subjects in source population | representative sample of unaffected (or of all) members of same source population; no individual matching | preferable for multiple exposures or if confounders not known; confounders controlled in analysis |
| *Unmatched institution-based* | all or representative sample of all affected subjects in eligible population | sample of unaffected members of same eligible population; no individual matching | preferable for multiple exposures or if confounders not known; confounders controlled in analysis |
| *Matched community- or institution-based* | affected members of eligible population | unaffected subjects chosen to be similar to cases on certain specified matching factors; from same eligible population | only if exposure specified and main confounders known in advance |

**Ex. 4.15.** Design of case–control studies. Some methods of selection of case and control groups in case–control studies. The list is not meant to be exhaustive

A community-based design has the advantage that if all cases of the disease of interest can be ascertained in the community, the case series can be fully representative. Moreover, the information from the control group may be much easier to interpret, as the controls will be healthy subjects representative of that community. The source population is also more closely related to other target populations, which will make the further generalization of the results more straightforward.

In a study based on a health care facility, for example comparing patients with a particular disease with patients with other conditions in the same hospital, a danger is that these other conditions may be related to the exposure under consideration. A useful protection with hospital-based case–control designs is to ensure that the control subjects are selected with a range of other diagnoses, as it is unlikely that the exposure under consideration will be related to all of them. Patients with diagnoses likely to be associated (positively or negatively) with the exposure factor under assessment should not be eligible as controls. Thus in a case–control study of venous embolism and hormone replacement therapy, data were presented for nine diagnostic categories of hospital controls, showing considerable variation in the frequency of use of hormone replacement therapy [27]. Also, the applicability of the results to the target population may be more difficult to assess in a hospital-based study.

From the above, the advantages of community-based case–control studies would seem to be considerable, but against these must be balanced the greater difficulty of carrying out such studies, and particularly of ensuring a high response rate in the control series. It is more difficult to obtain a high degree of cooperation from subjects in the community as they have less incentive to be involved in the study than have patients who have been treated. Further, some studies may require clinical information on comparison subjects that may not be easy to obtain from subjects chosen from the community.

It is usually valuable to achieve general comparability between cases and controls by balancing the numbers chosen in terms of gender, age group, and perhaps a few other demographic factors, such as place of residence or hospital. This is referred to as *frequency matching* and is mainly for efficiency, as will be discussed in Chapter 6. Controls can instead be chosen to be *individually matched* to the case series with regard to specified confounding factors, which are associated with both outcome and exposure. This is useful under certain circumstances, discussed in Chapter 6, but adds complexity to the study. In an individually matched design, the matching of the control subjects takes precedence over their other characteristics, but beyond this, institutional or community sources of controls may be used.

Finally, the control subjects need to be chosen so that the information on exposure can be obtained in a similar manner as in the case group. This may involve modification of the case or the control criteria.

## Examples of case–control studies

The association between cell phone use and brain cancer has also been assessed in several case–control studies, such as that by Muscat *et al.* [28] (**Ex. 4.16**). This uses a standard hospital-based case–control design to enrol cases and controls efficiently for what is a fairly rare disease. The cases were defined as patients aged 18–80 years who had been diagnosed with a primary brain cancer during the previous year, and were attending one of five hospitals in New York, Providence, and Boston. Controls were chosen as inpatients in the

A HOSPITAL-BASED CASE–CONTROL STUDY

**Ex. 4.16.** Selection of cases and controls in a hospital-based case–control study assessing the association between the use of cellular phones and the risk of brain cancer. From Muscat *et al.* [28]

same hospital, selected by checking each day's admissions and selecting the first patient who met the eligibility criterion of English language use and were of a suitable age, sex, race, and month of admission. These characteristics were set so that the control groups would eventually be similar in distribution on these factors to the case group, although they were not individually matched. Because there had been previous reports of links between radiofrequency exposures and lymphoma and leukaemia, patients with these conditions were excluded from the control group. The controls had diagnoses that fell into five major categories, and the use of cell phones is described for these five categories in the study results. This does suggest some variability, such as a lower rate of cell phone use in controls who had other cancers. Much of this difference is probably due to age, but it does suggest that selecting controls with a narrow range of diagnoses could be misleading. Cases and controls were then interviewed while in hospital by health professionals. This system had the advantage of giving high response rates. Of the 668 patients with brain tumours identified, 42 were not English-speaking, two had died, 55 were thought to be too ill to be approached, 75 agreed but were too ill to participate, and 25 declined to participate, giving a participation rate of 469/668 (70 per cent). The authors describe 571 subjects as eligible (omitting the 42 non-English-speakers and the 55 who were too ill), giving the response rate as 82 per cent (469/571). In the control subjects the response rate is given as 90 per cent. The high response rate is an advantage in this study. However, there are questions about whether the control group is representative of the general population in terms of cell phone exposure, and the validity of the information could be compromised as the interviewers were aware of the diagnosis of the subjects.

In contrast, in a case–control study of breast cancer in New Zealand assessing primarily oral contraceptive use, the investigators concentrated on obtaining a population-based series of both cases and controls [29] (**Exs 4.17** and **4.18**). This was a complex process. The cases were defined as all New Zealand resident women aged 25–54 who were diagnosed with breast cancer between 1983 and 1985; they could be identified from cancer registries. To obtain a representative population sample as a control series was more difficult. The most complete available population record was the electoral register, but this does not cover the entire population and does not give age. It was decided to collect the information by a telephone interview using a small number of trained interviewers at one site. Therefore both cases and controls had to have a listed telephone number, and the cases had to be on the electoral register to be comparable to the controls. Of 739 women identified within the age range from the cancer registers, 189 were excluded by not being on the electoral roll, not

THE CASE SERIES IN A CASE–CONTROL STUDY

| | |
|---|---|
| Source population | all New Zealand women aged 25–54 diagnosed with breast cancer between 1 July 1983 and 30 June 1985 |
| Eligible population | women aged 25–54, with histologically confirmed breast cancer notified to the NZ National Cancer Registry or to the Auckland Breast Cancer Study group between above dates ($n$=739); no previous breast cancer; on current electoral roll; whose telephone number was found; |
| $n = 550$ | exclusions = 189, eligible population = 550 |
| Participant population | had to have permission from their physician (28 not given) be identified in time to allow interview 4–8 months from diagnosis (49 too late) still alive (8 had died) well enough (4 too ill) exclusions (14 other exclusions) agreed to participate (14 refused) |
| $n = 433$ | participant population 433; exclusions 117 all participants gave usable information on oral contraceptive use |

Participants/eligible = 78.7%
Participants/source = 58.6%

**Ex. 4.17.** A case–control study. The source, eligible, and participant populations in the case series of a case–control study of breast cancer in New Zealand. From Paul *et al.* [29]

THE CONTROL SERIES IN A CASE–CONTROL STUDY

| | |
|---|---|
| Source population | all New Zealand women aged 25–54 and without diagnosed breast cancer |
| Eligible population | women on electoral register, aged 25–54, with a telephone number, with no history of breast cancer: selected by |
| $n = 1110$ | random sampling from register; estimate of number = 1110 |
| Participant population | still alive (10 had died) well enough (4 too ill) in New Zealand (12 overseas) no language difficulty (13 excluded) agreed to participate (99 refused) traced (75 not traced, of whom some were likely to be outside the age range) |
| $n = 897$ | participant population 897; exclusions 213 |

Participants/eligible = 80.8%
Participants/source  = unknown

**Ex. 4.18.** A case–control study. The source, eligible, and participant populations in the control group in a case–control study of breast cancer in New Zealand. From Paul *et al.* [29]

having a listed telephone number, or having had previous breast cancer, giving 550 eligible subjects. The approach to the breast cancer patients required consent from their doctor, fitness to be interviewed, an interview not more than 8 months after diagnosis, and the patient's consent. There were 433 women who participated, representing 79 per cent of the 550 eligible subjects, but only 59 per cent of the original source population. It is fairly typical of modern epidemiology that the least of the investigators' problems was failure of the subjects to agree to interview, with only 14 refusals; more women were excluded because their doctors did not give permission for them to be approached.

The control group sampling was further complicated by the lack of age information. The investigators had to take a random sample of women from the electoral rolls, exclude those for whom a telephone number could not be found, and then write to the women asking for their participation; they could determine age only if she responded, and previous breast cancer only when the interview was carried out. The eligible population cannot be precisely determined, but the best estimate is 1110 and the estimated participation rate is 81 per cent. This is a minimum estimate, as amongst the women not traced there are likely to be some who would have been ineligible because of age. Exclusions of controls because of illness or death were fewer than for cases, and of course a doctor's permission was not required. The voluntary response rate of eligible controls was 897/996 (90 per cent); this is lower than that of the cases, although is still very high. The lower response would be expected as the control subjects have less motivation to take part in a health study than the case subjects who have had a serious disease.

In both these designs, the emphasis in detailed design is, as it should be, on setting eligibility criteria and exclusion processes that are the same for the case and the control series. Both studies have considerable difficulties that could compromise the results, and it is not clear whether a hospital design is inherently better or worse than a community design. It is likely for instance that the case series interviewed in the brain cancer study represents a more complete series of cases than the case series interviewed in the breast cancer study. However, the control series in the breast cancer study is more likely to be representative of women in the general community.

## Comparison of study designs

Three of the studies reviewed here are summarized in **Ex. 4.19,** which shows for each where the group of prime interest and the comparison group diverge in terms of the participant, eligible, and source populations. The potential for substantial differences between the groups being compared clearly increases as we go from the randomized trial design to the case–control study.

EXAMPLES OF STUDY DESIGN

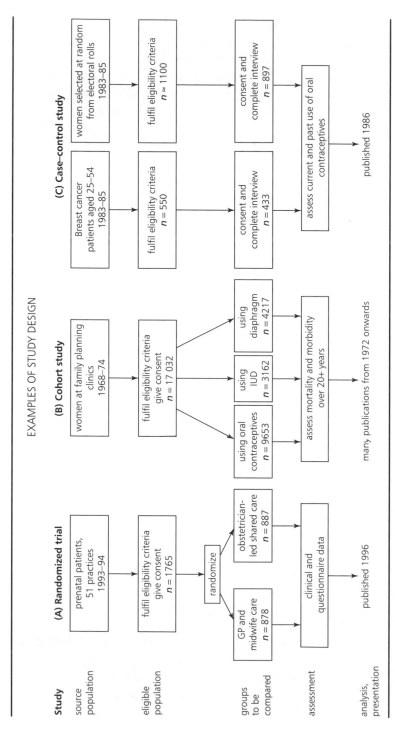

**Ex. 4.19.** Example of study design: (A) randomized clinical trial (Tucker et al. [18]); (B) prospective cohort study (Vessey et al. [23]); (C) case–control study (Paul et al. [29])

## Self-test questions (answers on p. 495)

**Q4.1** Define the target, source, eligible, and participant populations in the following study. To assess the role of magnetic fields in causing childhood leukaemia, children with leukaemia treated in a major referral centre were identified; those in a terminal stage of illness were excluded, and others were interviewed with a 60 per cent response.

**Q4.2** Suppose in the study just described, an association is found with a history of measles in the first year of life (odds ratio, 2.5). Summarize the concepts of internal and external validity with regard to this result.

**Q4.3** What effects can selection bias have on the results of a study?

**Q4.4** In selecting a case series for a case–control study, 1000 subjects with the disease in question are identified, and 900 fulfil the eligibility criteria of disease categorization and age. Of these, address information is incomplete on 60, and the doctors of 100 do not give permission for them to be approached. All the remaining subjects are approached for interview, and 500 consent; however, 10 per cent of those interviewed have missing data on the key variables for the analysis. Summarize the selection process, calculating the participation rate, voluntary response rate, and ratio of the participants to the eligible and the source populations.

**Q4.5** In a randomized trial of smoking cessation, smokers are randomly allocated to be offered an intervention or not. After 1 year, the frequency of smoking cessation in those randomized to no intervention was 20 per cent. Of those randomized to the intervention group, only half accepted the intervention, and their cessation rate was 50 per cent. The cessation rate in those randomized to the intervention but who did not accept the programme offered was 10 per cent. What is the most appropriate summary result from this study?

**Q4.6** What four criteria should be fulfilled by the exposed group in a cohort study?

**Q4.7** In a case–control study, cases are identified through general practitioners (family doctors) and interviewed by telephone. What selection principles apply to the controls?

**Q4.8** What is meant by a single-blind or double-blind trial?

**Q4.9** In the context of a cohort study of workers exposed to a particular chemical, how could an internal and an external control group be defined?

# References

1. Slanetz PJ, Moore RH, Hulka CA, *et al.* Physicians' opinions on the delivery of mammographic screening services: immediate interpretation versus double reading. *AJR Am J Roentgenol* 1996; **167**(2): 377–379.

2. Ellenberg JH, Nelson KB. Sample selection and the natural history of disease. Studies of febrile seizures. *JAMA* 1980; **243**: 1337.

3. The Toronto Leukemia Study Group. Results of chemotherapy for unselected patients with acute myeloblastic leukaemia: effect of exclusions on interpretation of results. *Lancet* 1986; **i**: 786–788.

4. Morris JN. *Uses of Epidemiology* (1st edn). Edinburgh: Livingstone, 1957.

5. Ziel HK, Finkle WD. Increased risk of endometrial carcinoma among users of conjugated estrogens. *N Engl J Med* 1975; **293**: 1167–1170.

6. Hulka BS, Grimson RC, Greenberg BG, *et al.* 'Alternative' controls in a case–control study of endometrial cancer and exogenous estrogen. *Am J Epidemiol* 1980; **112**(3): 376–387.

7. Morton LM, Cahill J, Hartge P. Reporting participation in epidemiologic studies: a survey of practice. *Am J Epidemiol* 2006; **163**(3): 197–203.

8. Edwards P, Roberts I, Clarke M, *et al.* Increasing response rates to postal questionnaires: systematic review. *BMJ* 2002; **324**: 1183.

9. Shapiro S, Venet W, Strax P, Venet L, Roeser R. Ten- to fourteen-year effect of screening on breast cancer mortality. *J Natl Cancer Inst* 1982; **69**: 349–355.

10. Multiple Risk Factor Intervention Trial Research Group. Multiple risk factor intervention trial: risk factor changes and mortality results. *JAMA* 1982; **248**: 1465–1477.

11. Fletcher SW, Black W, Harris R, Rimer BK, Shapiro S. Report of the International Workshop on Screening for Breast Cancer. *J Natl Cancer Inst* 1993; **85**: 1644–1656.

12. Tunis SR, Stryer DB, Clancy CM. Practical clinical trials: increasing the value of clinical research for decision making in clinical and health policy. *JAMA* 2003; **290**(12): 1624–1632.

13. Holmberg L, Anderson H. HABITS (Hormonal Replacement Therapy After Breast Cancer–Is It Safe?), a randomised comparison: trial stopped. *Lancet* 2004; **363**: 453–455.

14. Moher D, Schulz KF, Altman DG. The CONSORT statement: revised recommendations for improving the quality of reports of parallel-group randomised trials. *Lancet* 2001; **357**: 1191–1194.

15. Altman DG, Schulz KF, Moher D, *et al.* The revised CONSORT statement for reporting randomized trials: explanation and elaboration. *Ann Intern Med* 2001; **134**: 663–694.

16. Moher D, Jones A, Lepage L. Use of the CONSORT statement and quality of reports of randomized trials: a comparative before-and-after evaluation. *JAMA* 2001; **285**: 1992–1995.

17. Seaton ED, Charakida A, Mouser PE, Grace I, Clement RM, Chu AC. Pulsed-dye laser treatment for inflammatory acne vulgaris: randomised controlled trial. *Lancet* 2003; **362**: 1347–1352.

18. Tucker JS, Hall MH, Howie PW, *et al.* Should obstetricians see women with normal pregnancies? A multicentre randomised controlled trial of routine antenatal care by general practitioners and midwives compared with shared care led by obstetricians. *BMJ* 1996; **312**: 554–559.

19. **Baird PA, Yee IML, Sadovnick AD.** Population-based study of long-term outcomes after amniocentesis. *Lancet* 1994; **344**: 1134–1136.

20. **Key TJA, Thorogood M, Appleby PN, Burr ML.** Dietary habits and mortality in 11 000 vegetarians and health conscious people: results of a 17 year follow up. *BMJ* 1996; **313**: 775–779.

21. **Royal College of General Practitioners.** *Oral contraceptives and Health: An Interim Report from the Oral Contraception Study of the Royal College of General Practitioners.* New York: Pitman Medical; 1974.

22. **Beral V, Hermon C, Kay C, Hannaford P, Darby S, Reeves G.** Mortality associated with oral contraceptive use: 25 year follow up of cohort of 46 000 women from Royal College of General Practitioners' oral contraception study. *BMJ* 1999; **318**: 96–100.

23. **Vessey M, Doll R, Peto R, Johnson B, Wiggins P.** A long-term follow-up study of women using different methods of contraception-an interim report. *J Biomed Sci* 1976; **8**: 373–427.

24. **Vessey M, Painter R, Yeates D.** Mortality in relation to oral contraceptive use and cigarette smoking. *Lancet* 2003; **362**: 185–191.

25. **Vessey MP, Lawless M, McPherson K, Yeates D.** Neoplasia of the cervix uteri and contraception: a possible adverse effect of the pill. *Lancet* 1983; **ii**: 930–934.

26. **Johansen C, Boice JD, Jr., McLaughlin JK, Olsen JH.** Cellular telephones and cancer—a nationwide cohort study in Denmark. *J Natl Cancer Inst* 2001; **93**: 203–207.

27. **Daly E, Vessey MP, Hawkins MM, Carson JL, Gough P, Marsh S.** Risk of venous thromboembolism in users of hormone replacement therapy. *Lancet* 1996; **348**: 977–980.

28. **Muscat JE, Malkin MG, Thompson S,** *et al.* Handheld cellular telephone use and risk of brain cancer. *JAMA* 2000; **284**: 3001–3007.

29. **Paul C, Skegg DCG, Spears GFS, Kaldor JM.** Oral contraceptives and breast cancer: a national study. *BMJ* 1986; **293**: 723–726.

# Chapter 5

# Error and bias in observations

*Mathematics may be compared to a mill of exquisite workmanship, which grinds you stuff of any degree of fineness; but, nevertheless, what you get out depends on what you put in; and as the grandest mill in the world will not extract wheat-flour from peascod, so pages of formulae will not get a definite result out of loose data*

—T. H. Huxley: Geological reform; 1869

This chapter falls into two parts. First we will discuss the general principles of identifying and minimizing error and bias in observations, and in the second part we will look at how to measure and adjust for bias.

## Part 1. Identifying and minimizing error and bias
## Sources of error and of bias

In the previous chapter we saw that the choice of the subjects for inclusion in the study defines one of the two key factors 'exposure' or 'outcome'. In cohort studies and intervention trials, the subjects are defined by their exposure or intervention, and the remaining factor to be assessed is the outcome. In the case–control approach, the subjects are selected by their outcome and the remaining factor to be assessed is the exposure. As we have seen, the way in which the subjects are chosen defines the study and determines its external validity. For example, a study of the value of physiotherapy in rheumatoid arthritis may be seen on closer examination to be relevant only to patients of a certain age who have a particular form of rheumatoid arthritis. The eligibility criteria and the participation rate will affect the external validity, i.e. the applicability and usefulness of the results in a wider context.

In the next stage of assessing scientific work, either our own or that of others, we accept what has been done in terms of the subjects included in the study and the design used. We can then ask this central question: Do the results support a causal relationship between the exposure and the outcome, within the confines of the particular study?

If any association is shown within the study, it must be due to one (or more) of four mechanisms: *observation bias, confounding, chance,* or *causation*. In this chapter we shall deal with observation bias. Observation bias is relevant to the measurement of the dependent variable in the study, i.e. the outcome in studies of a cohort design and the exposure in studies of a case–control design.

The central issue is the relationship between the *true value* of the factor being assessed, outcome or exposure, and the value of the variable that is chosen to represent that factor in the study. In the intervention study of physiotherapy and rheumatoid arthritis, the outcome might be defined as an improvement in the function of the affected joints. How this improvement can be best assessed will be a major component of the study design; possibilities range from physiological measures such as hand grip to questionnaire assessments of degree of functional impairment. Expert knowledge is obviously required, and attention must be paid to the acceptability, reproducibility, and relevance of the measures considered. The variable measured in a study is often considerably far removed from the biological factor or event that is defined in the causal hypothesis.

Consider a case–control study assessing whether high vitamin C consumption is protective against heart disease. The causal hypothesis relates the occurrence of heart disease to the intake of vitamin C over a long time period many years before the clinical diagnosis. The variable used to represent this factor in the retrospective design may be the responses to a questionnaire on the frequency of consumption of a number of food items at a defined period in the recent past, converted through a formula into an estimate of vitamin C consumption. The variable appearing in the results as 'exposure' is considerably different from the biological 'exposure' in the hypothesis.

A good example is given by studies assessing the association between gastric cancer and infection with *Helicobacter pylori*, a bacterium that can survive within the stomach. The causal hypothesis relates to the occurrence of stomach cancer being increased in subjects who have had *H.pylori* infection, perhaps over a long time period many years before the clinical diagnosis of this tumour. In a case–control study, with recently diagnosed cases of stomach cancer and controls, the easiest way to assess *H.pylori* infection is to use a laboratory test for the presence of the bacterium at the time of the study. Many such studies have been done, usually showing an association with a modest relative risk of around 2–4. However, past exposure to *H.pylori* may not persist, and so such tests give only an inaccurate estimate of past exposure. Patients with certain characteristics shown by immunological tests are much more likely to clear the bacteria from their stomach mucosa and so produce a negative test. This misclassification of exposure can be minimized by studying only the subgroup of cases with immunological features likely to lead to persistence of the bacteria; one study using this method of control for misclassification showed increases in the observed odds ratio from 3.7, based on all cases, to 18.3, based on cases in which false-negative tests were unlikely [1].

## Error: non-differential classification

There are several influences that may cause differences between the true value of the factor being assessed and the *recorded value* of the variable chosen; these are shown in **Ex. 5.1.** We need to distinguish two different problems. First is the problem of 'error', which means *inaccuracy that is the same in the different groups of subjects being compared*. This is also referred to as 'non-differential' misclassification—it does not differ between the different groups of subjects.

Error includes several components (Ex. 5.1). If we assume that the true value is the usual value over a relevant time in an individual subject, the measurement used will have within-subject variation including true random variation, and also biological variations such as circadian or seasonal variations. All methods of measurement will have a degree of error as a function of the instrument used. Data have to be recorded, manually or electronically, for all

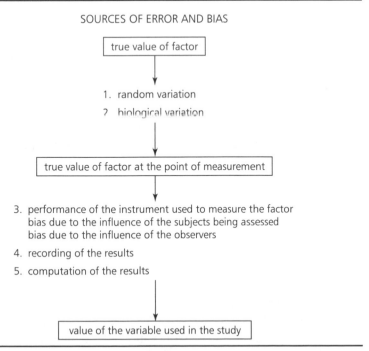

**Ex. 5.1.** Sources of error and of bias in the observed value of a variable compared with the true value of the factor it represents

studies, and in most studies raw data are converted in some way to give the final variable representing the factor under consideration.

To minimize error, methods of measurement and recording need to combine precision, reliability, and practicality, and the conduct of the study needs careful planning and monitoring. The details are specific to each topic and may be very complex; accurate assessments of exposures such as diet, electromagnetic fields, or social deprivation, and of outcomes such as cardiac function, mental state, or improved health, are all major topics in themselves. In general error is less of a problem than bias; therefore the general principle is that the *methods used will be applied in the same manner and with the same care to all the subjects in the study irrespective of the group to which they belong.* If this is done, then we will accept that a degree of error exists, but may be able to conclude that there is little possibility of systematic differences between the groups being compared.

Of course, error is important. The greater the error, the more 'noise' there is in the system, and therefore the more difficult it is to detect a true difference between the groups being compared. In the extreme situation, if the measurement used is so inaccurate that its value bears no relationship to the true value of the factor being assessed, we could not detect any differences between groups of subjects even if large differences exist. Thus, if physiotherapy is actually beneficial in improving joint function, a reasonably accurate method of assessing joint function will show this improvement, while a very inaccurate method will show no difference between treated and untreated groups of patients.

The effect of non-differential error will usually be to make the observed association closer to the null value than is the true situation. Except in some unusual situations, if a study shows a strong association, this association cannot be produced by error in the measurements used; on the other hand, if a study shows no association or a weak association, error in the observations may be disguising a much stronger association.

Studies of disease causation often produce only weak associations, with relative risks of the order of 2. The reason may be that the exposure variable measured is a very inaccurate estimate of the true biological factor concerned, because it is an indirect measurement. Many studies show that the incidence of breast cancer is increased in association with obesity, with fairly low relative risks, and this may be because obesity is an indicator, but an inaccurate indicator, of a specific dietary factor which is related to breast cancer incidence. Where the factor assessed is a closer estimate of the true biological agent, relative risks will be higher. The inhalation of certain types of wood dust is a cause of cancers in the nose and nasal sinuses; if we compare employees in an industry which uses wood with the general working population, we find a moderately increased relative risk, perhaps of 2–3; if we compare workers employed on dusty processes which use wood with the general working population, we find a much higher relative risk, perhaps 10 or more, while if we assess workers who personally have had exposure over many years to particular types of wood we find a relative risk of 100 or more. Thus in a study in France, a relative risk of 303 was found for workers with over 35 years exposure to hardwoods, while exposure to softwoods showed no increased risk [2]. The closer we come to the biological causal factor, the higher the relative risk will become.

The quality of information may depend on its source. A study in Vermont, USA, compared the data obtained from interviews with 857 men and their wives with regard to the wife's pregnancy history. There was disagreement on the numbers of live born children or on their dates of birth in 11 per cent of couples. Taking the history given by the wife as being accurate, husbands reported only 70–74 per cent of spontaneous abortions and low-birth-weight births, and only 35 per cent of induced abortions [3].

## Bias: differential misclassification

The other component of inaccuracy is bias, i.e. inaccuracy that is different in its size or direction in one of the groups under study than in the others. This is a much more serious problem, as bias can influence the results of a study in any direction. It can produce measurements of association that are exaggerated, and may produce strong associations when there is no true difference between the groups being compared.

### Examples of bias

Some quite dramatic examples of observation bias can be found. In a study to assess whether rheumatoid arthritis has a familial link, patients with the disease (cases) were asked whether their parents had suffered from arthritis, and their responses were compared with those of unaffected controls [4]. The results showed that the frequency with which parents were affected was much higher for the rheumatoid arthritis patients than for controls, with a high relative risk (**Ex. 5.2**). In a second comparison, another group of patients with rheumatoid arthritis were asked about arthritis in their parents, and independently the unaffected siblings of these rheumatoid arthritis patients were asked the same questions. Of course, the answers relate to the same parents, and therefore should be identical; however, these results also show that a higher frequency of parental arthritis was reported by the rheumatoid arthritis

REPORTING BIAS IN A CASE–CONTROL STUDY

|  | Patients with RA | Controls | Odds ratio |
|---|---|---|---|
| (A) Arthritis in parents |  |  |  |
| neither | 3 | 111 | 1.0 (referent) |
| one | 10 | 74 | 5.0 |
| both | 6 | 16 | 13.9 |
|  | 19 | 201 |  |
| (B) Arthritis in parents |  |  |  |
| neither | 11 | 20 | 1.0 (referent) |
| one | 23 | 17 | 2.5 |
| both | 6 | 3 | 3.6 |
|  | 40 | 40 |  |

**Ex. 5.2.** An example of subject recall bias. Results of case–control studies comparing patients with rheumatoid arthritis (RA) with unaffected controls in terms of whether their parents had arthritis, as reported by these respondents. Study A shows a strong positive association between RA and arthritis in parents. Study B also shows a positive association which, as it compares responses of RA patients and their unaffected siblings with regard to the same parents, must be due to variation in reporting. Knowledge of the results of study B will influence the interpretation of study A. From Schull and Cobb [4]

patients than by their unaffected siblings, and this result must be due to observation bias. Patients affected by a disease are more likely to know of family members with the same disease.

Studies of family history which depend upon asking mothers of babies with severe defects whether their relatives have had similarly affected babies have sometimes resulted in the conclusion that the disease occurred more commonly in the maternal than the paternal relatives. Such observations have led to hypotheses of complex inheritance patterns. These observations may be biased by the fact that mothers generally know more about the offspring of their own family than that of their husband's family, as can be seen if control families are investigated in the same way (**Ex. 5.3**). These data from a large family history study show that in the cousins of subjects with central nervous system malformations the reported frequency of similarly affected children was considerably higher in the mothers' relatives than in the fathers' relatives, suggesting a maternal inheritance pattern. However, the same type of investigation carried out on families of normal (control) babies showed a very similar degree of excess of malformations in the mothers' families compared with the fathers' families, which must be due to biased reporting [5]. These examples emphasize

| | Total | With CNSM | % affected |
|---|---|---|---|
| REPORTING BIAS IN A GENETIC STUDY OF CENTRAL NERVOUS SYSTEM MALFORMATIONS | | | |
| (A) Cousins of index subjects | | | |
| mother's siblings' children | 2327 | 26 | 1.12 |
| father's siblings' children | 2627 | 12 | 0.46 |
| (B) Cousins of control subjects | | | |
| mother's siblings' children | 1231 | 9 | 0.73 |
| father's siblings' children | 1333 | 4 | 0.30 |

**Ex. 5.3.** Recall bias in a genetic study. Table A compares the reported frequency of central nervous system malformations (CNSM) in cousins of an index series of 547 cases of these defects, and shows higher frequencies of CNS defects in maternal compared with paternal relatives (relative risk = 2.4). However, Table B shows the reported frequencies of CNSM in cousins of control births which did not have CNS defects, and shows a similar maternal–paternal difference (relative risk = 2.4). From Carter *et al.* [5]

that if the information is biased, the associations seen may be strong, and there is no point in applying statistical tests to biased data. The fact that the associations are statistically significant gives no protection against bias.

A notorious issue of observation bias arose with regard to a randomized trial comparing antibiotics and placebo in the treatment of otitis media in children, conducted in Pittsburgh, which resulted in a major conflict referred to as the 'Cantekin affair'. The first report of this trial, published in the *New England Journal of Medicine*, showed a doubling of the frequency of clinical resolution of the disease with antibiotic treatment, based on an outcome determined mainly by clinical examination [6]. However, other investigators in the trial thought that the ear examinations were open to observation bias, and submitted another analysis concluding that no benefit was seen, based on more objective tympanometric measurements [7]. They concluded that the clinical examination results for each ear were not done independently, and that they were not compatible with more objective measurements. In fact, the difference was more quantitative than qualitative: the clinical examination showed a larger effect, while the results based on tympanometry also showed a benefit, but smaller, and not statistically significant in the analysis published. Both groups of investigators agreed that no benefit was shown if a further endpoint, hearing tests, was used. There were allegations that some of the clinical investigators had been influenced by drug company funding. This conflict led to several investigations, which had criticisms of both main parties, and raised issues about the role of journal editors [8,9].

## Methods to minimize bias

The most important sources of bias are variation in the subject's response to the method of assessment, and variation in the observer's response (Ex. 5.1). The main principle in avoiding bias is to ensure that the same methods are used under the same circumstances by the same observers for all subjects involved in the study, and to employ double- or single-blind techniques as far as possible. In the study design the choice of outcome or exposure measures is important, and these must not only be relevant to the hypothesis, but be chosen to be objective, reproducible, and robust, i.e. likely to be little influenced by variations in the method of testing. We must guard against mistakes in both directions, however; while an outcome which is extremely difficult to measure and is open to highly subjective interpretation may be of little value, there is also the danger of choosing an outcome simply because it can be measured easily, even if it is not directly relevant to the hypothesis under test, or may even result in a distortion or change in that hypothesis. For example, we may want to know if a health education programme results in subjects changing their diet; but as this is very difficult to measure, we may choose to use something much simpler, such as the subjects' responses to factual questions about diet. This is perfectly appropriate if we accept that the hypothesis under test has now changed, and we are assessing only whether the educational programme results in increases in knowledge. However, we must not assume, unless we have good evidence, that an improvement in knowledge will be linked to a change in behaviour.

## Single- and double-blind methods

The best method of avoiding bias in measurements is to ensure that neither the subject nor the observer is aware of which group the subject is in, so that the study is *double-blind*. This is easiest to do in a prospective intervention trial. Thus to evaluate the effect of a new drug on the relief of symptoms from rheumatoid arthritis, a placebo drug can be made up which looks and tastes the same as the new drug, and the study is designed so that neither the subject nor the person making the observations of outcome is aware of whether the subject is taking the active drug or the placebo. Such a design should avoid most sources of subject and observer bias. Care has to be taken that the double-blindness is in fact preserved, and not broken either inadvertently through administrative lapses or through the active drug having some feature or side effect that makes its presence obvious. In the trial of treatment for acne described in Chapter 4 [10], the laser treatment procedure involved moving the laser instrument over the face, with the patients wearing opaque eye protection. The same procedure was followed for the controls, but with the instrument disconnected, to achieve patient blindness. The treatment outcome was assessed by a standardized examination with counting and classification of lesions, with the assessors unaware of which treatment had been given, to achieve observer blindness. The treatment was not usually perceptible, but two patients reported discomfort and would have been aware that they were receiving active treatment, so blindness cannot be assured.

In many other prospective designs, double-blindness is not possible. For example, if a comparison is being made between surgery and medical therapy for coronary artery disease, it is impossible to achieve double-blindness. A *single-blind* assessment, where the observer is unaware of the treatment given to the subject, may be possible. While the normal medical carers of the patient will be aware of the patient's treatment, outcome measures could be chosen as items which can be verified by an independent group of assessors on the basis of electrocardiograms, radiographs, and so on, or those in which observer bias is not an issue, e.g. total mortality. In the 1948 tuberculosis trial, those assessing the radiographs were kept unaware of the treatment the patient had received [11].

A randomized trial comparing specialist- and GP-led prenatal care was described in Chapter 4 [12]. There was potential observation bias in this trial. The trial obviously could not be single- or double-blind. Most of the clinical outcome information was based on routine clinical records, and so the validity of recording may differ in the two groups. For example, fewer women in the GP care group were recorded as having hypertension, proteinuria, or pre-eclampsia. This could be the real situation, despite the randomization, but could also indicate relative under-diagnosis or under-recording. The two groups had similar numbers of women with previously undiagnosed hypertension recorded at the time of admission in labour, giving some protection against this bias. An important section of the results is the self-report on satisfaction. This could be biased, as of course the women are only aware of the care system they have experienced. An important aspect is that the response rate to this questionnaire was quite good (78 per cent), and was virtually identical in each of the two groups.

The term 'triple-blind' has been used where the analysis of the trial is carried out by investigators with information on which study group each subject is in, without knowing which treatment was allocated to each group, which is often easy to achieve and is desirable. It is particularly important in interim analyses, which may modify the conduct of the study and even terminate it early. An example is a trial of homeopathic treatment for chronic fatigue syndrome, where control of potential bias is obviously important [13]. To add to the confusion, some authors separate blindness of the investigators who deal with entry to the study and treatment from those investigators who determine outcome; then, adding patient blindness and data analyst blindness produces a 'quadruple-blind' study; an example is a trial of prevention of renal dysfunction after cardiac surgery [14]. Less seriously, some have referred to higher levels of blinding as studies where, even after analysis, no-one knows what the results mean.

## Bias in cohort studies

In cohort studies, the subjects are selected in terms of their exposure, and the bias question applies to the outcome data. In observational cohort studies the subjects are usually aware of their exposure and the outcome may be assessed by the subjects' response to questionnaires or by routine clinical records. In such a situation, single- or double-blind outcome assessment may be impossible. It may be useful to compare the exposed and comparison groups in terms of the frequency with which routine examinations are done or outcomes are reported, who reports them, and the completeness and consistency of the observations. Comparability in these process measures will support comparability in the results. Another useful ploy is to look for specificity of the result, by showing that outcomes that are irrelevant to the causal hypothesis are similar in the groups being compared.

Two cohort studies of oral contraceptive use were described in Chapter 4 [15,16]. Both these studies were weak in terms of potential observation bias, as the outcome data were based on routine medical and clinical records. These could have been biased directly by knowledge of the method of oral contraceptive use, if certain conditions were looked for more carefully in women using a certain type of contraceptive method, and also indirectly, in that women using oral contraceptives might have visited a general practitioner or clinic more, or less, frequently than other women. For example, in the Royal College of General Practitioners' study, 18 per cent of all diagnoses were recorded on the prescription date of the oral contraceptive, suggesting that some complaints might have come to the general practitioner's notice only because the patient had to visit for the prescription [15]. Observation bias will be less likely if the assessment methods are more objective. In the Family Planning Association study, the association between oral contraceptive use and venous embolism was stronger where the evidence for the diagnosis was more objective [17], making bias less likely as an explanation. In this study, the morbidity information used was restricted to hospital referrals for inpatient or outpatient assessment, or inpatient or outpatient care, partly in order to avoid problems of observation bias.

# Bias in case–control studies; recall bias

As in a cohort study, in case–control studies the accuracy of case definition may need to be considered. For example, in a case–control study of pulmonary embolism and deep venous thrombosis, cases were categorized as having definite, probable, or possible venous thromboembolism on the basis of the diagnostic information available. The observed increased risk in association with the use of hormone replacement therapy was higher for definite and probable diagnoses than for possible diagnoses, which is consistent with a true effect [18].

In case–control studies, subjects are selected in terms of the outcome, and the main bias issue applies to the documentation of past exposure. In most case–control studies, information is obtained by interviewing cases and controls. The central issue is *recall bias* (or response bias), a differential response to questions between cases who have been diagnosed with disease and controls who have not. A good study design will ensure use of a well-designed standardized interview, a consistent approach by well-trained interviewers, and a supportive and non- judgemental atmosphere for the interview. However, a difference in the ability or willingness to report past events is likely, even if unconscious, on the part of the subject. Where the study concerns sensitive issues, this recall bias may be more marked.

For example, a meta-analysis (by methods to be described in Chapter 8) has brought together data on 83 000 women with breast cancer from 53 studies in 16 countries, relating breast cancer to a previous spontaneous or induced abortion (Ex. 5.4). These included cohort studies and case–control studies in which record linkage methods used information on abortion that had been recorded before the occurrence of the breast cancer; these studies may have random error in the data on abortions, but differential bias can be excluded. There were also case–control studies using retrospective interviews, where the data on abortions were collected from the women after the diagnosis of breast cancer in the cases; these studies are open to bias as well as random error. For spontaneous abortion, both types of study showed no association. For induced abortion, no increased risk was seen in cohort studies or in the case–control studies with information on abortion recorded before the occurrence of the breast cancer. However, the case–control studies using retrospective interviews showed a modest but statistically significant association with induced abortion which, given that no association was seen in the other studies, is due to recall bias. The women who have been diagnosed with breast cancer must have reported induced abortions more readily than the control women [19].

| | | Odds ratio for association of breast cancer with: | |
|---|---|---|---|
| EFFECT OF RECALL BIAS | | | |
| Time of recording of data on abortion | Number of studies* | Spontaneous abortion | Induced abortion |
| Prior to diagnosis of breast cancer | 12/13 | 0.98 | 0.93 |
| After diagnosis of breast cancer | 40/39 | 0.98 | 1.11 |
| * Number of studies of spontaneous / induced abortion, respectively | | | |

**Ex. 5.4.** Effect of recall bias. Results from a combined analysis of studies of breast cancer and both spontaneous and induced abortion. From Collaborative Group on Hormonal Factors in Breast Cancer [19]

A degree of blinding may be accomplished by doing the study on subjects with symptoms considered suggestive of the outcome under test, but who have not received a specific diagnosis. In the early study of lung cancer and smoking mentioned in Chapter 2 [20], bias in the smoking histories is made less likely because the smoking histories of patients thought to have lung cancer at the time of interview, but in whom the final diagnosis was not lung cancer, were similar to the controls and differed from the histories in confirmed cases. To study psychological factors in women with breast cancer, carrying out the interviews in screening clinics before examination allows comparison of women with breast cancer with those with normal results without the biases that might result from knowledge of the diagnosis. A control group may be chosen from subjects who have conditions of similar severity or nature to that of the cases; thus in a retrospective study looking at events during pregnancy in mothers of infants born with a specific congenital defect, the control group could be chosen as mothers of babies with a range of other defects, who would be expected to be influenced by the same factors affecting recall.

Observer variation is also difficult to control in a case–control study, as it is not easy to keep the observer unaware of the status of the interviewee. Simple precautions such as ensuring that cases and controls are assessed by the same observer or group of observers, and by the same methods used under the same circumstances, are of help. Some observations may be helpful in judging whether subject or observer bias may be a problem, such as recording the length of time taken for examinations or interviews, recording the interviewer's assessment of the cooperation of the subject and the degree of difficulty experienced with some of the key questions, and asking the subjects at the end of the interview whether they are aware of any relationship between their condition and some of the factors asked about. Similarly, the examiners or interviewers can be asked to record whether they became aware of the case or control status of the subject before or during the assessment. Such recordings give the possibility of analysing subsets of data for subjects who were aware or were not aware of the key hypothesis, and those in whom the observer did or did not know their status. Questions for which cases and controls would be expected to give similar answers may be useful.

If the study relies on a small number of interviewers, the results for each interviewer should be examined. In a large survey of women in the USA carried out by four different interviewers, no interviewer variation was seen for questions requiring recall of specific events, but the responses to questions involving subjective and personal information or requiring further probing from the interviewer varied between interviewers. As a result, results on the impact of support networks on psychological symptoms varied depending on which interviewers' data were used [21].

In the case–control study of breast cancer in New Zealand described in Chapter 4 [22], the information was collected by a standardized telephone interview, after an initial approach by letter. The standardization of the interview, and the fact that the interviewer did not know whether the interviewee was a cancer patient or a comparison subject, provides some protection against bias on the part of the interviewer. However, the major likely source of systematic observation bias is from the subjects themselves, who of course were well aware of whether they had been treated for breast cancer or not. A standardized, non-emotive, and systematic interview technique is the best protection against such bias. The bias could also be overcome if information on the exposure of interest, in this case oral contraceptive use, were obtained from other independent sources, such as medical records. However, doing this is often difficult in practice, and it is also unlikely that such sources would give comparable information on all the relevant confounding factors. In this study the investigators did assess general practitioners' records for women who reported recent use of prescribed contraceptives, and concluded that there was 'close agreement' between this information and that given by the women themselves.

## Practical issues in reducing bias and error

The design of methods of investigation that minimize error and bias is a large subject in its own right, and will not be dealt with fully here. However, it is useful to summarize some of the main approaches. Important issues include the *definition* of the items to be recorded, the choice of *methods of measurement*, the *standardization* of procedures, and *quality control* of all aspects of data gathering and processing. It is essential in any research study to define precisely the factor being assessed, even, one might say especially, when it appears simple; consider the definitional issues involved in items such as tumour stage, cardiac failure, pain relief, social class, diastolic blood pressure, high fat diet, or cellular atypia.

The 'instrument' used to assess the factor must then be chosen; we use this general term to include any means of assessment, such as a clinical examination, laboratory test, questionnaire, review of medical records, or observation. The way in which the instrument is to be applied must be standardized: by whom, when, how, and under what circumstances.

As an example of a difficult item to measure, the prevalence of stress disorder in 641 Australian Vietnam veterans was assessed. The lifetime prevalence of combat-related post-traumatic stress disorder assessed by a standardized interview format was 12 per cent, but when assessed by an interview which gave the interviewer the opportunity to interact more with the subject it was 21 per cent. Moreover, with the latter instrument, the prevalence found when the interviewer was a trained counsellor was up to twice as high as with non-counsellor interviewers, and was considerably greater for a female counsellor than for a male [23].

Quality control procedures should be developed to monitor the information collected throughout the study, and to produce useful data that will attest to its quality. These processes of definition, standardization, and quality control are relevant not only to the collection of information, but also to recording, coding, and computer entry. Quality control should include systematic checks for gross errors such as variables which are irreconcilable (e.g. males with menstrual problems), contradictory (e.g. non-matching age and date of birth), or outside an expected range, and systematic checks for inconsistencies, such as addresses or diagnoses from different sources; and rechecking of all or a sample of examination, interview, coding, and data entry procedures.

## Assessment of bias and error in a completed study

A checklist for the assessment of bias and error is given in **Ex. 5.5**. The questions can assess whether the variable recorded is a valid measurement of the biological factor that is relevant to the hypothesis under test. For each aspect of this measurement, a general question relates to the accuracy of the measurement, i.e. primarily to error, and a more specific question deals with differences in the assessment between the groups under test, and therefore relates primarily to bias. Bias is the more serious problem as it may affect internal validity; we concentrate on whether the methods used have been applied identically to all subjects in the study, and whether the subjects' responses to these methods are likely to have been similar. Error will always be present, but may

---

### ASSESSMENT OF OBSERVATION BIAS AND ERROR

| | |
|---|---|
| What is the definition of the factor being assessed? | Is it the same for each group? Is it appropriate to the hypothesis? |
| What is the method of assessment? instrument used observer making the assessment circumstances of use subjects' circumstances subjects' knowledge and cooperation | Are the methods of assessment similar for each group? Are the subjects, or the observers, aware of the grouping of the subjects when the assessment is made? How accurate and reliable is the method of assessment? |
| When is the observation made? in calendar time in relation to the hypothesis | Is it the same for each group? |
| How are the data handled? recording, coding computation | Are the methods the same for each group? |

---

**Ex. 5.5.** Bias and error. An outline scheme to assist in the consideration of issues of observation bias and error. The questions should be considered for the whole study, and specifically with regard to the comparability of the relevant groups: exposed and unexposed in cohort and intervention studies; affected and unaffected in case–control studies

be a serious problem, causing the results of the study to be influenced towards a null result. Often the assessments can only be made in a qualitative and subjective manner. We need to make a reasoned judgement as to whether the results can be accepted as valid. Good evidence on the validity, reproducibility, or consistency of the observations made is helpful, and so opportunities for such assessments should be taken when designing a study.

# Part 2. Measuring aspects of observation bias, and controlling for bias

## Measuring the consistency of information

It is important not only to collect data of good quality, but to be able to demonstrate its quality. The first criterion is *consistency*: data collected on more than one occasion or by more than one method or observer should be consistent. Checks for consistency can be made within an observation procedure such as an interview or clinical examination by repeating key items at different points in the procedure, and by assessing factors in more than one way. All or a sample of subjects can be reassessed; the likelihood of a true change over time must be considered in interpreting the results. Observer and instrument variation can be assessed on all or a sample of subjects, comparing data collected independently by a number of observers or by different methods. To capitalize on some of these techniques variables can be deliberately included in the study, chosen not because they are of intrinsic interest but because they should be stable over time, between interviewers, between subjects, and so on, and therefore variation in their recorded values can be used to assess the consistency of the information.

## A quantitative measure of consistency: kappa

This quantitative method of assessing consistency is applicable where two methods have been used on the same subjects (two observers, two occasions, or two procedures). **Exhibit 5.6** shows some data from a study that assessed the reproducibility of a self-administered questionnaire relating to risk factors for melanoma (a skin cancer) [24]. The data relate to subjects completing two questionnaires 1–3 years apart. For the question 'Have you ever had freckles?' (part A), 593 of the 646 respondents replied in the same way for each questionnaire (255 as 'yes', 338 as 'no'), giving an overall proportion with consistent responses $a = 593/646 = 0.918$. This quantity may be misleading, as even if there were no relationship between an individual's responses to the two surveys, substantial agreement would be expected by chance alone; this amount can be calculated in the manner shown. The logic is that as 0.433 of all subjects gave a 'yes' response on the first survey, and 0.438 on the second survey, if the two responses were unrelated, the expected proportion giving 'yes' responses on both occasions would be $0.433 \times 0.438 = 0.190$. Similarly, the expected proportion responding 'no' on both surveys is $0.567 \times 0.562 = 0.319$. The total expected agreement is the sum of the expected agreement for each category; here it is 0.508. If we take the excess of agreement over expected agreement by chance $(0.918 - 0.508)$, and divide it by the potential excess, which is $(1 - 0.508)$, we obtain a statistic known as kappa $(\kappa)$ [25]:

$$\kappa = (a - e)/(1 - e)$$

where $a$ is the proportion of subjects giving consistent responses and $e$ is the proportion with consistent responses expected by chance alone. Kappa has a range of +1 (complete agreement), to 0 (agreement equal to that expected by chance), to negative values (agreement less than that expected by chance). Here kappa is 0.83, which indicates good consistency.

Another question was about sunburn, with the number of times it occurred categorized into three groups (part B). The observed agreement is the proportion of subjects who give the same response in both surveys and so appear on the diagonal of the table, and is $57 + 312 + 74 = 443/593 = 0.747$.

CONSISTENCY OF INTERVIEW DATA

A:  Question: 'Have you ever had freckles?'

Second survey:

| | | Yes | | No | | Total | |
|---|---|---|---|---|---|---|---|
| | | Number | Prop. | Number | Prop. | Number | Prop. |
| First | Yes | 255 | | 25 | | 280 | 0.433 |
| survey | No | 28 | | 338 | | 366 | 0.567 |
| | Total | 283 | 0.438 | 363 | 0.562 | 646 | 1.000 |

Observed agreement           = (255 + 338)/646           = 0.918
Expected agreement by chance  = (0.433 × 0.438 + 0.567 × 0.562)   = 0.508

Kappa, $\kappa$, = (observed agreement − expected agreement)/(1 − expected agreement)
= (0.918 − 0.508)/(1 − 0.508)           = 0.833

B:  Question: Have you ever been sunburned causing erythema and pain for a few
days? If yes, how many times after the age of 19 years

Second survey:

| | | > 5 times | | 1–5 times | | never | | Total | |
|---|---|---|---|---|---|---|---|---|---|
| | | Number | Prop. | Number | Prop. | Number | Prop. | Number | Prop. |
| First | > 5 times | 57 | | 37 | | 4 | | 98 | 0.165 |
| Survey | 1–5 times | 30 | | 312 | | 36 | | 378 | 0.637 |
| | never | 3 | | 40 | | 74 | | 117 | 0.197 |
| | Total | 90 | 0.152 | 389 | 0.656 | 114 | 0.192 | 593 | 1.000 |

Observed agreement = (57 + 312 + 74)/593           = 0.747
Expected agreement by chance
= (0.165 × 0.152 + 0.637 × 0.656 + 0.197 × 0.192)   = 0.481

Kappa, $\kappa$, = (observed agreement − expected agreement)/(1 − expected agreement)
= (0.747 − 0.481)/(1 − 0.481)           = 0.512

Prop. = proportion of all subjects.

**Ex. 5.6.** Use of a re-interview technique to assess consistency of data. For questions
related to the aetiology of melanoma, subjects were re-interviewed after a period of
1–3 years, and the data on consistency were used to adjust the risk estimates in a
case–control study. From Westerdahl et al. [24]

This compares with the chance agreement of 0.481, calculated as shown, yielding a kappa value of 0.51. Thus there is much less consistency in the response
to this question than there was for the question on freckles. However, there are
two complications with this question. First, subjects who responded 'never' on
the first survey and 'more than five times' on the second survey, or vice versa,
show a greater level of disagreement than subjects whose responses were in

adjacent categories. The calculation shown is a simple unweighted calculation that does take into account different types of disagreement. A more appropriate formula is for *weighted kappa*, where 'weights' can be assigned to account for different degrees of disagreement, as described in texts such as Fleiss [26] and in many software packages. The weighted kappa result from this study was 0.54, somewhat higher than the value given by the simpler calculation. The other issue is that the true result may have changed; as the second survey was conducted later, more sunburns may have occurred, and we might expect a shift to the reporting of more sunburns in the second survey. However, examination of the overall proportions from the two surveys does not show any shift in this direction; in fact, the proportion of subjects reporting large numbers of sunburns in the second survey is slightly lower than in the first survey, and so a real augmentation of experience is unlikely to explain the discrepancy in the interview results.

The variance of kappa can be calculated and used to test whether the observed agreement is statistically significantly better than that expected by chance alone. Confidence limits can be calculated (see Chapter 7 for a general explanation of confidence limits, and Appendix Table 10 for their calculation). The index can also be generalized to apply to studies with many categories of result and many observers, and to take account of different degrees of disagreement.

These measures of agreement have several limitations. First, their interpretation is subjective. Harlow and Linet [27] reviewed the agreement between questionnaire data and medical records for a large number of items, and suggested that kappa values above 0.80 should be regarded as showing very good agreement, 0.60–0.80 good agreement, 0.40–0.60 moderate, and values under 0.40 fair to poor agreement. This simple categorization has been used frequently but is only a rough guide; it is more important to assess the impact of the degree of inconsistency. The consistency of some common clinical assessments has been shown to be quite low, with kappa values of 0.3–0.7; many are in the range 0.4–0.6. Secondly, the kappa value will vary with the prevalence of the condition, being difficult to interpret where the prevalence is very low or very high [28,29]. If the prevalence is very low, kappa may be low even if the consistency is high; an example will be shown in the next section.

However, consistency results may indicate the best of several ways of assessment. In studies of the value of routine skin screening, the quality of information obtained by interview is important. In a study in Australia, subjects were asked if they had had an examination of their skin by a doctor in the last 3 years, and in another question if they had had an examination in the last 12 months, and the responses were checked against doctors' records. The kappa value for the 3-year question was 0.87, showing very good agreement, but it was only 0.27 for the question on 12 months. This difference was attributed to *telescoping*, i.e. patients tend to remember events as being more recent than they were; many subjects reported an examination within the last 12 months when in fact it had been more than 12 months in the past. This comparison led to a decision that an analysis based on reported three-yearly screening would be better for further studies [30].

## Assessment of the accuracy of information: sensitivity, specificity, and predictive value

If one method of assessment can be regarded as definitive, often termed a *gold standard*, the accuracy of any other method can be assessed against it. For example, a screening or diagnostic test can be compared against the final diagnosis achieved after full investigation. A measure of overall consistency is not so useful here, as the consequences of a positive and a negative result will be very different.

*Sensitivity* and *specificity* together describe the performance of a test against the 'true' result, but can be calculated only where the true result is known for all subjects. The *sensitivity* of the test measures its accuracy in identifying truly affected subjects. In the example shown in **Ex. 5.7**, the sensitivity is 77 per cent: the screening test identified 77 per cent of all affected subjects; the other 23 per cent gave a normal test result, and were *false negatives* [31]. *Specificity* is the accuracy in identifying subjects who are truly unaffected; here the specificity is 96.2 per cent, meaning that 96.2 per cent of unaffected subjects had a normal screening test result. The other 3.8 per cent were *false positives*.

A kappa statistic is of little value here. It only assesses overall consistency, whereas the implications of sensitivity and specificity are quite different. Also, the simple kappa statistic is not useful where prevalence is low. In Ex. 5.7, 96 per cent of subjects overall are classified correctly, but the low prevalence means that the likelihood of correct classification by chance is also high (95.6 per cent). Calculation of the kappa value gives a result of 0.11, which is not very informative.

In routine screening and diagnostic applications, subjects giving a positive result to the first test will be investigated further; thus the *predictive value positive* will be the most easily measured parameter. It is a very relevant one, showing the proportion of all those testing positive, and suffering the consequences of worry and further testing, who do have the condition being sought. Here, 262 subjects had positive tests, which required further investigation, and 17 (6.5 per cent) were confirmed as positive. The predictive value increases with both the

---

ASSESSMENT OF ACCURACY OF DATA (1)

|  |  | True result | | Total |
|  |  | Affected | Unaffected |  |
| --- | --- | --- | --- | --- |
| Screening result | Abnormal | 17 | 245 | 262 |
|  | Normal | 5 | 6176 | 6181 |
|  | Total | 22 | 6421 | 6443 |

Sensitivity = proportion of affected subjects giving a positive test
= 17/22 = 77%

Specificity = proportion of unaffected subjects giving a negative test
= 6176/6421 = 96.2%

Predictive value positive = proportion of subjects with positive tests who are affected
= 17/262 = 6.5%

---

**Ex. 5.7.** Assessment of accuracy of data by comparison with a fully accurate method: the validity of antenatal screening for neural tube defects by a measurement of α-fetoprotein in maternal serum at 16–22 weeks' gestation compared with the presence of a neural tube defect assessed after delivery. The test is only the first step in the screening process; the ultimate result was that terminations were carried out on 16 affected and two unaffected pregnancies. For open neural tube defects, the sensitivity was 17/18 (94 per cent). From Wald *et al.* [31]

sensitivity and the specificity of the test, and, for given levels of these, also increases as the true prevalence of the condition in all those tested increases. The *predictive value negative*, the proportion of all those with a negative test who in fact are disease free, may need specific research to measure it, as all persons who test negative will need to be further assessed so that those with disease can be identified. In the example, the predictive value negative is 6421/6443 (99.66 per cent). However, note that, because of the low prevalence of disease, this impressive specificity still means that there are 245 mothers with false-positive results, compared with only 17 true positives; all 262 need further investigation.

A test that is very sensitive will miss few cases of disease; it has a high negative predictive value, i.e. a negative result is reliable. This has been described in clinical terms by the mnemonic SNOUT: if a Sensitive test is Negative it rules OUT disease. Equally, a test that is very specific means that few people without disease will have positive tests and so the positive predictive value is high, i.e. a positive test is reliable. The mnemonic is SPIN: if a SPecific test is Positive, it rules IN disease. The ideal balance depends on the purpose of the test. For example, to test donated blood for HIV virus, we need to know that a negative test result will give virtual certainty of the safety of the sample.

The test has to be highly sensitive to rule out a hazard. However, if we were testing an individual patient for HIV, the most important thing is to avoid giving a false-positive report, and so we want the reliability of the positive test to be virtually perfect, to rule in disease; therefore the test has to be very specific [32].

Defining a screening or diagnostic test involves both the technique and the cut-off point used. For a given test and a given prevalence of abnormality in those tested, if the cut-off point is made more extreme (e.g. a higher concentration of α-fetoprotein in serum), the sensitivity will fall (as more affected subjects will give a normal test) but the specificity will rise (as fewer unaffected subjects test positive). The optimum balance between sensitivity and specificity depends on the consequences of each.

## ROC curves

One way to describe the effects of changing the cut-off is by a *receiver operating characteristic* (ROC) curve. These curves, or plots, were developed in the context of radar signal detection to separate signals from noise, and the radio terminology has persisted. An ROC plot is a graph of the sensitivity of the test against 1 – specificity, i.e. the true-positive rate against the false-positive rate. **Exhibit 5.8** shows data for different cut-off points of measurements of prostate-specific antigen (PSA) in blood, giving the sensitivity and specificity for the detection of prostate cancer in men. Two ROC curves shown, one relating to all prostate cancer and the other to only aggressive cancers, with a pathological appearance giving a Gleason score of 7 or higher. A completely uninformative test would show a straight line from lower left to top right. A test that is better than random classification shows a curve above the line; the area under that curve indicates the probability that a subject with the disease has a higher measurement than a subject without the disease. The ideal test will produce a curve going close to the top left-hand part of the graph. These curves show that the test is clearly better than chance, and is better for more aggressive cancers. The graphs show the sensitivity obtained when an acceptable level of specificity is chosen, and vice versa. The ideal cut-off will depend on the consequences of false-positive and false-negative results. For example, if it is acceptable for 15 per cent of men to receive a positive-test result and go through the necessary further tests which that implies, the test at 0.15 for 1 – specificity will detect about 50 per cent of men with aggressive prostate cancer, while 50 per cent will have lower levels and be reported as 'normal'. It is clear that if the cut-off was set to detect a high proportion of aggressive prostate cancers, such as 80 per cent, many men (nearly 40 per cent of those tested) would have false positive results. The authors of this

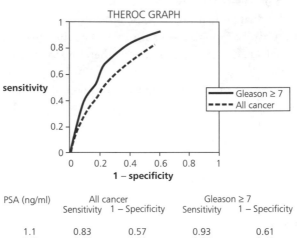

THEROC GRAPH

| PSA (ng/ml) | All cancer | | Gleason ≥ 7 | |
|---|---|---|---|---|
| | Sensitivity | 1 – Specificity | Sensitivity | 1 – Specificity |
| 1.1 | 0.83 | 0.57 | 0.93 | 0.61 |
| 1.6 | 0.67 | 0.38 | 0.85 | 0.42 |
| 2.1 | 0.55 | 0.27 | 0.75 | 0.31 |
| 2.6 | 0.45 | 0.19 | 0.66 | 0.23 |
| 3.1 | 0.37 | 0.15 | 0.54 | 0.18 |
| 4.1 | 0.28 | 0.08 | 0.43 | 0.11 |
| 6.1 | 0.06 | 0.03 | 0.15 | 0.03 |
| 8.1 | 0.03 | 0.01 | 0.06 | 0.01 |
| 10.1 | 0.01 | 0.01 | 0.02 | 0.01 |

**Ex. 5.8.** ROC plot (receiver operating characteristic): plot of sensitivity versus 1 – specificity, and data for various cut-off points of PSA concentration, for PSA blood level compared with presence of any prostate cancer, and presence of aggressive prostate cancer (Gleason grade 7 or higher). Reproduced with permission from Thompson *et al.*, JAMA, 294, 66–70; copyright 2005, American Medical Association, all rights reserved [33]

study commented that the results challenge the assumption that there is a 'normal' PSA level, and that they show that there is no clearly defined cut-off point [33].

Curves can be compared by calculating the area under the curve (AUC) as a proportion of the total area of the graph; a 'better' test gives a higher AUC. Here the AUC was 0.78 for aggressive prostate cancer, but lower (0.68) for all cancer. Extensive further mathematical analysis can be done [34].

The ROC plot is valuable for comparing different tests. For example, to compare the new technique of digital mammography with the established method of film mammography (the difference is analogous to the difference between a digital camera and one using film), nearly 50 000 women in the USA and Canada were screened by both methods, in random order, and each set of images was assessed independently by two radiologists, using a seven-point scale for reporting the suspicion of malignancy. The analysis used ROC curves and the assessment of the AUC as the main statistic. While the two methods were similar in performance overall, digital mammography was superior in women under the age of 50, as shown by the area under the ROC curve being greater. It was also better for women with dense breast tissue, and for women before or close to menopause [35].

## Other measures of consistency of observations

The assessment of the consistency or inconsistency of observations is a large topic with extensive literature. The kappa method is described here because it is mathematically simple, and the effects of non-differential misclassification can be adequately explained by its use. However, there are many other methods, which are computationally more complex although similar in concept. One widely used measure is the *intra-class correlation coefficient*, which is derived from an analysis of variance. It is the ratio of the variance attributed to the different observation methods (e.g. two or more observers or episodes of observation) to the total variance, which is this plus the intra-subject variance. Like kappa, the range is from 1 to zero. A value of 1 means that all the variance in the data is equal to the variation between subjects and none of it is due to variation between observers, which means that there is no misclassification. Fuller discussion of these and other methods is given by, for example, Armstrong *et al.* [36].

## Effects of error (non-differential misclassification) on study results

Clearly, misclassification of the exposure or the outcome will affect the results of a study. Error (non-differential misclassification) is misclassification of the same degree and direction in the different groups being compared. It will lead to a dilution of the effect, i.e. the observed odds ratio or other measure of association will be closer to the null value than is the true situation. (There are some exceptions to this, which will be mentioned later.) The extent of this bias may be considerable. We will describe the effects of non-differential misclassification on odds ratio estimates in a simple study design.

### Approximate result based on kappa:

Two approximate results are very useful. For a simple study of any design with a $2 \times 2$ format, comparing diseased and non-diseased subjects, and exposed or unexposed subjects, for non-differential misclassification there is an approximate relationship between the observed and the true odds ratios and the value of kappa [37]:

$$OR_O = \kappa \, (OR_T - 1) + 1$$

where $OR_O$ is the observed odds ratio and $OR_T$ is the true odds ratio. The extremes of this formula show that if kappa is 1.0, perfect assessment, the observed OR equals the true OR, and if kappa is zero, i.e. the measure of exposure is no better than chance, the observed OR is 1.0 irrespective of the true association.

For example, if the true odds ratio in a case–control study is 3.0, and the measure of exposure used has a kappa value of 0.8 compared with the true measure of exposure, the observed odds ratio will be about $0.8 (3.0 - 1) + 1 = 2.6$.

If we know kappa (from a study of consistency of data), we can adjust an observed odds ratio to give an estimate of the true odds ratio. The formula is

$$OR_T = (\kappa + OR_O - 1)/\kappa.$$

The study shown in Ex. 5.6 was related to a case–control study showing an odds ratio of 1.51 between having had freckles and developing melanoma. Using the kappa value of 0.83 gives an estimated true odds ratio of $(0.83 + 1.51 - 1)/0.83 = 1.61$, i.e. modestly increased.

## Approximate result based on continuous exposure measures

Information on the reproducibility or validity of an exposure measurement is often expressed as the correlation between measurements over the range of the variable. For a continuous measure, such as caloric intake, number of cigarettes smoked per day, or level of blood pressure, the extent of non-differential misclassification can be expressed as the *validity coefficient v*, which is the correlation between the observed measure of the exposure and its true value [36]. The relationship between the observed odds ratio $OR_o$ related to a unit change in the measured variable and the true odds ratio $OR_T$ is given by the square of this validity coefficient:

$$OR_O = OR_T^{v^2}$$

or

$$OR_O = \exp (v^2 \ln OR_T)$$

and

$$OR_T = \exp \overline{(\ln OR_O/v^2)}$$

Suppose that a study shows an odds ratio of 1.50 with a unit increase in obesity, as measured in a field survey, and the correlation between that measurement of obesity and the true value, assessed by comparing the field measurement with an ideal measurement on an adequate sample of subjects, is 0.7. Then the true odds ratio is $\exp(\ln 1.5/0.49) = 2.29$.

The validity coefficient will often be unknown, as the true value of the quantity may be difficult or impossible to measure (e.g. exposures in the past). Often all that is available is information from repeated measurements. The correlation between two measures of an exposure is the *reliability coefficient r*. Under ideal conditions this is equal to the square of the validity coefficient, and so *r* can be substituted for $v^2$ in the above equations. However, in practice such a measure should be assumed to be the upper limit, or most optimistic estimate, of validity.

For example, suppose a study assessing a relationship of adult disease to alcohol consumption in the teenage years yields an odds ratio of 2.0. There is no method of measuring the true value of this variable, but repeated measures using the same questionnaire will give a reliability coefficient. If this were 0.80, the revised estimate of the true odds ratio would be exp(ln 2.0/0.80) = 2.38.

## Use of estimates of sensitivity and specificity to calculate the effects of non-differential misclassification

We have seen how the effects of non-differential misclassification on study results can be estimated using an overall measure of agreement, kappa. Information of the sensitivity and specificity of the measures can also be used to estimate the effects of the misclassification. We will discuss this in the context of case–control studies, although the main results apply to all study designs.

The odds ratio seen in a study is related to the true odds ratio in a way that depends on sensitivity, specificity, and the prevalence of exposure prevalence in the control group. The arithmetic required to adjust observed results using known values of sensitivity and specificity is simple, if rather tedious. The sensitivity and specificity estimates are applied to the observed data to produce estimated 'true' data giving the numbers of exposed and unexposed cases and controls, and then the 'true' odds ratio is calculated from these data.

Non-differential misclassification means that sensitivity and specificity are known or assumed to be the same in cases and controls. Non-differential misclassification will move the observed odds ratio closer to the null value, i.e. it will dilute the effect, but the observed association will be in the correct direction as long as the sum of sensitivity and specificity is greater than 1.

**Exhibit 5.9** shows a hypothetical example of a case–control study where the observed odds ratio is 2.67. If the sensitivity of the exposure assessment is 0.86 and the specificity is 0.93, and these figures apply to both cases and controls (i.e. the misclassification is non-differential), the estimated true odds ratio must be higher than the observed ratio. The calculations show that it is considerably higher (3.66). We shall discuss the lower part of Ex. 5.9 later in this chapter.

---

### ADJUSTMENT OF RESULTS OF A CASE–CONTROL STUDY FOR MISCLASSIFICATION OF THE EXPOSURE MEASUREMENT

*Observed results of study*

|  | cases | controls |  |
|---|---|---|---|
| exposed | 200 | 100 | |
| unexposed | 300 | 400 | |
| total | 500 | 500 | odds ratio = 2.67 |

For each of the case and control groups:
estimated 'true' number of exposed subjects = $[O - (1 - spec)N]/(sens + spec - 1)$
where $O$ = observed number, $N$ = total, sens = sensitivity, spec = specificity.
Estimated number of unexposed subjects by subtraction from total.

*Non-differential misclassification: sensitivity and specificity equal in cases and controls*

|  | cases | controls |
|---|---|---|
| sensitivity | 0.86 | 0.86 |
| specificity | 0.93 | 0.93 |

calculated 'true' numbers

|  | cases | controls |  |
|---|---|---|---|
| exposed | 209 | 82 | |
| unexposed | 291 | 418 | |
| total | 500 | 500 | odds ratio = 3.66 |

*Differential misclassification: sensitivity and/or specificity different in cases and controls*

|  | cases | controls |
|---|---|---|
| sensitivity | 0.86 | 0.70 |
| specificity | 0.93 | 0.98 |

calculated 'true' numbers

|  | cases | controls |  |
|---|---|---|---|
| exposed | 209 | 132 | |
| unexposed | 291 | 368 | |
| total | 500 | 500 | odds ratio = 2.00 |

---

**Ex. 5.9.** Calculation of estimated 'true' results, adjusted for misclassification: hypothetical example of observed results of a case–control study with independent information on the sensitivity and specificity of the exposure measure

A table illustrating the relationship between the true and the observed odds ratios with non-differential misclassification is shown in **Ex. 5.10**. This shows that the effect on the odds ratio can be quite considerable. As mentioned, the extent of the reduction towards the null of the observed odds ratio depends on the sensitivity and specificity values, and also on the prevalence of exposure. For example, if sensitivity and specificity are both 90 per cent, which would be regarded as quite good in most circumstances, and the prevalence of exposure

## EFFECTS OF MISCLASSIFICATION OF EXPOSURE ON THE OBSERVED ODDS RATIO

| prevalence of exposure in controls | sensitivity | specificity | True odds ratio | | | |
|---|---|---|---|---|---|---|
| | | | 2.0 | 3.0 | 5.0 | 10.0 |
| 0.2 | 0.9 | 0.9 | 1.7 | 2.3 | 3.4 | 5.8 |
| | | 0.8 | 1.5 | 1.9 | 2.8 | 4.5 |
| | | 0.6 | 1.3 | 1.6 | 2.1 | 3.1 |
| | 0.8 | 0.9 | 1.6 | 2.1 | 3.0 | 4.8 |
| | | 0.8 | 1.4 | 1.8 | 2.4 | 3.6 |
| | | 0.6 | 1.2 | 1.4 | 1.8 | 2.4 |
| | 0.6 | 0.9 | 1.5 | 1.8 | 2.4 | 3.4 |
| | | 0.8 | 1.3 | 1.5 | 1.9 | 2.4 |
| | | 0.6 | 1.1 | 1.2 | 1.3 | 1.5 |
| 0.5 | 0.9 | 0.9 | 1.7 | 2.3 | 3.3 | 4.8 |
| | | 0.8 | 1.6 | 2.2 | 3.0 | 4.2 |
| | | 0.6 | 1.5 | 1.9 | 2.4 | 3.2 |
| | 0.8 | 0.9 | 1.6 | 2.0 | 2.6 | 3.4 |
| | | 0.8 | 1.5 | 1.9 | 2.3 | 2.9 |
| | | 0.6 | 1.3 . | 1.6 | 1.8 | 2.2 |
| | 0.6 | 0.9 | 1.4 | 1.7 | 2.0 | 2.3 |
| | | 0.8 | 1.3 | 1.5 | 1.7 | 1.9 |
| | | 0.6 | 1.1 | 1.2 | 1.3 | 1.4 |

**Ex. 5.10.** Observed odds ratios in a case–control study with non-differential classification, for given true odds ratio, sensitivity and specificity of exposure assessment, and prevalence of exposure in the control group

in the control group is 20 per cent, a true association with an odds ratio of 5.0 would relate to an observed odds ratio of only 3.4.

These calculations should be used only as a general guide. In most situations the information on the sensitivity and specificity of the measurements of exposure or outcome in studies is limited, and is often obtained from other studies. The estimates of sensitivity and specificity will themselves have sampling errors dependent on the numbers of observations used to produce them. Therefore, although it is possible to use tables such as Ex. 5.10 or calculations to estimate the odds ratio from an observed odds ratio, such estimates must be treated as approximate. Mathematical adjustment of the observed results of a study is usually used in published studies, if at all, only as a discussion point for interpretation.

## Further effects of non-differential misclassification

We will mention some further issues with misclassification; but these are of less general relevance.

## Situations in which non-differential misclassification can bias results away from the null: reversal of effect with extreme misclassification

As stated already, non-differential misclassification will almost always reduce the estimate of association towards the null value. There are some extreme situations where this generalization does not hold, which will be described briefly. In a case–control study where exposure is being assessed, if there is no misclassification, so that sensitivity and specificity are both 100 per cent, there is no bias; the observed odds ratio will equal the true odds ratio. As the sensitivity or the specificity of the exposure assessment is reduced, the odds ratio shifts towards the null value until, when the sum of sensitivity and specificity is equal to 1.0, the observed odds ratio will be 1.0. This will happen for any value of the true odds ratio. This situation is the equivalent of the exposure assessment being no better than labelling cases and controls as being exposed or unexposed by a random process. If the sum of sensitivity and specificity is less than 1 (i.e. sensitivity and specificity average less than 50 per cent), the assessment of exposure is worse than chance assignment, and the odds ratio can show an association in the opposite direction to the true association. Therefore very severe misclassification can reverse the direction of an association. This situation also applies to non-differential misclassification of the exposure in a cohort study.

## Effects of non-differential misclassification of the outcome in cohort studies

In a cohort design, subjects are selected on their exposure and the outcome is assessed. The effects of non-differential misclassification of the outcome depend differently on sensitivity and specificity. A reduction in sensitivity from the ideal of 100 per cent will have no effect of the relative risk estimate, but will reduce the observed risk difference. A reduction in specificity will reduce both the relative risk and risk difference estimates [38]. Even at very low levels of sensitivity and specificity the direction of the true association will not be reversed.

## Effects if there are more than two categories

If the exposure is in more than two categories, the effects of non-differential misclassification may be more complex. If there are categories of unexposed, moderately exposed, and highly exposed, and the true situation is that the risk increases across that gradient, the effect of misclassification will be to reduce the observed association in the highly exposed group (as it will contain more individuals who are not actually highly exposed), but it could either increase or decrease the observed risk in the moderately exposed category. Thus the effects of non-differential misclassification for exposures in more than two categories may be complex, and can sometimes result in a bias of the trend estimate away from the null.

## Non-independent errors

A further situation in which non-differential error can produce biases away from the null is where the errors in the ascertainment of the exposure and of the outcome are not independent. For example, in a survey using several interviewers and subjective data, interviewer differences in assessing exposure and outcome may produce related effects. Such situations need special caution, but the effects will be specific to the situation.

## Misclassification of confounders

Confounding will be discussed in Chapter 6. The ability to adjust for the affects of confounding will depend on the accuracy of measuring the confounder. If the confounder is only approximately measured, the ability to control its true confounding affect is limited. It follows that the non-differential misclassification of a confounding variable will reduce the degree to which the confounding can be controlled. An example will be given in Chapter 6.

## Effects on the numbers of subjects needed in a study

A useful application of this, and the situation in which the calculation of observed values from assumed true values is useful, is in the estimation of the size of a projected study. As will be discussed in Chapter 7, this estimation depends on the odds ratio that is assumed to apply. As the observed odds ratio will be closer to the null than the true ratio because of misclassification, it is prudent to take this into account by using the projected observed odds ratio when calculating sample sizes.

The situations are of interest. However, it is still a reasonable assumption that in the great majority of studies, imperfect assessment of exposure and outcome will show itself in decreases in both sensitivity and specificity, and the inaccuracy of assessments is likely to reduce the observed risk ratio and risk difference estimates towards the null.

## Differential misclassification

Differential misclassification can produce bias in either direction, and of almost any magnitude; the observed measure of association can be higher or lower than the true result. In case–control studies, odds ratio and relative risk estimates will tend to be increased (further from the null) if the sensitivity is higher and/or the specificity is lower for the measure of exposure assessment in cases than for controls.

---

## COMPARISONS OF RESULTS USING TWO DATA SOURCES

*Antidepressants in last 2 years*

| Breast cancer cases | | | | Controls | | | |
|---|---|---|---|---|---|---|---|
| | Pharmacy record | | | | Pharmacy record | | |
| | Yes | No | Total | | Yes | No | Total |
| Self-report: yes | 24 | 2 | 26 | Self-report: yes | 17 | 5 | 22 |
| Self-report: no | 19 | 145 | 164 | Self-report: no | 14 | 129 | 143 |
| Total | 43 | 147 | 190 | Total | 31 | 134 | 165 |

| | | | | | |
|---|---|---|---|---|---|
| Prevalence of use, self-report | 13.7% | | Prevalence of use, self-report | 13.3% |
| Prevalence of use, pharmacy | 22.6% | | Prevalence of use, pharmacy | 18.8% |

| | | | | | |
|---|---|---|---|---|---|
| | Sensitivity | 0.56 | | Sensitivity | 0.58 |
| | Specificity | 0.99 | | Specificity | 0.97 |

|  |  |
|---|---|
| Odds ratio using self-report data | 1.03 |
| Odds ratio using pharmacy records | 1.26 |

*Statins in last 2 years*

| Cases | | | | Controls | | | |
|---|---|---|---|---|---|---|---|
| | Pharmacy record | | | | Pharmacy record | | |
| | Yes | No | Total | | Yes | No | Total |
| Self-report: yes | 18 | 2 | 20 | Self-report: yes | 12 | 2 | 14 |
| Self-report: no | 6 | 164 | 170 | Self-report: no | 2 | 149 | 151 |
| | 24 | 166 | 190 | | 14 | 151 | 165 |

| | | | | | |
|---|---|---|---|---|---|
| Prevalence of use, self-report | 10.5% | | Prevalence of use, self-report | 8.5% |
| Prevalence of use, pharmacy | 12.6% | | Prevalence of use, pharmacy | 8.5% |

| | | | | | |
|---|---|---|---|---|---|
| | Sensitivity | 0.75 | | Sensitivity | 0.86 |
| | Specificity | 0.99 | | Specificity | 0.99 |

|  |  |
|---|---|
| Odds ratio using self-report data | 1.27 |
| Odds ratio using pharmacy records | 1.56 |

**Ex. 5.11.** Results based on two data sources: results for the association between breast cancer and use of prescribed drugs in the previous 2 years based on self-report and on pharmacy records that are regarded as more valid. From Boudreau *et al.* [39]

The misclassification being 'differential' means that the sensitivity and/or specificity is different for cases and controls. In the example in the lower part of Ex. 5.9, sensitivity is 0.86 for cases but 0.70 for controls, and specificity is 0.93 for cases but 0.98 for controls, and the 'true' odds ratio is 2.00, lower than the observed value of 2.67. Therefore in this example, differential misclassification causes the observed odds ratio to be exaggerated. Of course, examples can be produced where differential effects have a wide range of outcomes. Tables similar to that in Ex. 5.10 can be generated by the same calculations, but with different values of sensitivity and/or specificity for cases and for controls.

As a real example, Boudreau *et al.* [39] performed a case–control study of breast cancer in Washington State in members of a health plan with its own pharmacies. The primary source of information on the use of medical drugs was interviews, but the interview data could be checked against pharmacy records, which were accepted as a gold standard. As shown in **Ex. 5.11**, the prevalence of use of antidepressants was considerably underestimated in the interview, with only 13.7 per cent of breast cancer patients reporting use in the previous 2 years, compared with 22.6 per cent reported by pharmacy records. However, this considerable inaccuracy was largely non-differential; the prevalence of use was under-reported by both breast cancer cases and controls. The table shows that the sensitivity of self-report was 56 per cent in cases and 58 per cent in controls, while the specificity was 99 per cent in cases and 97 per cent in controls. The odds ratio of the association between antidepressant use and breast cancer based on self-reported data is 1.03, while the odds ratio using pharmacy records is 1.26.

With regard to the past use of statins, the accuracy of the information appears to be better. The prevalence of use in cases based on self-report was 10.5 per cent compared with 12.6 per cent based on pharmacy records, and in the control group was 8.5 per cent by both sources. The difference between self-report and pharmacy records is considerably smaller than that for antidepressants, but is more differential. The sensitivity of self-report was 75 per cent in cases but 86 per cent in controls, although the specificity was 99 per cent in each group. The self-reported data give the association between past use of statins and breast cancer as an odds ratio of 1.27, again below the odds ratio of 1.56 that is given by the pharmacy records.

## Self-test questions (answers on p. 498)

Q5.1 Which should be considered first in interpretation of a study: chance variation, observation bias, or confounding?

Q5.2 What is the essential distinction between error and bias?

Q5.3 What is the effect of error (non-differential error) on the results of a study?

Q5.4 What is the effect of observation bias on the results of a study?

Q5.5 What do the terms single-blind, double-blind, and triple-blind imply?

Q5.6 What are the main practical methods available to reduce bias and error?

**Q5.7** In a study in which a yes/no question was asked on two occasions, 60 per cent of subjects answered 'yes' on each occasion, 20 per cent answered 'no' on each occasion, 10 per cent answered 'yes' on the first test and 'no' on the second, and 10 per cent answered 'no', then 'yes'. Calculate:

  (a) The proportion showing agreement.

  (b) The expected agreement by chance.

  (c) Kappa.

**Q5.8** If the study in Q5.7 showed an odds ratio of 1.8 for the association between the factor assessed and outcome, what would the true odds ratio be?

**Q5.9** For general purposes, how would kappa values of 0.9, 0.7, 0.5, and 0.2 be interpreted?

**Q5.10** A screening test applied to 1000 subjects identified 100 of them as positive. On further investigation, 50 of these were found to have the disease being tested for. In subsequent follow up, 10 of the subjects who tested negative developed the disease within a reasonably short time. Calculate the sensitivity, specificity, and predictive value positive of the test.

**Q5.11** A survey using a simple portable method of measuring haemoglobin level shows an odds ratio of 1.2 for the association of disease with a unit change in haemoglobin level. The correlation between this field measurement and the best laboratory method is 0.9. What is the estimated true odds ratio?

**Q5.12** In a case–control study with a dichotomous exposure variable, 50 per cent of cases and 25 per cent of controls are exposed. For the exposure measurement, the sensitivity is 0.80 and specificity 0.95. Assuming non-differential misclassification, what is the true odds ratio?

# References

1. Brenner H, Arndt V, Stegmaier C, Ziegler H, Rothenbacher D. Is *Helicobacter pylori* infection a necessary condition for noncardia gastric cancer? *Am J Epidemiol* 2004; **159**: 252–258.

2. Leclerc A, Martinez CM, Gerin M, Luce D, Brugere J. Sinonasal cancer and wood dust exposure: results from a case–control study. *Am J Epidemiol* 1994; **140**: 340–349.

3. Fikree FF, Gray RH, Shah F. Can men be trusted? A comparison of pregnancy histories reported by husbands and wives. *Am J Epidemiol* 1993; **138**: 237–242.

4. Schull WJ, Cobb S. The intrafamilial transmission of rheumatoid arthritis. III: The lack of support for a genetic hypothesis. *J Chronic Dis* 1969; **22**: 217–222.

5. Carter CO, David PA, Laurence KM. A family study of major central nervous system malformations in South Wales. *J Med Genet* 1968; **5**: 81–106.

6. **Mandel EM, Rockette HE, Bluestone CD, Paradise JL, Nozza RJ.** Efficacy of amoxicillin with and without decongestant-antihistamine for otitis media with effusion in children. Results of a double-blind, randomized trial. *N Engl J Med* 1987; **316**: 432–437.

7. **Cantekin EI, McGuire TW, Griffith TL.** Antimicrobial therapy for otitis media with effusion ('secretory' otitis media). *JAMA* 1991; **266**: 3309–3317.

8. **Rennie D.** The Cantekin affair. *JAMA* 1991; **266**: 3333–3337.

9. **Silverman WA.** *Where's the Evidence? Debates in Modern Medicine.* Oxford: Oxford University Press, 1998.

10. **Seaton ED, Charakida A, Mouser PE, Grace I, Clement RM, Chu AC.** Pulsed-dye laser treatment for inflammatory acne vulgaris: randomised controlled trial. *Lancet* 2003; **362**: 1347–1352.

11. **Medical Research Council.** Streptomycin treatment of pulmonary tuberculosis. *BMJ* 1948; **ii**: 769–782.

12. **Tucker JS, Hall MH, Howie PW,** *et al.* Should obstetricians see women with normal pregnancies? A multicentre randomised controlled trial of routine antenatal care by general practitioners and midwives compared with shared care led by obstetricians. *BMJ* 1996; **312**: 554–559.

13. **Weatherley-Jones E, Nicholl JP, Thomas KJ,** *et al.* A randomised, controlled, triple-blind trial of the efficacy of homeopathic treatment for chronic fatigue syndrome. *J Psychosom Res* 2004; **56**: 189–197.

14. **Burns KE, Chu MW, Novick RJ,** *et al.* Perioperative *N*-acetylcysteine to prevent renal dysfunction in high-risk patients undergoing CABG surgery: a randomized controlled trial. *JAMA* 2005; **294**: 342–350.

15. **Royal College of General Practitioners.** *Oral Contraceptives and Health: An Interim Report from the Oral Contraception Study of the Royal College of General Practitioners.* New York: Pitman Medical, 1974.

16. **Vessey M, Doll R, Peto R, Johnson B, Wiggins P.** A long-term follow-up study of women using different methods of contraception-an interim report. *J Biomed Sci* 1976; **8**: 373–427.

17. **Vessey MP.** Some methodological problems in the investigation of rare adverse reactions to oral contraceptives. *Am J Epidemiol* 1971; **94**: 202–209.

18. **Daly E, Vessey MP, Hawkins MM, Carson JL, Gough P, Marsh S.** Risk of venous thromboembolism in users of hormone replacement therapy. *Lancet* 1996; **348**: 977–980.

19. **Collaborative Group on Hormonal Factors in Breast Cancer.** Breast cancer and abortion: collaborative reanalysis of data from 53 epidemiological studies, including 83 000 women with breast cancer from 16 countries. *Lancet* 2004; **363**: 1007–1016.

20. **Doll R, Hill AB.** A study of the aetiology of carcinoma of the lung. *BMJ* 1952; **ii**: 1271–1286.

21. **Johannes CB.** Interviewer effects in a cohort study: results from the Massachusetts Women's Health Study. *Am J Epidemiol* 1997; **146**: 429–438.

22. **Paul C, Skegg DCG, Spears GFS, Kaldor JM.** Oral contraceptives and breast cancer: a national study. *BMJ* 1986; **293**: 723–726.

23. **Grayson DA, O'Toole BI, Marshall RP,** *et al.* Interviewer effects on epidemiologic diagnosis of posttraumatic stress disorder. *Am J Epidemiol* 1996; **144**: 589–597.

24. Westerdahl J, Anderson H, Olsson H, Ingvar C. Reproducibility of a self-administered questionnaire for assessment of melanoma risk. *Int J Epidemiol* 1996; **25**: 245–251.
25. Cohen J. A coefficient of agreement for nominal scales. *Educ Psychol Meas* 1960; **20**: 37–46.
26. Fleiss JL. *Statistical Methods for Rates and Proportions* (2nd edn). New York: John Wiley, 1981.
27. Harlow SD, Linet MS. Agreement between questionnaire data and medical records. The evidence for accuracy of recall. *Am J Epidemiol* 1989; **129**: 233–248.
28. Sackett DL, Haynes RB, Guyatt GH, Tugwell P. *Clinical Epidemiology: A Basic Science for Clinical Medicine* (2nd edn). Boston, MA: Little Brown, 1991.
29. Brennan P, Silman A. Statistical methods for assessing observer variability in clinical measures. *BMJ* 1992; **304**: 1491–1494.
30. Aitken JF, Youl P, Janda M, *et al.* Validity of self-reported skin screening histories. *Am J Epidemiol* 2004; **159**: 1098–1105.
31. Wald NJ, Cuckle HS, Boreham J, *et al.* Antenatal screening in Oxford for fetal neural tube defects. *Br J Obstet Gynaecol* 1979; **86**: 91–100.
32. Institute for Clinical Evaluative Sciences. The jargon decoder: interpreting diagnostic tests. If you expect me to be sensitive, then don't ask me to be so specific. *Informed* 1998; **4**: 1–2.
33. Thompson IM, Ankerst DP, Chi C, *et al.* Operating characteristics of prostate-specific antigen in men with an initial PSA level of 3.0 ng/mL or lower. *JAMA* 2005; **294**: 66–70.
34. Zweig MH, Campbell G. Receiver-operating characteristic (ROC) plots: a fundamental evaluation tool in clinical medicine. *Clin Chem* 1993; **39**: 561–577.
35. Pisano ED, Gatsonis C, Hendrick E, *et al.* Diagnostic performance of digital versus film mammography for breast-cancer screening. *N Engl J Med* 2005; **353**: 1773–1783.
36. Armstrong BK, White E, Saracci R. *Principles of Exposure Measurement in Epidemiology.* Oxford: Oxford University Press, 1992.
37. Thompson WD, Walter SD. Variance and dissent. A reappraisal of the kappa coefficient. *J Clin Epidemiol* 1988; **41**: 949–958.
38. Rothman KJ, Greenland S. *Modern Epidemiology* (2nd edn). Philadelphia, PA: Lippincott–Raven, 1998.
39. Boudreau DM, Daling JR, Malone KE, Gardner JS, Blough DK, Heckbert SR. A validation study of patient interview data and pharmacy records for antihypertensive, statin, and antidepressant medication use among older women. *Am J Epidemiol* 2004; **159**: 308–317.

# Chapter 6

# Confounding

*Thus it is easy to prove that the wearing of tall hats and the carrying of umbrellas enlarges the chest, prolongs life, and confers comparative immunity from disease; for the statistics shew that the classes which use these articles are bigger, healthier, and live longer than the class which never dreams of possessing such things.*

—George Bernard Shaw: Preface to 'The Doctor's Dilemma'; 1906

## Part 1. Confounding: definition and examples

Confounding is the most challenging issue in the interpretation of studies. This chapter is in three parts. In part 1 we will define confounding and show what effects it can produce. In part 2 we will deal with how confounding can be controlled. In part 3, we will consider some further applications of the logic of confounding.

One of the central concepts of science in general, and biology in particular, is that of the tightly controlled experiment. In the classic laboratory experiment, the investigator uses laboratory rats that have been bred under controlled conditions for many generations, are housed in identical physical environments, are fed and handled in the same way, and are then randomly allocated into the required groups. Observations are then made in a standardized manner, with the observer being 'blind' as to the allocation of the animal. The objective is to achieve a situation where the groups of animals differ in terms of only one factor, the exposure factor under consideration, and therefore there is no alternative but to assume that a difference in the measured outcome between the groups of animals is due either to that exposure factor or to chance. The randomization of animals from a common pool protects against there being other factors that differ between the groups, and the standardized and blind assessment procedure protects against bias in the observations of outcome.

In observational studies on humans such tight control is not possible, for scientific or more commonly for ethical or logistic reasons. Human subjects will differ from one another much more than the laboratory animals will, and we can only attempt to control a few aspects of their environment and activities. The challenge is to conduct studies of free-living human subjects that will still have a high degree of validity.

We have seen already that the results of a study, in terms of the differences between the groups being compared, may be due to any of four mechanisms: bias, confounding, chance, or causation.

Confounding is defined as (**Ex. 6.1**) *a distortion of an exposure–outcome association brought about by the association of another factor with both outcome and exposure.*

To understand confounding, let us consider some situations intuitively. Suppose that we need to assess if there is a causal association between the use of oral contraceptives by women and the occurrence of myocardial infarction. There are two standard designs: a cohort study comparing oral contraceptive users with non-users, and a case–control study comparing women with myocardial infarction with an unaffected comparison group.

The issue we are to deal with now is: can an observed association between oral contraceptive use and myocardial infarction be influenced by differences between the two groups of women in terms of other factors? Consider first the issue of smoking. There is ample evidence that people who smoke have an increased risk of myocardial infarction. There is also evidence, in some communities at least, that women who use oral contraceptives smoke more than women who do not. Now consider the effect of these two associations on the results of these studies. Consider the situation where the null hypothesis is in fact the truth, i.e. there is no causal association between oral contraceptive use

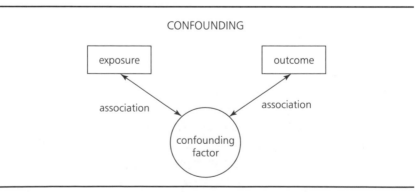

CONFOUNDING

**Ex. 6.1.** Confounding, showing the two associations which are necessary for it to occur

and myocardial infarction. In the cohort study, because the oral contraceptive users smoke more than the non-users, they will have a higher risk, shown by a higher incidence rate, of myocardial infarction. In the case–control study, because smoking is a causal factor for myocardial infarction, the prevalence of smoking will be greater in the myocardial infarction patients than in the comparison patients; and, because smoking is associated with oral contraceptive use, oral contraceptive use will also be more common in the myocardial infarction patients.

Thus both studies will give a result suggesting a positive relationship between oral contraceptive use and myocardial infarction, even if there is no true causal relationship (**Ex. 6.2**). If the true situation is that oral contraceptive use increases the risk of myocardial infarction, this confounding effect will mean that the true effect is overestimated. If the true situation is that oral contraceptive use decreases the risk of myocardial infarction, this confounding effect will mean that the true protective effect will be underestimated or not detected.

In this situation smoking is a confounding factor. Confounding is produced by the two simultaneous and independent properties: smoking is associated

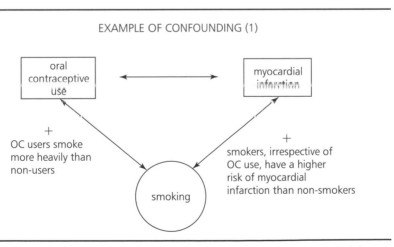

EXAMPLE OF CONFOUNDING (1)

oral contraceptive use

myocardial infarction

+
OC users smoke more heavily than non-users

smoking

+
smokers, irrespective of OC use, have a higher risk of myocardial infarction than non-smokers

**Ex. 6.2.** An example of confounding: any comparison of the risks of myocardial infarction in oral contraceptive (OC) users and in non-users (cohort design), and any comparison of the prevalence of past OC use in myocardial infarction patients and in unaffected subjects (case–control design), will be influenced by the associations of both OC use and myocardial infarction with smoking, which is a confounding factor. The measured association between OC use and myocardial infarction will overestimate the true association with the outcome in this study, and independently smoking is associated with the exposure.

The definition of confounding involves a definition of the study hypothesis, because it may be that smoking and oral contraceptives are both causal factors for myocardial infarction. Therefore if we were studying the relationship between smoking and myocardial infarction in women, we should have to consider oral contraceptive use as a potential confounding factor.

The effects of a confounding factor can be in either direction. In the situation given, the exposed group (oral contraceptive users) has a *higher* prevalence of smoking, and smoking is associated with an *increase* in risk of myocardial infarction. The net result of this confounding will be to give an apparent *excess* risk of myocardial infarction in the oral contraceptive users. In another situation, consider the relationship of oral contraceptive use to myocardial infarction in women and the effect of obesity as a confounding factor (**Ex. 6.3**). Suppose that oral contraceptive users are *less* obese than non-users, but that obesity gives an *increased* risk of myocardial infarction. In this situation the 'exposed' group of oral contraceptive users will be less obese than the group of non-users, and because of this their risk of myocardial infarction will be *reduced*. If the null hypothesis of no association between oral contraception and myocardial infarction is true, the study will give

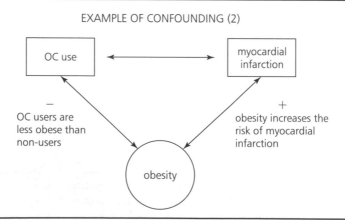

EXAMPLE OF CONFOUNDING (2)

**Ex. 6.3.** Negative confounding: if obesity increases the risk of myocardial infarction, and oral contraceptive (OC) users are less obese than non-users, the measured association between OC use and myocardial infarction will underestimate the true association

a spurious indication of a protective effect. If there is a real increase in the risk of myocardial infarction in oral contraceptive users, the study will underestimate this risk, and may not show it at all, if it fails to take into account the counteracting effect of the difference in obesity between contraceptive users and non-users.

How do we know if the two associations critical to confounding exist? The issue is not whether the associations exist in general, for example whether it is true in general that oral contraceptive users are less obese than non-users. That would be a difficult claim to substantiate, as the relationship is likely to vary between women of different ages, in different countries, and so on. That is not important. The crucial issue is: does the association exist within the study population, within the data used in the analysis? Thus, if within the data set given by a particular study it is true that oral contraceptive users are less obese than non-users, and that obese subjects have a higher incidence of myocardial infarction, then obesity will be a confounding factor in the relationship between oral contraceptive use and myocardial infarction. The only other proviso is that the obesity–oral contraceptive and obesity–infarction associations must apply independently from the oral contraceptive–infarction relationship, i.e. obesity must be associated with oral contraceptive use even in women without infarction, and obesity must be related to infarction even in women who do not use oral contraceptives. This may seem difficult logic, but should be clearer after some examples are presented.

Therefore a factor is a confounding factor only when the *two* associations exist—when *the factor is associated with both the exposure and the outcome* under assessment. Oral contraceptive users and non-users may differ in terms of many other factors; for example, they may differ in their exposure to hair dyes, with oral contraceptive users more frequently using hair dyes. Do we have to consider hair dye use as a confounder in assessing the study? The answer is, only if hair dye use is itself related to myocardial infarction. If we have asked questions about hair dye use in our study, we can assess this by looking at the women who are not exposed to oral contraceptives, and within that subpopulation see if there is an association between hair dye use and myocardial infarction. If there is not, there is no need to consider hair dye use as a confounder. Similarly, there may be factors related to the outcome but not to the exposure. For example, the risk of myocardial infarction is increased in women who have certain types of familial hypercholesterolaemia. This will be a confounding factor only if in the study in question the prevalence of hypercholesterolaemia differs between oral contraceptive users and non-users.

## Confounding in cohort and intervention studies

Because an understanding of confounding is so important, we shall look at a number of simple examples, using both hypothetical and real data. Consider the hypothetical example in **Ex. 6.4** which shows the results of a cohort study in which subjects with low exercise levels are compared with subjects with high exercise levels; the outcome under investigation is the incidence of myocardial infarction in a given follow-up period.

Table A shows the simplest form of the results, showing a strong association with low exercise people having a relative risk of 4.2 compared with high exercise people. However, let us assume that the subjects vary in obesity, and that obesity and exercise are related; obesity is less common in the high exercise subjects than in the low exercise subjects. Subtables $B_1$ and $B_2$ show the results in an identical format to the first table, separately for obese subjects and non-obese subjects. Subtable $B_1$ shows that the relative risk for low compared with high exercise in subjects who are obese is 3.0. Subtable $B_2$ shows that the relative risk for low compared with high exercise in subjects who are not obese is also 3.0. Therefore, irrespective of obesity, the best estimate of the effect of exercise is clearly 3.0. Why then did we get the result of 4.2 in the first table for all subjects? The reason

| | Myocardial infarctions | Person-years | Incidence/1000 |
|---|---|---|---|
| CONFOUNDING IN A COHORT STUDY (1) | | | |
| *Table A: all subjects (n = 8000 person-years)* | | | |
| Low exercise | 105 | 4000 | 26.25 |
| High exercise | 25 | 4000 | 6.25 |
| Relative risk = 26.25/6.25 = 4.2 | | | |
| | | | |
| *Subtable B₁: obese subjects (n = 4000)* | | | |
| Low exercise | 90 | 3000 | 30.0 |
| High exercise | 10 | 1000 | 10.0 |
| Relative risk = 3.0 | | | |
| | | | |
| *Subtable B₂: non-obese subjects (n = 4000)* | | | |
| Low exercise | 15 | 1000 | 15.0 |
| High exercise | 15 | 3000 | 5.0 |
| Relative risk = 3.0 | | | |

**Ex. 6.4.** Confounding: a cohort study assessing the association between the incidence of myocardial infarction and exercise, where obesity is a confounding factor (hypothetical data)

is that obesity is a confounding factor. Obesity is itself a risk factor for myocardial infarction, and this can be seen by comparing the risks for obese subjects for a given level of exercise (Subtable $B_1$) with those for non-obese subjects with the same level of exercise (Subtable $B_2$). For low exercise subjects, the incidence rates per 1000 are 30.0 in obese and 15.0 in non-obese subjects; for high exercise subjects, the corresponding rates are 10.0 and 5.0. Moreover, obesity is related to exercise level, as comparison of the subtables shows that low exercise subjects are much more obese in terms of their distribution by person-years of experience; for the low exercise group, 75 per cent of the person-years apply to obese subjects, while for the high exercise group the proportion is 25 per cent.

The relationships between these factors, low exercise, obesity, and the outcome of myocardial infarction, are shown diagrammatically in **Ex. 6.5**. Low exercise is a risk factor for myocardial infarction, with a true relative risk of 3.0. Obesity is also a risk factor for myocardial infarction, with a relative risk of 2.0; this result is derived from a comparison of Subtables $B_1$ and $B_2$. However, because low exercise and obesity are positively related to each other, the apparent relative risk of low exercise, based on simply comparing all low exercise subjects with all high exercise subjects, is 4.2. Further, we can add the data in Subtables $B_1$ and $B_2$ to compare all obese subjects with all non-obese subjects; we obtain the apparent risk ratio of 3.3 for the crude relationship between obesity and myocardial infarction. Thus in this situation there are two independent risk factors for myocardial infarction, low exercise and obesity, which are positively correlated with each other; therefore each acts

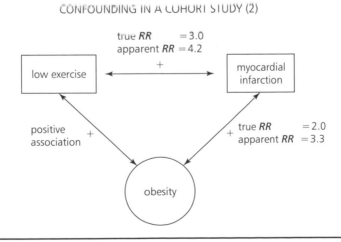

CONFOUNDING IN A COHORT STUDY (2)

**Ex. 6.5.** Confounding: the associations which exist in Ex. 6.4. *RR* = relative risk

| CONFOUNDING: TREATMENT OF RENAL CALCULI | | | | |
| --- | --- | --- | --- | --- |
| | Successes | Failures | Total patients | Successes (%) |
| All stones (n = 700) | | | | |
| open surgery | 273 | 77 | 350 | 78 |
| percutaneous nephrolithotomy | 289 | 61 | 350 | 83 |
| Stones < 2 cm (n = 357) | | | | |
| open surgery | 81 | 6 | 87 | 93 |
| percutaneous nephrolithotomy | 234 | 36 | 270 | 87 |
| Stones ≥ 2 cm (n = 343) | | | | |
| open surgery | 192 | 71 | 263 | 73 |
| percutaneous nephrolithotomy | 55 | 25 | 80 | 69 |

**Ex. 6.6.** Confounding: a comparison of two surgical methods of treating renal calculi, showing success rates (percentage of patients with no stones at 3 months after treatment). The summary of this paper states 'success was achieved in 273 (78 per cent) of patients after open surgery, 289 (83 per cent) after percutaneous nephrolithotomy, ...'. However, in fact the success rates for open surgery are higher, not lower, than those for the percutaneous technique. The main result of this paper concerns a third method, extracorporeal shock-wave lithotripsy, which was followed by higher success rates than those shown. From Charig et al. [1]

as a confounding factor when the relationship of the other to myocardial infarction is assessed.

Consider now a real example of rather simple confounding, shown in **Ex. 6.6.** This is derived from a 1986 paper in the *British Medical Journal*, which amongst other comparisons (a third method, lithotripsy, was also assessed) compared the success rate for two different surgical procedures in the treatment of renal calculi [1]. The upper table shows the results as they were described in the summary of the paper. For each surgical technique, open surgery and percutaneous nephrolithotomy, 350 patients were assessed, and the success rates were 78 per cent with open surgery and 83 per cent with percutaneous nephrolithotomy. In this study patients were categorized into those who had stones of less than 2 cm in diameter, and those with larger stones. For patients with small stones, the success rate of open surgery was better than that of the other technique: 93 per cent compared to 87 per cent. For patients with larger stones, open surgery also had a higher success rate: 73 per cent compared to 69 per cent. Thus, for either of the two groups of patients, open surgery gave better success rates. An erroneous impression of a lower success rate is created from the pooled data, because open surgery was used much more often on patients with large stones, and those patients had a lower success rate irrespective of the technique used. (As an aside, when this error was pointed out and a more sophisticated analysis suggested, the authors rejected this as '… it would only confound the clinicians' [2]. In fact, no complex analysis is needed, just a cross tabulation as in Ex. 6.6.)

In this situation, the confounding factor has produced a reversal in the direction of a relationship: while percutanoeus nephrolithotomy in fact had the higher success rate, the uncontrolled confounding by size of stone gave results showing a higher success rate with open surgery. While there is nothing different in this than in other confounding effects, such a reversal of effect is sometimes called Simpson's paradox. Simpson was a statistician who discussed confounding with a hypothetical example in a 1951 paper [3]. He showed how confounding would occur unless the factor involved was independent of either the exposure or the outcome, but he did not show or emphasize a reversal of effect.

Often the confounding factor will have more than two categories. A further example of real data (**Ex. 6.7**) shows the relationship between physical activity and mortality from coronary heart disease in the prospective study of long-shoremen (dockworkers) in California, noted in Chapter 3 [4]. Table A in **Ex. 6.7** shows the total data comparing light or moderate exercise level workers with heavy exercise level workers, and shows a relative risk of 3.4 in the light exercise group. However, as one might predict, there was considerable confounding by age in this study. Workers doing the lighter physical work tended to be older than those doing the heavier work. Therefore their high relative risk could have been because they were older, rather than a direct effect of their lower exercise levels. Thus, in Table B the results are subdivided into four age groups. The relative risks for each age group range from 1.1 to 2.0. We can see that the true effect of exercise averaged over all workers must be some figure between these numbers, and cannot be as high as the observed crude relative risk of 3.4, which is produced partly by the difference in age distribution. It is not intuitively obvious what the best single estimate of the effect of exercise would be; that will be discussed later.

## Confounding in case–control studies

The logic of confounding in case–control studies is identical to that in cohort studies, but the arithmetic is slightly different. **Exhibit 6.8** shows a simple hypothetical example of a case–control study comparing patients with skin cancer with controls, the exposure of interest being eye colour in two categories, blue and brown.

| Activity level | Deaths | Man-years | Rate/10 000 | Relative risk |
|---|---|---|---|---|
| CONFOUNDING IN A COHORT STUDY | | | | |
| *Table A. All ages* | | | | |
| Light or moderate | 532 | 65 000 | 81.8 | 3.4 |
| Heavy | 66 | 27 700 | 23.8 | 1.0 (referent) |
| | | | | |
| *Table B. Age 35–44* | | | | |
| Light or moderate | 3 | 5900 | 5.1 | 1.1 |
| Heavy | 4 | 8300 | 4.8 | |
| | | | | |
| *Age 45–54* | | | | |
| Light or moderate | 62 | 17 600 | 35.2 | 1.9 |
| Heavy | 20 | 11 000 | 18.2 | |
| | | | | |
| *Age 55–64* | | | | |
| Light or moderate | 183 | 23 700 | 77.2 | 1.7 |
| Heavy | 34 | 7400 | 45.9 | |
| | | | | |
| *Age 65–74* | | | | |
| Light or moderate | 284 | 17 800 | 159.6 | 2.0 |
| Heavy | 8 | 1000 | 80.0 | |

**Ex. 6.7.** Confounding: data from a cohort study of mortality from coronary heart disease and exercise. Confounding by age distorts the association between physical activity and mortality from heart disease. In Table A, a comparison of men with light or moderate physical activity with those with heavy activity gives a relative risk of 3.4. Table B shows that (1) mortality rises with age and (2) the proportion of men doing light or moderate work rises with age. Age is a confounding factor, and its effect gives an increase in the observed relative risk between light activity and CHD mortality. This excess is shown as the relative risks within each of four age bands are all much lower than the crude estimate of 3.4. From Paffenbarger and Hale [4]. See also Chapter 3, p. 60. The situation can be represented as:

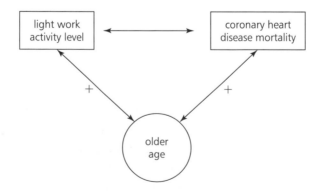

CONFOUNDING IN A CASE–CONTROL STUDY (1)

|  | Cases | Controls |
|---|---|---|
| *Table A. All subjects (n = 1000)* |  |  |
| Blue eyes | 257 | 200 |
| Brown eyes | 243 | 300 |
| Total | 500 | 500 |

Odds ratio = (257 × 300)/(243 × 200) = 1.59

| *Subtable B₁ Dark hair colour (n = 550)* |  |  |
|---|---|---|
| Blue eyes | 57 | 100 |
| Brown eyes | 143 | 250 |
| Total | 200 | 350 |

Odds ratio = (57 × 250)/(143 × 100) = 1.00

| *Subtable B₂ Light hair colour (n = 450)* |  |  |
|---|---|---|
| Blue eyes | 200 | 100 |
| Brown eyes | 100 | 50 |
| Total | 300 | 150 |

Odds ratio = (200 × 50)/(100 × 100) = 1.00

**Ex. 6.8.** Confounding in a case–control study: a hypothetical example examining the relationship of eye colour to skin cancer

In Table A, the results for 500 cases and 500 controls are shown, giving an odds ratio of 1.59 for blue compared with brown eyes. However, hair colour has been shown to be a risk factor for skin cancer, so Subtables $B_1$ and $B_2$ show the association between disease and eye colour for subjects with dark or light hair colour separately. For those with dark hair the odds ratio is 1.0, showing no association, and for those with light hair it is also 1.0. Clearly the best estimate of the association of eye colour with skin cancer is an odds ratio of 1.0, showing no association. We have an apparent association between blue eyes and skin cancer, with an odds ratio of 1.59, although there is no true association. The apparent excess risk in individuals with blue eyes is because of a positive association between blue eyes and light skin colour. This association can be seen by comparing Subtables $B_1$ and $B_2$ in terms of the control subjects: the proportion of control subjects with light hair colour who have blue eyes is 67 per cent (100/150), while the proportion of those with dark hair who have blue eyes is only 29 per cent (100/350)

Subtables $B_1$ and $B_2$ can also be used to look at the relationship between hair colour and skin cancer. The apparent odds ratio, comparing all light-haired

CONFOUNDING IN A CASE CONTROL STUDY (2)

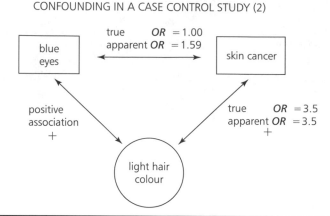

**Ex. 6.9.** Confounding: a diagram showing the relationships present in the data given in Ex. 6.8

with all dark-haired subjects, is $(300 \times 350)/(200 \times 150) = 3.5$. The true odds ratio is obtained by examining hair colour within the categories of eye colour. For subjects with blue eyes, the odds ratio for the relationship between light hair colour and skin cancer is $(200 \times 100)/(100 \times 57) = 3.5$; for subjects with brown eyes it is $(100 \times 250)/(50 \times 143) = 3.5$. Therefore adjusting for eye colour makes no difference to the association between hair colour and skin cancer, showing that eye colour is not a confounder in the relationship between hair colour and skin cancer. The reason eye colour is not a confounder is that although it is associated with hair colour, it is not itself a risk factor for skin cancer, as shown by its true odds ratio with skin cancer being 1.0. The associations are shown diagrammatically in **Ex. 6.9**. In fact, the calculation of odds ratio for hair colour within the categories of eye colour was unnecessary. Given that there is no association between eye colour and skin cancer, once hair colour is controlled, we can deduce that eye colour cannot be a confounder because it does not fit the definition of a confounder; it is not associated with the outcome under study. Therefore the crude odds ratio relating hair colour to skin cancer will not be affected by controlling for eye colour. A further example of confounding in a case–control study, based on real data, will be shown in Ex. 6.23.

# Part 2. Methods for the control of confounding

Having understood what confounding is, we can consider the methods available to deal with it. There are only five methods available, as shown

---

METHODS OF CONTROLLING CONFOUNDING

| In the design of the study | restriction |
| | matching |
| | randomization |
| In the analysis of the study | restriction |
| | stratification |
| | multivariate methods |

---

**Ex. 6.10.** The methods of controlling confounding: one or more may be used

in **Ex. 6.10**. In the *design* of a study we can *restrict* the participation in the study to certain individuals; we can decide to *match* individuals in the comparison group to individuals in the group of interest; and we may have the option of doing a *randomized* intervention study. Irrespective of what has been done at the design stage, when we come to the *analysis* we may again use *restriction* to certain individuals in the data set; we may divide the data into subgroups by categories of the confounding factor, which is the process known as *stratification*; or we may use *multivariate* mathematical methods to take into account the effect of more than one confounding factor simultaneously. In practice a combination of these methods is usually used. We will discuss each of these five methods.

## Control of confounding: restriction

Let us go back to our example of a study of oral contraception and myocardial infarction, and consider how we could avoid being misled by the effect of smoking. One way would be to include only women who had never smoked in the study population. We could do this with either a cohort or a case–control design, and we refer to this method as 'restriction'. It is clearly an effective method, as it leaves no possibility of confounding, but obviously the disadvantage is that the study then becomes specific to the relationship between oral contraceptive use and myocardial infarction in non-smokers, and we cannot generalize the study beyond that target population. (Of course, this restriction only controls for active smoking by the woman herself, not for exposure to smoking by other people. Indeed, a study restricted to never-smokers would be a good design to assess the effects of passive smoking, as the major confounding factor of active smoking is removed).

Suppose instead we do the entire study on women who smoke or have smoked. Can there still be confounding by smoking in comparing, for example, a cohort of oral contraceptive users who smoke with non-oral contraceptive users who smoke? The answer is that there is still potential for confounding. The fact that all the women in the study smoke does not mean that they all smoke the same amount, and if smoking has a dose–response relationship with myocardial infarction, and if the amount or duration of smoking is different in users and non-users, there is still potential for confounding. However, if we restrict the entire study to women who had all smoked, for example, 10–20 cigarettes per day for 5–10 years, the extra specification in the design will reduce the extent of any confounding. However, such a precise restriction would be cumbersome to apply in a practical study.

All studies involve some restriction, if only for practical reasons. The source and eligible populations will be restricted in terms of calendar time, geographical location, and frequently other factors such as age. Restriction should be considered if it is clear that within the study there may be relatively small groups of individuals whose results may be appreciably different from those of the main study population, and for whom the study is unlikely to provide much useful information because of the small numbers. A frequent situation is that of a racial or ethnic group which contributes only a small proportion of subjects. It may have substantially different outcome rates and exposure histories, but there is little value in including such subjects if their total number is likely to be too small for independent consideration.

## Randomization

We have dealt with restriction first because some degree of restriction applies to all studies. We deal with randomization next because it has many advantages over the other methods, and therefore there is a major distinction between randomized and non-randomized studies, both in design and evaluation. If a randomized intervention study is feasible, it has many advantages and should be considered first. However, it is only relevant for certain situations: prospective intervention studies assessing the effects of an ethical, practical, and acceptable intervention which is potentially beneficial and not likely to be harmful. Thus while of prime importance in assessing the effectiveness of clinical or public health interventions, randomization is not relevant to most issues regarding the causes of disease and cannot be applied to retrospective studies.

The principle of randomization is that from a pool of study entrants, subjects are randomly assigned to each of the intervention and non-intervention groups. The definition of *random* is that each subject in the study has the same chance of being allocated to any particular group, and that the chance of a particular individual being allocated to one group is not influenced by the allocation of any other individual. It is not simply an unsystematic or haphazard assignment. Methods based on an apparently random process, like tossing a coin, will work in principle, but in practice are too open to the possibility of conscious or unconscious manipulation. Randomization is normally done by reference to numbers generated to be completely random obtained either from a computer program or from a table of such numbers available in a standard statistical text.

The allocation sequence must be random, and the integrity of the process must be protected, and seen to be protected. Each study participant, and the staff working with them, should complete all the study entry requirements before their assignment to an intervention group is made. Subjects should be invited to participate in the study, be confirmed as eligible according to the study protocol, and should give informed consent; and their participation should be recorded. Only then should their allocation to a specific intervention group be given. The assignment and the decision about eligibility should not be changed after the assignment has been revealed. To achieve this, the randomization process is best administered independently from the recruitment of the subjects. The randomization should be done by someone who is not involved in subject recruitment, such as a statistician or pharmacist; in large trials it is often done by staff in an independent office. A record should be kept of all subjects assessed and considered eligible for trial entry, showing whether they gave consent to the trial, and then whether they were randomized. All subjects randomized should be considered as trial participants from the time of randomization.

The essential logic is that random allocation makes it *likely* that the two groups created will be similar with respect to any particular variable. The essential limitation of randomization is that it is a method based on probability. Therefore its chances of success will be great only if substantial numbers of subjects are used, and we can never be *certain* that randomization will provide equivalent groups. In the extreme, randomization in a study of only two individuals may protect against investigator bias in the assignment, but does not reduce the differences between the two subjects. In a large randomized study, it is highly likely that the groups created by randomization will be comparable with respect to specific factors. However, if the numbers in each group are relatively small (a reasonable guideline might be less than 100), then it is quite likely that purely by chance the groups will still vary. If they vary in terms of a factor which is strongly related to the outcome in the study, that factor will be a confounding factor, and we must deal with that in the analysis. The practical message is that randomization is a valuable technique, which with reasonable numbers of subjects should work in most situations; but we should not assume that simply because randomization has been used, the groups being compared cannot differ in terms of any confounding factor. Just as in any other study, data on the factors likely to be the main confounders should be used to compare the groups to make sure they are similar. If they are not, even in a randomized study, other methods of analysis such as stratification or multivariate methods may also be used to take account of any differences of confounding factors.

## The value of randomization

**Exhibit 6.11** shows the value of randomization. In a study previously mentioned in Chapter 2, the provision of iron rather than aluminum cooking pots to families was assessed as a method of reducing anaemia and improving growth in children in Ethiopia [5]. A randomized controlled trial was used, the randomization being by household, with one child per household participating. It might be expected that any comparison other than by randomization would result in the families using iron pots and those using aluminium pots differing in terms of a wide range of characteristics, which could be themselves related to child development. Exhibit 6.11 shows that the groups created by the

| RANDOMIZATION TO PRODUCE EQUIVALENT GROUPS | Randomized to iron pots ($n = 195$) | Randomized to aluminium pots ($n = 212$) |
|---|---|---|
| Age (months, mean and std deviation) | 31.3 (14.6) | 30.5 (15.7) |
| Male/female (numbers) | 99/96 | 106/106 |
| Weight (kg, mean and SD) | 11.6 (2.3) | 11.9 (2.3) |
| Length (cm, mean and SD) | 87.2 (8.5) | 88.0 (8.7) |
| Ill in week preceding study | 57 (29%) | 70 (33%) |
| Diarrhoea in week preceding study | 35 (18%) | 40 (19%) |
| Mother literate | 72 (37%) | 68 (32%) |
| Mother ill in last 7 days | 50 (26%) | 49 (23%) |
| Access to clean water | 148 (76%) | 157 (74%) |
| Adequate sanitation | 57 (29%) | 72 (34%) |

**Ex. 6.11.** The benefits of randomization: in a trial in Ethiopia assessing whether the use of iron pots or aluminum pots affected anaemia and weight gain in children, households were randomly allocated to receive either iron or aluminum pots, and one child per household participated in the study. These data show the similarity of the two groups in regard to characteristics at the time of randomization. SD = standard deviation. From Adish *et al.* [5]

randomization process are very similar in terms of the age, sex, height, and weight of the children, their recent medical history, characteristics of the mother, and household access to clean water and sanitation.

We can look at these two groups of subjects and consider whether, if they were subsequently treated in an identical manner, we should expect their outcomes to be the same; there is little in the table that would suggest otherwise. Randomization is the simplest way to achieve such equivalent groups. In principle, we could have a design where the first family seen was allocated an iron pot, and was matched to another family on the features shown in Ex. 6.11 which would be given an aluminium pot, but such a study would be difficult or impossible. The results of this study were that children in households using iron pots had a greater rise in haemoglobin concentration, and gained more in both weight and height over a 12-month period, and it was concluded that the provision of iron cooking pots may be a useful way to prevent iron deficiency anaemia in similar less developed countries [5].

There is one advantage of randomization that is shared by no other technique. This is that randomization, given reasonably large numbers of subjects, is likely to produce groups that are similar even with respect to variables that we have not anticipated, defined, or measured. Suppose that after the study just described is completed, evidence appears that an infection common in this community is a strong predictor of childhood anaemia. The study would have been better if that infection had been assessed, and if it were shown that the groups were similar in terms of it. However, even without those data, as the original study was randomized and had adequate numbers, we can be reasonably sure that the distribution of the two groups in terms of this unmeasured factor would have been similar.

## The limits of randomization: pre-stratification

The amount of confounding produced by a factor depends on the strength of its association with the outcome, and the strength of its association with the exposure. Consider a comparison of two treatments for lung cancer. The outcome, mortality, will vary greatly with the extent (stage) of the disease; because this association (stage-outcome) is very strong, stage may have a major confounding effect even if the difference in stage distribution between the treatment groups is small. It is not appropriate to assess confounding by applying a statistical test to compare the stage distribution in the two treatment groups. Stage could be an important confounder even if the difference in stage between the two groups is not statistically significant. Papers describing randomized trials should have a table such as Ex. 6.11 showing the distribution of relevant factors in the randomized groups, but statistical tests should not be used. This is recommended in the CONSORT statement [6], which was discussed in Chapter 4 (Ex. 4.8, p. 96).

It follows from this that where some major confounding factors can be predicted in advance, it may be better not to rely only on the randomization procedure to produce similar groups. A more reliable procedure is to group the eligible subjects within categories of the strong confounder, and randomize within these categories. Thus in the above example we could classify all study entrants by stage of disease, and randomize within each stage, thus ensuring that the stage distribution of the treatment groups will be virtually identical. This is a combination of randomization and stratification, and is sometimes referred to as *randomization within blocks*, or *pre-stratification*. For example, in a trial of perineal pain relief after childbirth, women were randomized within four strata, determined by parity (first birth and later births) and mode of birth (spontaneous and instrumental) as these factors were important with regard to perineal trauma and pain [7]. However, randomized trials are often difficult and time consuming in practice; simple designs have great advantages in clinical studies, and pre-stratification should be used cautiously. It is often used to randomize within centres in multicentre studies, ensuring that each centre treats similar numbers of subjects on each of the alternative therapies.

## Difficulties with randomized studies

A randomized trial makes heavy demands on participants, health care professionals, and those involved indirectly such as service managers and support staff. Randomization is often difficult to use for reasons of logistics or informed consent. For example, Cook *et al.* [8] describe a randomized trial comparing two drugs for the management of heroin withdrawal. The trial required support from a charitable foundation and from the manufacturers of the drugs, logistical support in hospital bed capacity and laboratory services, and the support of hospital staff and the patients themselves. All these presented difficulties so that the trial could not be completed.

The design of trials has to balance the ideal scientific design with practical considerations. For example, to evaluate a new method of encouraging smoking cessation in pregnant women, it may be administratively much easier to offer the new programme to all women in a particular clinic, and compare them with women in a different clinic, than to allocate women randomly in each clinic. Such a systematic allocation method is weaker than randomization, as there is a greater chance of the groups chosen differing in terms of relevant factors, and analytical methods need to take account of the group allocation (as will be discussed later).

Questions of informed consent may be a critical influence on study design. In a randomized trial in Australian general practice assessing a new method of assessing skin lesions, the choice was between a study design in which individual patients were randomized, and one where general practices were randomized. If patients within each practice were randomized, the general practitioner would need to discuss both the new and the conventional assessment systems and the randomized design with each potential participant, and obtain their written consent. If practices were randomized, the general practitioners would need to give their own consent to being involved in the study, but in their opinion, and that of the ethics committees, formal consent from individual patients would not be required as both management options could be used in ordinary practice. While this ethical distinction is debatable, the result was that a study involving individual randomization was impractical because of the time it would require busy general practitioners to discuss the randomization process with each patient. The trial based on randomization of practices was carried out, with enthusiastic support from practitioners and patients [9].

Randomization achieves its objectives by a random process. The principle is that it is *likely* that the groups produced by randomization will be equivalent. However, some differences between the groups will remain, and on some occasions these differences may be substantial and important. **Exhibit 6.12** shows a

| RANDOMIZED GROUPS MAY DIFFER | | |
|---|---|---|
| | Randomized to diet + tolbutamide $n = 204$ (% of subjects ) | Randomized to diet + placebo $n = 205$ (% of subjects) |
| Age > 55 | 48.0 | 41.5 |
| Digitalis use | 7.6 | 4.5 |
| Angina | 7.0 | 5.0 |
| ECG abnormality | 4.0 | 3.0 |
| Cholesterol > 300 mg /100 ml | 15.1 | 8.6 |
| Fasting glucose > 110 mg/100 ml | 72.1 | 63.5 |
| Relative body weight > 1.25 | 58.8 | 52.7 |
| Arterial calcification | 19.7 | 14.3 |
| Hypertension | 30.2 | 36.8 |

**Ex. 6.12.** The limits of randomization: this study compared four regimes for the management of diabetes; here the subjects randomized to diet + tolbutamide (an oral glucose-lowering agent) are compared with those randomized to diet + placebo. From University Group Diabetes Program [10]

table of baseline characteristics for subjects in an important randomized study of the treatment of diabetes, comparing those randomized to receive diet and tolbutamide (an oral glucose-lowering agent) with those randomized to receive diet plus a placebo; the outcome of interest was subsequent deaths, of which many were from cardiovascular disease [10]. Comparing these two groups shows that the patients randomized to receive tolbutamide were older and more frequently had a history of digitalis use or angina, and higher proportions had an electrocardiograph abnormality, high cholesterol levels, high glucose levels, increased relative body weight, and arterial calcification assessed by a radiograph of the lower limb. On the other hand, there was a lower proportion with a history of hypertension. With these data, we cannot be confident that if the two treatments used had identical effects, the two groups would show the same results in terms of subsequent mortality. Several of these factors could have considerable effects on subsequent mortality, and the differences between the groups appear substantial.

Sometimes this is loosely referred to as a 'failure of randomization', but that is an inappropriate term. The randomization process has been carried out correctly, but being a probabilistic technique it does not guarantee that the groups will be similar in terms of all factors. Statistical tests show that all but one (cholesterol levels) of these differences are not statistically significant at the conventional 5 per cent level, i.e. differences of this or greater magnitude would be expected to occur on more than 5 per cent of occasions. However, this is not the relevant issue. The relevant issue is whether the differences are sufficiently large to influence the subsequent outcome rates in the two groups; a small difference in a factor which is strongly related to outcome will be important. Thus in Ex. 6.12 we have a randomized study in which there are important differences between the groups being compared. The results of this study showed that total deaths, and particularly deaths from cardiovascular disease, were substantially higher in the group treated with tolbutamide than in the placebo group. The crucial question is whether this difference in mortality can be attributed to the tolbutamide, or whether it is due to the other factors that differ between the two groups. As will be shown later in this chapter, other analytical techniques can be used to address this question.

## Analysis of randomized trials

In most randomized trials not all individuals complete the treatment to which they have been randomized. Some patients may start the treatment but not complete it; they may decide to discontinue, either for reasons related to the treatment (e.g. side effects) or for other reasons (e.g. change of residence),

ANALYSIS OF A RANDOMIZED TRIAL (1)

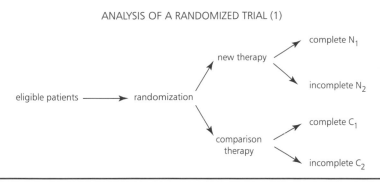

**Ex. 6.13.** Compliance: a randomized trial in which not all subjects complete the treatment course offered. Which groups should be compared?

or their clinical situation may change so that a change in treatment is indicated. Some patients may be randomized but not even commence treatment. **Exhibit 6.13** represents a clinical trial in which patients are randomized into two treatment groups, but only some of the patients complete the course of treatment offered. The question is: to assess the effect of the new therapy, which groups of patients should be compared?

One simple answer is to compare patients who received the new therapy with those who did not. The only group who received the new therapy is group $N_1$—those who were allocated the new treatment and completed it. Therefore we could compare group $N_1$ with either all other subjects ($C_1 + C_2 + N_2$), with all subjects allocated to the comparison treatment ($C_1 + C_2$), or with those allocated to the comparison treatment who completed it (group $C_1$).

However, if any of these comparisons is used, the value of randomization in controlling confounding is lost because the comparisons are no longer being made between randomized groups. There may be very considerable differences between the subjects who complete the new treatment ($N_1$), and those who withdraw or do not receive it ($N_2$). A classic example of this is shown in a randomized double-blind trial comparing lipid-reducing drugs with placebo, which was carried out in the USA between 1966 and 1969 [11] (**Ex. 6.14**). The outcome was mortality from any cause over the following 5 years. The mortality rate in those patients who were allocated to the lipid-lowering agent clofibrate, and actually consumed over 80 per cent of the allocated dosages, was 15.0 per cent. This rate could be compared with the mortality rate in all patients allocated to the placebo, which was 19.4 per cent, showing a statistically

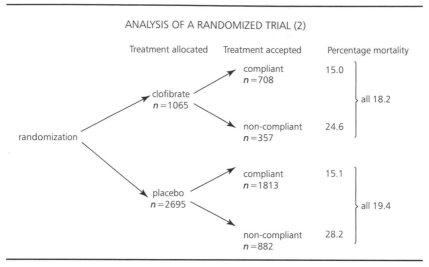

ANALYSIS OF A RANDOMIZED TRIAL (2)

Treatment allocated    Treatment accepted    Percentage mortality

clofibrate
n=1065

compliant
n=708    15.0

non-compliant
n=357    24.6

all 18.2

randomization

placebo
n=2695

compliant
n=1813    15.1

non-compliant
n=882    28.2

all 19.4

**Ex. 6.14.** Compliance in a randomized trial: the results show the mortality rates from all causes after 5 years follow-up in patients randomized to either a lipid-lowering agent (clofibrate) or a placebo, in terms of their compliance with the drug regime. 'Compliant' means taking > 80 per cent of the allocated drug. From Coronary Drug Project Research Group [11]

significant difference in favour of clofibrate. However, the patients who were randomized to clofibrate but did not take it had a much higher mortality (24.6 per cent). Of course, this is consistent with a beneficial effect of the drug; we would expect patients who did not take the drug adequately to have a higher mortality than those who took it well. However, it would be dangerous to ascribe these results to the pharmacological effects of the drug. The point is dramatically illustrated by the mortality experience in relation to compliance with the placebo; those who took more than 80 per cent of the allocated doses of the placebo had a mortality of 15.1 per cent, and those who took less had a mortality rate of 28.2 per cent. The correct analysis of the randomized groups shows that the mortality rate in all those randomized to clofibrate was 18.2 per cent, similar to the rate in all those randomized to placebo (19.4 per cent). Any other comparison gives an incorrect result because of the confounding effects of factors related to compliance. The results also show that irrespective of what drug is prescribed, subjects who follow the instructions carefully have a lower mortality rate than those who do not. This cannot be ascribed to any pharmacological action, but reflects the influence of factors that are related to compliance, which are confounding factors in the association between the drug allocated and outcome. The correct analysis is referred to as *intention to treat* analysis; we compare the groups defined by the initial treatment offered.

## Management and explanatory trials

The trial shown in Ex. 6.14 shows the dangers of making any other comparison in a randomized trial except between the groups chosen by randomization. This is despite the fact that, in many trials, the proportions of patients who fulfil all the protocol criteria, particularly that of maintaining the allocated therapy for its full course, may be relatively small.

This issue is important in both clinical and community-based studies. In the first randomized trial of breast cancer screening, women who were members of a health maintenance plan in New York were randomly allocated into two groups [12]. One group continued their normal medical care. Women in the other group were offered an innovative programme of screening for breast cancer, using mammography and clinical examination. About two-thirds of those offered this programme participated. The relevant outcome is death from breast cancer, and so the appropriate randomized analysis shows the effect of *offering* a breast cancer screening programme, with a two-thirds acceptance rate, on breast cancer mortality. After some 10 years of follow-up, there was a reduction of around 30 per cent in breast cancer mortality. This randomized trial shows the effect of offering a programme of screening. It does not measure the reduction in mortality risk for an individual who agrees to participate, except that this must be higher than the difference shown. Estimates of this can be made, but are uncertain because they depend on how those who participated in the programme differed from those who declined the offered screening with regard to their underlying risk of death from breast cancer.

One could argue that analysis by comparison of randomized groups, while effective in controlling confounding, is likely to be inefficient, as there is a considerable dilution effect because many subjects in the intervention group are not actually receiving the intervention. However, in considering this we have to go back to the question of what the trial is actually for, and how the results will be applied. It is a naive supposition that all patients will follow a doctor's advice, or that everyone will participate in a planned intervention. In many situations, unless the intervention results in an improved outcome, given that a substantial proportion of subjects will not accept it in full, it will not be useful. We can distinguish between trials which address the *management* question—what is the effect of prescribing a certain therapy, or offering an intervention, in a practical situation?—and those whose aim is *explanatory*— irrespective of the practical issues involved, what is the effect of the intervention in ideal circumstances, in subjects who do accept it? This distinction between management and explanatory trials is important in the design and interpretation of randomized trials.

Both types of trial are legitimate; the dangers arise if the results from a study designed or analysed as an explanatory trial are interpreted in management terms. For example, iron deficiency anaemia in adolescence may affect cognitive function, and so iron supplementation could protect or improve cognitive function. A randomized trial of iron supplementation carried out on high school girls in the USA assessed this, and showed that, after 8 weeks, the girls who received iron supplementation performed better on tests of verbal learning and memory than girls in the control group [13]. However, girls who were clinically anaemic were excluded from the trial, other vitamins or iron supplements were prohibited, many strategies were used to ensure compliance, and the outcome measures used were research tools; most important, the analysis was based on only the girls who completed treatment rather than being an intention to treat analysis. As pointed out in an accompanying editorial, this is an explanatory study which gives the results under ideal conditions, and therefore demonstrates the potential rather than the practical value of iron supplementation [14]. A management study, to assess directly whether iron supplementation would have clinically relevant benefits in practice, would need to use realistic rather than ideal methods of ensuring compliance, less stringent eligibility criteria, and a more relevant endpoint and time of assessment, and in particular include in the analysis all subjects randomized.

Randomized trials are often designed to guide clinical or health policy decisions, and the terms *pragmatic* or *practical* clinical trials have been used for trials designed to facilitate such decision-making. These have some features that contrast with more explanatory orientated trials, which may concentrate on a highly selected group of subjects. Practical trials relevant to policy-making should be based on relevant interventions, and include a diverse population of study participants, recruited from different practice settings, with data collected on a broad range of health outcomes [15].

If a management trial, correctly analysed by intention to treat, shows no effect, this could be because the intervention did not work or because too few subjects accepted it. A controversial example, which also shows the dangers of incorrect analysis, is a randomized trial of prostate cancer screening. Men aged 45–80 years sampled from the electoral rolls in Quebec City, Canada, were randomly allocated in a 2:1 ratio either to receive an invitation to a screening programme using annual measurements of serum prostate-specific antigen (PSA) and digital rectal examination, or to be in a non-invited control group.

This is a standard randomized design. The outcome was the death rate from prostate cancer in the 11 years after randomization, reported in two main papers [16,17].

The results based on this randomization (**Ex. 6.15**) show a relative risk of 1.08, i.e. an 8 per cent increase in deaths in the group offered screening. However, in contrast, the summary of the more recent paper reports a relative risk of 0.38, i.e. a 62 per cent reduction in mortality. The earlier paper showed a similar reduction, and the authors concluded that their study 'demonstrates, for the first time, that early diagnosis and treatment permits a dramatic decrease in deaths from prostate cancer' [16]. The large mortality reduction is based on a comparison between men who were randomized to screening and were screened, and those randomized to no screening who were not screened (groups $N_1$ and $C_1$ in the terminology of Ex. 6.13, shown earlier). This analysis restricted to compliant subjects is shown in Ex. 6.15, and gives the relative risk of 0.38. In the earlier paper, the main comparison was between all the men who were screened, whether they were invited for screening or not, and all other men in the study who were not screened (groups $N_1 + C_2$ versus groups $N_2 + C_1$ in Ex. 6.13); this gave a similar large reduction.

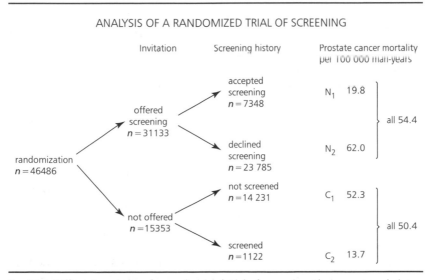

ANALYSIS OF A RANDOMIZED TRIAL OF SCREENING

**Ex. 6.15.** Different analyses of a randomized trial of screening: the correct analysis, maintaining the randomized groups, gives a relative risk of 54.4/50.4 = 1.08. Other comparisons lose the advantage of the randomization. From Labrie *et al.* [17]

In both these analyses, the benefits of the randomized design have been lost. In the body of the recent paper an analysis on an 'intent to screen' basis was also made and the lack of effect recognized, but this is given little importance. In this trial, few men invited for screening were actually screened (23 per cent), so that the randomized trial has lost most of its ability to detect an effect of screening because of misclassification (in addition, 7 per cent of the men randomized to the non-invited group were screened, but this is a smaller problem). However, this does not give validity to the non-randomized comparisons which, presented in papers with the title of a randomized trial, are misleading. It is surprising that such a fundamentally flawed analysis was published in a reputable and peer-reviewed journal on a topic of great practical importance. The problems in the analysis have been pointed out in correspondence [18,19].

## Stratification

To discuss the next method of controlling confounding, let us go back to the example of studies of oral contraceptives and myocardial infarction, and the problem of confounding by smoking. As we have seen, we could use restriction to avoid confounding by smoking. This could lead to a series of restricted studies, one looking at non-smokers, one at smokers of a certain quantity, and so on. However, this situation can be achieved in one study. We could include oral contraceptive users and non-users in the study without any limitations, but with careful recording of each woman's smoking history. Then in the analysis, we divide the data, and compare oral contraceptive users who have never smoked with non-users who have never smoked, and so on throughout the various levels of smoking. This procedure is *stratification*, as strata or layers of data are formed. The stratification is done on the basis of the suspected confounding factor. This is the most important and widely used method of controlling confounding. It is used in the majority of studies either on its own or in combination with other methods.

Indeed, if you have worked through this chapter, you have already used stratification several times. In Ex. 6.4 we demonstrated the effect of stratification by obesity in a study relating exercise to myocardial infarction. In Ex. 6.6, we stratified by the size of the renal stone in the study comparing surgical methods in the treatment of renal stones. In Ex. 6.7, we used four age groups to control confounding by age in a cohort study. In Ex. 6.8, we used stratification by hair colour in a case–control study relating eye colour to skin cancer. In each of these examples, we went as far as dividing the data into strata, and looking at the measure of association (relative risk or odds ratio) within each stratum of the confounder, and we also made some comments about the range of these results. The extra process, which we will now consider, is how to use the stratified data to produce a *single overall estimate* of effect that has been *adjusted* for the effects of the confounding factor.

## Stratification in cohort and intervention studies: Mantel–Haenszel method

The results from the cohort study relating exercise to deaths from heart disease previously shown in Ex. 6.7 are summarized in **Ex. 6.16**, Subtable A,

---

STRATIFICATION IN A COHORT STUDY: MANTEL–HAENSZEL ANALYSIS

*Subtable A: Data stratified by the confounder (age)*

| Age group | Exposed (light exercise) | | | Unexposed (heavy exercise) | | | Relative Risk |
|---|---|---|---|---|---|---|---|
| | Deaths | Man-years (thousands) | Rate/1000 | Deaths | Man-years (thousands) | Rate/1000 | |
| | $a_i$ | $N_{1i}$ | $a_i/N_{1i}$ | $c_i$ | $N_{0i}$ | $c_i/N_{0i}$ | |
| 35–44 | 3 | 5.9 | 0.51 | 4 | 8.3 | 0.48 | 1.06 |
| 45–54 | 62 | 17.6 | 3.52 | 20 | 11.0 | 1.82 | 1.94 |
| 55–64 | 183 | 23.7 | 7.72 | 34 | 7.4 | 4.59 | 1.68 |
| 60–74 | 284 | 17.8 | 15.96 | 8 | 1.0 | 8.00 | 1.99 |
| All ages | 532 | 65 | 8.18 | 66 | 27.7 | 2.38 | |

Crude relative risk (no adjustment for age) = 8.18/2.38 = 3.44

*Subtable B. Calculation of summary relative risk, adjusted for the confounder, by the Mantel–Haenszel method*

| Age group | Total man-years ($T_i$) | $a_i N_{0i}/T_i$ | $c_i N_{1i}/T_i$ |
|---|---|---|---|
| 35–44 | 14.2 | 1.75 | 1.66 |
| 45–54 | 28.6 | 23.85 | 12.31 |
| 55–64 | 31.1 | 43.54 | 25.91 |
| 65–74 | 18.8 | 15.11 | 7.57 |
| Sum | | 84.25 | 47.45 |

Mantel–Haenszel relative risk = (84.25/47.45) = 1.78

---

**Ex. 6.16.** Stratification in a cohort study: the study shown in Ex. 6.7 gives, on simple analysis, a misleading result because of confounding by age (subtable A). Stratification by age avoids this. One method of calculating a summary relative risk measure, adjusting for the stratification, is shown in subtable B for the four age groups. The summed data for all ages give a relative risk of 3.44, but this is misleading as it is confounded by age; the age-specific relative risks range from 1.06 to 1.99.

A practical difficulty arises when data are divided into a number of strata. The numbers of subjects in one stratum may be small, and therefore the outcome measure, such as the relative risk, for that stratum will be imprecise; therefore the relative risk estimates may vary considerably among the strata. There are two issues. First, can we assume that there is a *constant* measure of association, such as relative risk, which can be applied to all strata? At this point we will simply point out that differences based on small numbers are unlikely to be important (such as the youngest age group in Ex. 6.16), and we should be concerned only about substantial differences between the relative risks in different strata. In the next chapter we will present statistical methods to test whether the assumption of a constant relative risk for all the strata is justified. Then, if we assume that the true relative risk is likely to be the same in all strata, we can use the data for all strata to produce a single estimate of relative risk, which is adjusted for the effects of the confounding factor.

This adjusted relative risk will be some type of average of the relative risks in the different strata. There are several methods of producing an overall estimate, which use different methods of averaging. Indeed, one method would be a simple arithmetic average of the relative risks for each stratum. However, this would assume that they are equally precise, and in our example the relative risk for the youngest age group is based only on seven deaths in total, and intuitively we should give it less importance than the relative risks in the other groups.

A more appropriate method of averaging is to give each stratum an importance related to the amount of information or, in other words, the numbers in the stratum. One widely used method is shown in **Ex. 6.17**, and applied in Ex. 6.16 in Subtable B. The formula for the adjusted relative risk has the same structure as the formula for the relative risk in one stratum. The numerator is the sum of the numerator terms derived from each stratum, and the denominator is a sum of the denominator terms derived from each stratum. The result gives a *weighted average* of the relative risks, in which the weights given to each stratum relate to the amount of information within each stratum. This adjusted relative risk is a reasonable summary value of the overall relative risk, adjusting for the confounding effect of the stratification factor, in this case, age. Here this adjusted relative risk is 1.78, which is compatible with the age-specific relative risks. This particular method is derived from a method first developed for use in case–control studies, and is referred to as the

---

MANTEL–HAENSZEL ESTIMATION OF RELATIVE RISK

In each subtable $i$, stratified by the potential confounder:

|  | Cases | Total subjects or person-years |
|---|---|---|
| exposed | $a_i$ | $N_{1i}$ |
| unexposed | $c_i$ | $N_{0i}$ |

$T_i$ = total in the subtable

Relative risk for this subtable = $(a_i/N_{1i})/(c_i/N_{0i}) = a_iN_{0i}/c_iN_{1i}$

The Mantel–Haenszel estimate of relative risk uses the data from all subtables, but gives an estimate of the unconfounded relative risk:

$$\text{given by } \frac{\sum_i a_iN_{0i}/T_i}{\sum_i c_iN_{1i}/T_i}$$

where $\sum_i$ indicates summation over all the subtables

---

**Ex. 6.17.** Stratification: calculation of the Mantel–Haenszel estimate of the summary relative risk in a stratified analysis

Mantel–Haenszel method [20]. (The algebraic notation used in Exs. 6.16 and **6.17** is the same as that used previously in Chapter 3, except that we indicate the data within one stratum by a subscript 1 for the first stratum, 2 for the second, etc., which is shown in general terms by the subscript $i$).

Stratification can be used in any study design, including randomized trials. We emphasized earlier that while randomization is likely to produce evenly balanced groups, it does not always do so. In Ex. 6.12, some information from a randomized trial of tolbutamide and placebo in the management of diabetes was given, which suggested some substantial differences in the groups being compared. **Exhibit 6.18,** Subtable A, gives the main results of that study, showing death rates from all causes of 14.7 per cent in the tolbutamide-treated patients and 10.2 per cent in the placebo-treated patients, giving a relative risk of 1.44. We can use stratified analyses to assess whether these differences are influenced by the differences in the baseline characteristics shown in Ex. 6.12. In Ex. 6.18, Subtable B, the stratification by arterial calcification is shown. Arterial calcification is a true confounder; it is more common in the tolbutamide-treated group than in the placebo-treated group, and within each treatment group the death rate is higher in the subjects with arterial calcification. However, both within subjects with arterial calcification and within those without arterial calcification, the death rate is higher in the tolbutamide-treated subjects.

---

STRATIFIED ANALYSIS OF A RANDOMIZED TRIAL

*Subtable A. Main results (n = 409)*

| Treatment | Deaths | Survivors | Total | % dead | Relative risk |
|---|---|---|---|---|---|
| Tolbutamide | 30 | 174 | 204 | 14.7 | 1.44 |
| Placebo | 21 | 184 | 205 | 10.2 | 1.0(R) |

*Subtable $B_1$. Stratified: arterial calcification present (n = 68)*

| Treatment | Deaths | Survivors | Total | % dead | Relative risk |
|---|---|---|---|---|---|
| Tolbutamide | 13 | 26 | 39 | 33.3 | 1.93 |
| Placebo | 5 | 24 | 29 | 17.2 | |

*Subtable $B_2$. Stratified: arterial calcification absent (n = 333)*

| Treatment | Deaths | Survivors | Total | % dead | Relative risk |
|---|---|---|---|---|---|
| Tolbutamide | 16 | 143 | 159 | 10.1 | 1.09 |
| Placebo | 16 | 158 | 174 | 9.2 | |

Relative risk adjusted for arterial calcification
$$= (13 \times 29/68 + 16 \times 174/333)/(5 \times 39/68 + 16 \times 159/333) = 1.32$$

---

**Ex. 6.18.** Stratified analysis of a randomized trial: main results of the trial shown in Ex. 6.12 (subtable A), and results stratified for arterial calcification (subtables $B_1$ and $B_2$), and adjusted relative risk calculated by the modified Mantel–Haenszel method (Ex. 6.17). From University Group Diabetes Program [10]. As often occurs, some data are missing: eight subjects are omitted from the stratified analysis as data on arterial calcification were missing. The crude relative risk for the two subtables combined is 1.42

The best estimate of the relationship between tolbutamide treatment and mortality, adjusted for the differences in prevalence of arterial calcification, is given by the Mantel–Haenszel relative risk calculation, which gives a relative risk of 1.32. We compare this with the original relative risk of 1.44 in Subtable A. The conclusion is that the crude increased risk in the tolbutamide group ($RR = 1.44$) is reduced by stratifying for arterial calcification, but is not abolished, and most of the excess risk is still maintained ($RR = 1.32$). Analyses of this form can be carried out for each of the variables listed in Ex. 6.12. However, it is clear that this method of analysis is still unsatisfactory, as although it is easy to adjust for each of the variables singly, we are still not answering the more general question: does the difference in mortality between tolbutamide- and placebo-treated patients persist when we take into account the effect of *all* the factors on which we have baseline information? That issue requires more complex analysis which will be shown later in this chapter.

## Direct standardization

Another method of taking a weighted average of stratum-specific relative risks is direct standardization, which is frequently used in large data sets such as vital statistical data from whole countries or communities. It is most frequently applied to age, often within the 18 5-year age groups from 0–4 years to 85+ years, or to sex, or to ethnic group. It is simply another form of averaging of stratified data, and can be applied to any confounder. For each group being compared, the stratum-specific rates are multiplied by the number of subjects or person-years in that stratum of a 'standard population'. This standard population may be an intuitively relevant population (such as the whole country in a particular year), or an arbitrary or even artificial population.

**Exhibit 6.19** shows the use of direct standardization to compare incidence rates for two populations, taking account of the differences in age distribution. The data show the incidence rates of cancer of the stomach in men recorded between 1993 and 1997 by cancer registries in India (Mumbai) and Sweden, showing total rates and age-specific rates [21]. The crude incidence rates are 3.6 per 100 000 person-years in India and 17.2 per 100 000 person-years in Sweden, giving an incidence ratio of 17.2/3.6 = 4.8, i.e. the crude incidence rate is nearly five times higher in Sweden than in India. To adjust for age, we will use the 'world standard population', an arbitrary population developed by the World Health Organization for this purpose which approximates the age distribution of the whole world population. For each age group the observed rate is multiplied by the world standard population number for that age group, and then the results are summed and divided by the total world standard population. The direct age-standardized incidence rates produced in this way are 6.4 per 100 000 person-years in India and 8.6 per 100 000 person-years in Sweden. The ratio of these is only 1.35, showing that the incidence rates, once adjusted for the differing aged populations, are only modestly higher in Sweden than in India. Stomach cancer, like most cancers, increases greatly in incidence with increasing age. The Indian population is younger than the world standard population, and so its crude incidence rate is low and its age-standardized incidence rate is higher than the crude rate. The Swedish population is considerably older than the world standard population, and so its crude rate is high and adjustment produces an age-standardized rate which is lower than the crude rate. Most of the difference in crude rates between the two countries is due to the older age distribution in Sweden, rather than to the

## AGE STANDARDIZATION

*Cancer of the stomach in men; data from cancer registries, 1993–1997*

| Age | India (Mumbai) | | | | | | Sweden | | | | | |
|---|---|---|---|---|---|---|---|---|---|---|---|---|
| | Cases | Person-years | Incidence per 100 000 person-years | World standard population | Rate*std population | | Cases | person-years | Incidence per 100 000 Person-years | World standard population | Rate*std population |
| 0–4 | 0 | 2 606 530 | 0.0 | 12 | 0.0 | | 0 | 1 491 716 | 0.0 | 12 | 0.0 |
| 5–9 | 0 | 2 873 805 | 0.0 | 10 | 0.0 | | 0 | 1 454 119 | 0.0 | 10 | 0.0 |
| 10–14 | 0 | 2 814 265 | 0.0 | 9 | 0.0 | | 0 | 1 290 659 | 0.0 | 9 | 0.0 |
| 15–19 | 2 | 2 830 345 | 0.1 | 9 | 0.6 | | 1 | 1 313 792 | 0.1 | 9 | 0.7 |
| 20–24 | 4 | 3 351 470 | 0.1 | 8 | 1.0 | | 1 | 1 465 616 | 0.1 | 8 | 0.5 |
| 25–29 | 13 | 3 092 025 | 0.4 | 8 | 3.4 | | 3 | 1 607 164 | 0.2 | 8 | 1.5 |
| 30–34 | 18 | 2 678 690 | 0.7 | 6 | 4.0 | | 16 | 1 591 005 | 1.0 | 6 | 6.0 |
| 35–39 | 36 | 2 388 920 | 1.5 | 6 | 9.0 | | 20 | 1 497 476 | 1.3 | 6 | 8.0 |
| 40–44 | 61 | 1 918 280 | 3.2 | 6 | 19.1 | | 46 | 1 515 350 | 3.0 | 6 | 18.2 |
| 45–49 | 89 | 1 532 425 | 5.8 | 6 | 34.8 | | 83 | 1 653 006 | 5.0 | 6 | 30.1 |
| 50–54 | 145 | 1 194 715 | 12.1 | 5 | 60.7 | | 149 | 1 488 244 | 10.0 | 5 | 50.1 |
| 55–59 | 145 | 817 305 | 17.7 | 4 | 71.0 | | 192 | 1 133 210 | 16.9 | 4 | 67.8 |

| Age | Mumbai cases | Mumbai population | Mumbai rate | Mumbai rate×wt | Sweden cases | Sweden population | Sweden rate | Std weight | Sweden rate×wt |
|---|---|---|---|---|---|---|---|---|---|
| 60–64 | 146 | 624 025 | 23.4 | 93.6 | 291 | 984 656 | 29.6 | 4 | 118.2 |
| 65–69 | 161 | 372 010 | 43.3 | 129.8 | 480 | 947 266 | 50.7 | 3 | 152.0 |
| 70–74 | 114 | 225 650 | 50.5 | 101.0 | 712 | 907 764 | 78.4 | 2 | 156.9 |
| 75+ | 129 | 240 825 | 53.6 | 107.1 | 1756 | 1 405 204 | 125.0 | 2 | 249.9 |
| Totals | 1063 | 29 561 285 | | 635.2 | 3750 | 21 746 247 | | 100 | 860.0 |

Crude incidence rate = 1063/295.61285 = 3.60     = 3750/217.46247 = 17.24

Age-standardized incidence rate = 635.2/100 = 6.35     = 860/100 = 8.60

*Incidence rate ratio (Sweden:India)*

Crude = 17.24/3.60 = 4.80

Age-standardized = 8.60/6.35 = 1.35

**Ex. 6.19.** Age standardization of incidence rates: data for two populations (Mumbai and Sweden), adjusted by direct standardization using the World Health Organization 'world standard' arbitary population. Data from *Cancer Incidence In Five Continents, Vol. VIII*. [21]

modest difference in the incidence rates of stomach cancer within age groups. Of course, other factors, such as the completeness of diagnosis and recording, also have to be considered.

Direct standardization can be applied to any stratified data where the stratum-specific rates are known. **Exhibit 6.20** shows direct age standardization applied to the study of exercise and heart disease shown earlier. The death rates are calculated within each age group and then, for both the light and the heavy exercise group, these rates are multiplied by the standard population, which here is taken as the total number of man-years of observation in each age group. The product of the actual death rate and the standard population number gives an 'expected' number of deaths in each stratum. For each exercise group, the total of these expected numbers is the number of deaths which would have occurred if the distribution by age had been the same as that of the standard population. As the same standard population has been applied to each of the exercise groups, comparison of these expected numbers removes

---

### STRATIFICATION IN A COHORT STUDY: DIRECT STANDARDIZATION

| Age group | Standard population | Exposed (light exercise) | | Unexposed (heavy exercise) | |
|---|---|---|---|---|---|
| | | Observed death rate | Expected deaths in std. pop. | Observed death rate | Expected deaths in std. pop. |
| | $S_i$ | $r_{ei}$ | $S_i r_{ei}$ | $r_{ui}$ | $S_i r_{ui}$ |
| 35–44 | 14.2 | 0.51 | 7.2 | 0.48 | 6.8 |
| 45–54 | 28.6 | 3.52 | 100.7 | 1.82 | 52.1 |
| 55–64 | 31.1 | 7.72 | 240.1 | 4.59 | 142.7 |
| 65–74 | 18.8 | 15.96 | 300.0 | 8.00 | 150.4 |
| Sum | 92.7 | | 648.1 | | 352.0 |

Age-standardized incidence rate =
(sum expected deaths) / (sum standard population) = 6.99 (exposed); 3.80 (unexposed)
Age standardized relative risk = 6.99/3.80 = 1.84

**Ex. 6.20.** Stratification in a cohort study: direct standardization. The stratified data are the same as in Ex. 6.16. Here a standard population is chosen as the total man-years at risk in each age group, and to this is applied the age-specific death rates in each of the exposure groups, to give the numbers of deaths expected in each exposure group if each had had the same age distribution. The ratio of these expected numbers is the standardized relative risk

the confounding effect of age (unless there is so much variation within the age strata used that there is still some confounding, in which case narrower age strata should be used). The ratio of these expected numbers gives the age-standardized relative risk, which here is 1.84. This is not numerically the same as the Mantel–Haenszel relative risk, which as shown in Ex. 6.16 was 1.78, because a different weighting system has been used. In the example given, the Mantel–Haenszel estimate is probably preferable, as its weighting system takes into account the different amount of information in each stratum, whereas the age-standardization system does not necessarily do this. In large data sets, such as routine vital statistics, there is so much data available that this is not really a problem, and that is where direct standardization is most frequently used.

## Indirect standardization

Another method of standardization is indirect standardization, which gives results often referred to as a standardized mortality ratio (SMR) or standardized incidence ratio (SIR). This method is frequently used to compare one smaller group with a larger group that includes it, for example to compare rates in one occupational group with those of the whole country. **Exhibit 6.21** shows an example where 12 deaths from lung cancer occurred in an occupational group (male cooks) over 4 years in New Zealand. To assess this, we calculate the 'expected' number of lung cancers, i.e. the number that would arise if the death rates for the standard population (here, all employed men) applied to the cooks. For each age group, we multiply the age-specific rate in the standard population by the numbers of person-years in each age group for the cooks (basically the number of cooks, obtained from census data, multiplied by 4 years) to give an expected number of deaths in that age group. We then add the expected numbers, here giving 7.1 'expected' deaths. The ratio of the observed number of deaths to this expected number of deaths shows how the actual mortality experience varies from that expected, adjusted for age. This is often expressed as a percentage, so that a value above 100 shows a higher mortality rate in the study population than in the standard population. In our example, the (age) standardized mortality rate (SMR) is 1.69, or 169 per cent. For this calculation, the only required data for the cooks is the number of cooks (or person-years) in each age group and the total number of deaths. It is not necessary to know the number of deaths within each age group, which is needed for direct standardization or a Mantel–Haenszel analysis. However, this indirect standardization method is not so useful, as although it produces a comparison of each specific population with the reference standard population, it is not so simple to compare

---

### CALCULATION OF A STANDARDIZED MORTALITY RATIO

Total observed number of events (deaths from lung cancer) = 12

Expected number of deaths if stratum-specific rates were same as the standard population is calculated as follows:

| Strata of confounder (age group) | Number of person-years $P_i$ | Mortality rate in standard population per 100 000 $R_i$ | Expected number of deaths = $R_i \times P_i$ |
|---|---|---|---|
| 25–34 | 7557 | 0.8 | 0.06 |
| 35–44 | 4023 | 4.8 | 0.19 |
| 45–54 | 2961 | 47.9 | 1.42 |
| 55–64 | 2043 | 265.8 | 5.43 |

Total expected number = sum of expected numbers = 7.10

Standardized mortality ratio = observed / expected = 1.69

---

**Ex. 6.21.** Calculation of a standardized mortality ratio: the data needed are the total number of events in the 'special' population. Here the special population is male 'cooks and related workers' aged 25–64 in New Zealand, 1983–1986. The expected number is calculated by applying the age-specific rates for a 'standard' population, here all employed males in New Zealand, 1983–1986, to the age-specific population at risk for the special occupational group

the SMR of one specific group with that of another group. To make a comparison between two specific groups, it is better to use direct standardization or the Mantel–Haenszel method.

## Stratification in case–control studies

To apply stratified analysis in a case–control study, we follow the same principle: we divide the data into strata defined by levels of the confounding factor, and calculate the measure of association, usually the odds ratio, for each stratum. As the same issues of small numbers and consequent instability of estimates apply in case–control studies as in cohort studies, we need a method of producing a summary measure of association. The most widely used method is the Mantel–Haenszel estimate of odds ratio, described in a now classic paper [20]. This is a weighted average of the stratum-specific odds ratios, with the weights being dependent on the numbers of observations in each stratum, as shown in **Ex. 6.22.**

---

### MANTEL–HAENSZEL ESTIMATION OF ODDS RATIO

In each subtable $i$, stratified by the potential confounder:

|  | Cases | Controls |
|---|---|---|
| exposed | $a_i$ | $b_i$ |
| unexposed | $c_i$ | $d_i$ |

$T_i$ = total in the subtable

Odds ratio for this subtable $= a_i d_i / b_i c_i$
The Mantel–Haenszel estimate of odds ratio uses the data from all subtables, but gives an estimate of the unconfounded odds ratio:

$$\text{given by } \sum_i (a_i d_i / T_i) \Big/ \sum_i (b_i c_i / T_i)$$

where $\sum_i$ indicates summation over all the subtables

---

**Ex. 6.22.** Stratification: calculation of the Mantel–Haenszel estimate of the summary odds ratio in a stratified analysis

**Exhibit 6.23** shows some simplified, but real, data from a case–control study comparing patients with malignant melanoma (a skin cancer) with community-based controls [22]. Table A shows a positive association of melanoma with a history of severe sunburn, giving an odds ratio of 1.40. This association could be due to the trauma of the sunburn, the sun exposure involved, or the individual's susceptibility to sunburn. In the subtables, we control for susceptibility to sunburn. Both in subjects who burn easily and in those who do not, the odds ratio for the association between sunburn history and melanoma is lower than that in the crude analysis; the Mantel–Haenszel estimate gives 1.19 as the unconfounded odds ratio. Thus the crude odds ratio of 1.40 is produced partially by confounding by tendency to sunburn, which is also related to melanoma. Statistical tests on these data will be shown in Chapter 7 (Ex. 7.8).

## Effect modification

In the example in Ex. 6.23, the odds ratios in individual strata are so similar that there is no obvious utility in the summary estimate. However, with many subtables with small numbers of observations in each, the stratum-specific odds ratios will be unstable, but the summary estimate provides a stable measure of the overall odds ratio which is not affected by confounding by the factor which has been stratified. Of course, if the odds ratios in the different

---

### STRATIFICATION IN A CASE–CONTROL STUDY

| | Cases | Controls |
|---|---|---|
| *Table A: all subjects (n = 924)* | | |
| Exposed: severe sunburn | 136 | 98 |
| Unexposed: mild sunburn | 343 | 347 |
| Total | 479 | 445 |

Odds ratio = (136 × 347)/(98 × 343) = 1.40

| | Cases | Controls |
|---|---|---|
| *Subtable $B_1$: subjects who sunburn easily (n = 595)* | | |
| Severe sunburn | 119 | 76 |
| Mild sunburn | 227 | 173 |
| Total | 346 | 249 |

Odds ratio = (119 × 173)/(76 × 227) = 1.19

| | Cases | Controls |
|---|---|---|
| *Subtable $B_2$: subjects who do not sunburn easily (n = 329)* | | |
| Severe sunburn | 17 | 22 |
| Mild sunburn | 116 | 174 |
| Total | 133 | 196 |

Odds ratio = (17 × 174)/(22 × 116) = 1.16

Mantel-Haenszel estimate of odds ratio

$$= \frac{119 \times 173/595 + 17 \times 174/329}{76 \times 227/595 + 22 \times 116/329}$$
$$= 1.19$$

---

**Ex. 6.23.** Stratified analysis of a case–control study comparing patients with malignant melanoma with community controls with regard to history of sunburn, and adjusting for tendency to sunburn. Simplified from Elwood *et al.* [22]

strata are very different from each other, it may be misleading to use a summary estimate.

In a case–control study relating smoking to carcinoma of the uterine cervix, the overall data show an odds ratio of 6.6 (**Ex. 6.24**). When the data are subdivided by age, the odds ratios show great variation, from 27.9 at age 20–29, to 5.9 at age 30–39, and 2.8 at ages over 40 [23]. This large variation in the association between cervical cancer and smoking demonstrates *effect modification* (also called *interaction*). Effect modification can occur without confounding. To assess confounding by age, we can use a Mantel–Haenszel estimate, calculated

EFFECT MODIFICATION

*Table A: all ages*

| | | Cases | Controls | Odds ratio |
|---|---|---|---|---|
| All ages: | smokers | 130 | 45 | |
| | non-smokers | 87 | 198 | 6.6 |

*Subtable B: data stratified by age*

| | | | | |
|---|---|---|---|---|
| Age 20–29 | smokers | 41 | 6 | |
| | non-smokers | 13 | 53 | 27.9 |
| Age 30–39 | smokers | 66 | 25 | |
| | non-smokers | 37 | 83 | 5.9 |
| Age 40+ | smokers | 23 | 14 | |
| | non-smokers | 37 | 62 | 2.8 |

Mantel–Haenszel odds ratio, adjusted for age = 6.3

**Ex. 6.24.** Effect modification: in this case–control study relating smoking to cancer of the cervix in women, the crude odds ratio (table A) is 6.6, and the Mantel-Haenszel odds ratio, adjusted for age, is 6.3; there is little confounding by age. However, age modifies the effect; the odds ratios for smoking in the different age groups are very different. Data from Lyon *et al.* [23]

by the method already shown in Ex. 6.22, which gives an odds ratio after age adjustment of 6.3. This is close to the crude odds ratio of 6.6, and shows that there is very little confounding by age in these data.

This example illustrates the difference between confounding and effect modification. If a factor is acting solely as a confounding factor, it will bias the overall association between exposure and outcome in the data set, and this can be accomplished without any variation in the measure of association between different strata. The examples given so far demonstrate this. In Ex. 6.23, the odds ratio between melanoma and sunburn history was confounded by tendency to sunburn, but there was no substantial effect modification, i.e. the association was virtually the same amongst subjects who sunburnt easily and those who did not. In the study of exercise levels and heart disease in Ex. 6.20, there was also substantial confounding by age, but little evidence of any effect modification, i.e. the relative risks comparing light and heavy exercise workers were similar in the different age groups. In contrast, in the current example in Ex. 6.24, there is relatively little confounding, but there is very clear effect modification. A similar result was seen in the randomized trial analysis in Ex. 6.18 where the relative risk between tolbutamide treatment and mortality was

1.44 in the crude form, and 1.32 after adjustment for arterial calcification, showing only a small degree of confounding. However, the relative risk for subjects with arterial calcification ($RR = 1.93$) was substantially higher than for the subjects without such calcification ($RR = 1.09$), showing effect modification. We shall explore the example of cervical cancer and smoking further in Chapter 7, Ex. 7.9.

**Exhibit 6.25** shows results from a cohort analysis of the case fatality rate from SARS (severe acute respiratory syndrome) in Hong Kong [24]. The overall

---

### CONFOUNDING AND EFFECT MODIFICATION

Fatality rate in SARS (severe acute respiratory syndrome), comparing males with females, in Hong Kong

*Table A: all ages*

|  |  | cases | deaths | survivors | fatality rate (%) | male: female relative risk |
|---|---|---|---|---|---|---|
|  | Males | 776 | 170 | 606 | 21.9 | 1.66 |
|  | Females | 979 | 129 | 850 | 13.2 |  |
|  | Total | 1755 | 299 | 1456 | 17.0 |  |

*Subtable B: data stratified by age*

|  |  | cases | deaths | survivors | fatality rate (%) | male: female relative risk |
|---|---|---|---|---|---|---|
| age 0–44 | Males | 425 | 27 | 398 | 6.4 | 2.27 |
|  | Females | 607 | 17 | 590 | 2.8 |  |
| age 45–74 | Males | 249 | 77 | 172 | 30.9 | 1.45 |
|  | Females | 295 | 63 | 232 | 21.4 |  |
| age ≥ 75 | Males | 102 | 66 | 36 | 64.7 | 1.02 |
|  | Females | 77 | 49 | 28 | 63.6 |  |

Mantel–Haenszel relative risk, adjusted for age = 1.35

---

**Ex. 6.25.** Combined confounding and effect modification: comparison of male and female case fatality rates from SARS in Hong Kong. The death rates are higher in males, particularly at younger ages (effect modification by age), and the overall crude relative risk of 1.66 is partially due to confounding by age, shown by the adjusted relative risk being only 1.35. From Karlberg *et al.* [24]

fatality rate was considerably greater in men than in women, with a relative risk of 1.66. Stratification by age demonstrates both confounding and effect modification. As shown in Ex. 6.25, some of the difference in mortality rates is due to the older age distribution of the men, allied to the increasing death rate with increasing age. This is shown by the Mantel–Haenszel relative risk, adjusted for age, being 1.35, i.e. lower than the crude relative risk. Examination of the results within age groups shows that there is also effect modification, with the higher death rate in men being more pronounced in the younger age groups, and there being no substantial difference between the death rates in men and women at ages 75 years and over.

Thus in an exposure–outcome relationship, a third factor may act as a confounding factor or an effect modifier, may have both effects, or may have neither effect.

## Matching

Another method of avoiding confounding is to choose the comparison sub-jects for a study so that they are similar to the case or exposed subjects with regard to specified confounding factors, and then analyse the study appropri-ately. For example, in a cohort study assessing the risk of myocardial infarction in women who use oral contraceptives, factors such as age and cigarette smoking might be important confounders. If, for each woman using oral contraceptives entering the study, we select a comparison woman who is not using oral contraceptives but is the same age and has the same smoking history, we will create two groups of subjects who are similar in terms of these two factors. Therefore within our study there will be no association between age or smok-ing status and oral contraceptive exposure, and thus these two factors will not be confounding. This process is referred to as matching.

Matching is a much more complex technique than it appears, and the applications and value of the method are very commonly misunderstood. This misunderstanding often arises from a lack of appreciation of the other meth-ods of controlling confounding, particularly stratification, so that the specific advantages and disadvantages of matching are not recognized. More subtly, difficulties arise because matching has three different purposes: it can be used to increase the *efficiency* of the study, to *control confounding*, or to improve the *comparability* of the information collected.

### Frequency matching to increase efficiency

With regard to *efficiency*, i.e. the amount of information that is gained in relation to the size of the study, the value of matching is quite simple. In the example here, it is likely that most women using oral contraceptives will be between 16 and 45 years old. There is no value in enrolling as comparison subjects women who are 60 years old or, even more obviously, enrolling men in the study. Ideally the ratio of comparison subjects to exposed subjects in each age range should be reasonably constant. An age group in which there are many oral contraceptive users and very few non-users, or vice versa, will give unreliable information because of the small numbers in one category (in the extreme, a group with no exposed or no controls gives no information). The same process can be used for other factors such as smoking history. Thus to increase efficiency, matching can ensure that the groups of subjects being compared are similar in terms of the most important potential confounding factors in the study. This can be achieved by 'frequency matching'; the study is designed so that the distribution of the groups of subjects being compared is similar in terms of major confounding factors. This is an easily applied, useful, and widely used technique, particularly for such characteristics as age and sex. Frequency matching should be considered only as a method of ensuring reasonable efficiency, and should not be regarded as a method of controlling confounding, because it involves only approximate matching and does not ensure total comparability. The confounding factors, both those on which frequency matching has been done and others, need to be controlled by methods such as stratification or multivariate analysis. The analysis is done in the same way as in unmatched studies. Indeed, the advantage of frequency matching is to increase the efficiency of stratification and multivariate methods to control confounding.

## Individual matching to control confounding

The second form of matching, 'individual matching', is a precise technique. Rather than simply ensuring broad comparability between the groups being compared, comparison subjects are chosen to match particular index subjects with regard to one or more specified confounding factors. The purpose is not only to improve efficiency, but also to control for the confounding effects of these factors.

There is an important distinction between the use of this technique in cohort or intervention studies and in case–control studies. In cohort and intervention studies, precise matching by important confounding factors will control for the effects of those factors. An analysis done in the same way as in an unmatched cohort study will give estimates of relative and attributable risks which can normally be regarded as free from the confounding effects of the variables on which matching has been done. A caution applies, as during the time course of the study subjects may withdraw or be lost to follow-up, and so the initial matched situation will be compromised. This can be dealt with by stratifying or using multivariate methods to deal with any confounding, or in some studies it may be necessary to censor the whole matched set of subjects at the same time, that is, to terminate their follow-up (see Chapter 7).

In a case–control study, controls are selected by matching them to the cases on specified factors. This will give an efficient study, but to control confounding it is necessary to analyse the study by special methods that keep the data in matched form, i.e. consider each matched group of cases and controls as a unit. As long as this is done correctly, the combination of matching and using a matched analysis should control confounding by the matching factors. The analysis is basically a stratified analysis in which each matched case–control set forms one stratum, or the equivalent multivariate analysis. This is necessary because matching can in fact introduce confounding by the matching factors, and this confounding needs to be controlled. If a matched case–control study is not analysed correctly, the result may be invalid.

The simplest form of analysis is given by a fixed one-to-one matching ratio, where one matched control is chosen for each case, as shown in **Ex. 6.26** [25].

---

### ONE-TO-ONE MATCHING IN A CASE–CONTROL STUDY

*A. Distribution of 120 case-control pairs by smoking history*

|  |  | Controls | |
|---|---|---|---|
|  |  | Smokers | Non-smokers |
| Cases | smokers | 31 | 30 |
|  | non-smokers | 7 | 52 |

Matched odds ratio = 30/7 = 4.3

*B. An incorrect unmatched analysis of the same 240 individuals*

|  | Cases | Controls |
|---|---|---|
| smokers | 61 | 38 |
| non-smokers | 59 | 82 |
|  | 120 | 120 |

Unmatched odds ratio = $(61 \times 82)/(59 \times 38) = 2.2$

---

**Ex. 6.26.** One-to-one matching in a case–control study: this yields a simple analysis. Here 120 male patients with nasal or nasal sinus cancer (a very rare cancer), seen in one clinic over a 38-year period, were matched to male controls with a range of other non-smoking related cancers by age and year of diagnosis. Table A shows a matched analysis; the odds ratio is based only on the pairs with different exposures. Table B shows the unmatched analysis of the same data; this analysis is incorrect as it loses the value of the matched pair comparison, and produces a substantially different odds ratio. From Elwood [25]

Note the format of the table: it shows the *numbers of pairs* classified by exposure and by outcome. The odds ratio is simply the ratio of the number of discordant pairs where only the case is exposed to the number of discordant pairs
where only the control is exposed. On the null hypothesis, these numbers will
be equal. The (incorrect) unmatched table in the familiar 2 × 2 format uses
exactly the same data, but the value of the matching is lost. If the matching
factors, as in this example, have a strong confounding effect, the odds ratio
based on an unmatched analysis is confounded and is substantially different
from the matched unconfounded odds ratio. It will be biased towards the
null, as shown here. Where another fixed ratio of controls to cases (such as
3:1) is used, the analysis is also relatively simple, but where the matching ratio
is variable it becomes complex. Analyses of a fixed-ratio matched study are
shown in Appendix Tables 5 and 6. Matched analyses also become complex if
it is necessary to adjust for further confounding factors after the matched
design is set up. Normal stratification procedures are difficult to use, as the
matched groups must be kept intact. However, 'conditional' multivariate
statistical techniques will allow a matched design to be handled in an analysis
that controls other confounding factors; this will be discussed later in
this chapter.

## Matching to increase comparability of data

A further use of matching is to ensure comparability in terms of the information collected. In a case–control study where some case subjects are
interviewed in a hospital and others in their own homes, it is logical to
ensure that the comparison subjects are matched for method of interview,
and ideally the interviews are conducted on a single-blind basis. This was
done in a case–control study of venous embolism and hormone replacement therapy, where most interviews took place in hospital, but 23 per cent
were done after discharge [26]. Similar considerations arise if several investigators or centres are involved. However, stratification or other methods
may also be used.

## Advantages of matching

What then are the advantages of matching? There are three main situations in
which matching may be useful, but these advantages always have to be compared to the disadvantages of matching when designing a study.

First, matching is useful where there is a complex confounding factor.
Matching has particular value where there is an important confounding
variable that cannot be easily measured or easily defined. Examples include

complex social factors, medical care factors, environmental exposures, or circumstances in childhood; these might be controlled by matching with neighbours, other patients, coworkers, or siblings, respectively. For example, to assess associations with emotional and behavioural problems, girls with anorexia nervosa were compared with their unaffected siblings, giving control for a range of family and childhood factors [27]. Similarly, to assess the relationship of smoking with Parkinson's disease, using sibling controls may control for other environmental exposures [28].

Studies comparing individuals who are twins with their co-twins, where they differ on the exposure or outcome of interest, can be a very powerful design. Thus an international case–control study comparing women with breast cancer at ages under 50 with their unaffected twin sisters showed associations with childhood weight, height, and time of breast development [29], and in a prospective cohort study twins with moderate alcohol consumption (compared with those with lower consumption) showed a reduced incidence of type 2 diabetes than their same-sex co-twins, despite the similarity in genetic and early life factors [30]. Comparison between monozygotic (identical) and dizygotic (non-identical) twins is a fundamental technique in assessing the contribution of genetic and environmental factors. Using a twin registry in Sweden, smokers were compared with their non-smoking co-twins; from 9319 pairs of twins, 1924 pairs who differed in their smoking habits were found; the prevalence of cough and bronchitis was higher in the smoking twins, and the prevalence ratio was similar for non-identical and for identical twin pairs, showing that the association with smoking could not be explained by a genetic confounding factor [31].

Secondly, matching is useful where the study has a fixed and limited number of cases, and therefore maximizing efficiency is critical. This may arise from either a particularly rare exposure or a particularly rare outcome. For example, in the 1960s some eight cases of vaginal adenocarcinoma were diagnosed in young women in Boston, Massachusetts. Vaginal cancer was previously virtually unknown in young women, and this particular disease was of an unusual histological type. To study the possible causes, the most efficient design is one in which causal factors are assessed using comparison subjects who are closely matched for the main confounders. To study the aetiology of this condition, for each patient with vaginal adenocarcinoma, four comparison subjects were chosen who were matched on sex, date of birth (within 5 days), hospital of birth, and ward or private type of service [32]. The same consideration of maximizing efficiency also applies if collecting data from the study subjects is expensive, so that the number of subjects needs to be kept a small as possible. For example, if there is a set of subjects with stored blood or tissue samples, careful matching can be done so that fewer samples need to be used for expensive chemical or genetic tests. Thus to assess the relationships of breast cancer with plasma levels of carotenoids and other indicators, stored blood samples collected up to 10 years before diagnosis from over 70 000 subjects in three cohort studies in Sweden were used. For each of 624 breast cancer cases, two controls matched for age, date of blood sample, and sampling centre were selected, and so biochemical analyses were done only on these samples [33].

## Disadvantages of matching

Matching is a technique that involves both practical and conceptual difficulties. It has several disadvantages compared with other methods of controlling confounding. In a conventional study with new subject recruitment, to obtain each appropriate matched comparison subject, several potential comparison subjects may have to be approached and initial information gathered, making the study more expensive and difficult to set up. If the subjects can be selected from an existing data bank with information already available on the matching factors, this is not a problem, and matching is more often used in those circumstances. The matched design is prone to loss of data; if one member of a matched pair does not participate in or complete the study, the whole matched group usually has to be excluded. A further disadvantage has been referred to, that the analysis becomes complex if other factors have to be considered or if the matching ratio is variable.

The most important disadvantage of matching is that the matching factor cannot itself be assessed in the analysis in terms of its relationship to the outcome. Therefore matching should be used only for factors that are known to be important risk factors and thus important confounders, and should not be used if it is necessary to assess the relationship between the matched factor and the outcome in the study. Therefore matching is inappropriate for an exploratory study to answer a general question as to what are the causes of the outcome in question.

The further disadvantages of matching are in its inappropriate use resulting in overmatching, which will now be discussed.

## Unnecessary matching: 'overmatching'

If the study involves matching on a factor which is not a true confounder, this is often referred to as 'overmatching', although 'unnecessary matching' is a clearer description. It may occur in two situations. Suppose in a case–control study the subjects are matched on a factor which is associated with the exposure, but which is not itself associated with the outcome; therefore it is not a confounding factor, and it is unnecessary to control its effects. Because the matching factor is associated with exposure, the controls are chosen in a way that will make them more similar to the cases in terms of exposure. The differences in exposure between potential case and control subjects in the source population will be reduced in the study subjects, and an (incorrect) unmatched analysis will lead to an underestimate of the true outcome–exposure association. If a correct analysis is done, stratifying for the matching variable, using multivariate methods, or using an analysis on matched sets, the result of the unnecessary matching will be to increase the proportion of all case–control sets that are concordant for exposure. As these sets do not contribute to the estimate of odds ratio, the study results will not be biased, but the study will be less efficient as fewer sets of observations are contributing to the results. In the extreme, if the matching factor is very closely associated with the exposure, the study will have no ability to assess the exposure. In a cohort study, unnecessary matching also leads to inefficiency, but the study results will still be valid as specific analytic methods are not needed.

As an example, consider a case–control study assessing the relationship between passive exposure to tobacco smoke and lung cancer. Should lung cancer subjects and controls be matched on their personal smoking experience? As this is a major risk factor and is associated with passive smoking, it needs to be controlled, and matching with a correct analysis would give a powerful study. Should subjects be matched for the size of their family, or for the number of fellow workers they have? These factors are not themselves risk factors for lung cancer, but may be associated with passive smoking; matching would be detrimental. If we wish to guard against the possibility of family size being a risk factor, perhaps by being an indicator of other exposures, it would be better to deal with it by stratification or multivariate analysis. Then we have freedom to assess if it is a risk factor, or a confounding factor; if we match on family size, we do not have flexibility. The error here is in matching for a factor which is associated with the exposure, but is not an independent risk factor for the outcome and so is not a confounder. However, matching for this factor can make it a confounding factor, which then has to be controlled in the analysis.

Unnecessary matching will also occur if the matching factor is not a confounding factor because it is part of a causal pathway linking exposure and outcome. In this situation, different methods of analysis may not help, as the study is fundamentally flawed. Consider a case–control study to assess the causes of bladder cancer in a workforce where records of both a chemical exposure and previous bladder cytology are available for the employees; if the association between the chemical exposure and bladder cancer is to be assessed, should subjects be matched on prior cytology findings? If they are, and the true causal chain is

chemical exposure → abnormal cytology → bladder cancer,

a matched study will probably show no difference in chemical exposure. To conclude from such results that chemical exposure is not linked to bladder cancer is wrong. In such situations, the study design is not so much wrong, as misapplied. The design used in fact tests a different hypothesis: is chemical exposure related to bladder cancer irrespective of prior cytology findings? This may be a question worth asking, although probably only in specific subgroups; for example, if chemical exposure increases the risk of bladder cancer in subjects with previous abnormal cytology, it may indicate a tumour-promotion effect, increasing the risk of progression from abnormal cytology to invasive cancer. In these situations the interpretation cannot be made solely on the data; it requires assumptions regarding the causal model and is dependent on whether the third factor is a confounding factor or not. If subjects are chosen without matching, and information on the third factor is collected, analyses can be done with and without control for that factor, and its associations with exposure and outcome can be assessed. If matching has been used, this flexibility is lost. The risks of unnecessary matching again show that matching should be used only after careful consideration, including knowledge about the confounding factors relevant to a given situation.

Another situation of overmatching is where matching is done on a factor which is itself affected by either the exposure or outcome in the study. This includes symptoms and signs produced either by the exposure or the outcome, including early indications of disease. Again, the issue is that these factors are not true confounders. For example, in a cohort study of smokers, if smokers and non-smokers are matched in terms of a history of cough, the effect of smoking on the subsequent incidence of lung cancer would be underestimated. This situation particularly applies to studies of the effects of drugs, where the dominant confounder is the underlying disease for which the drugs are prescribed. This is referred to as *confounding by indication*. A strong association between a drug and a disease may arise if the drugs are prescribed for clinical signs or symptoms which are associated with the early stages of the disease, so-called *protopathic bias*. For example, in the assessment of the association between aspirin use and Reye's syndrome (an encephalitis-like illness mainly affecting children, usually after a viral illness), such an association could arise because aspirin was prescribed to children who had symptoms which were early manifestations of Reye's syndrome. This is reverse causation: the putative outcome (disease) causes the exposure. A further case–control study concluded that the association was not explicable by such a mechanism, and strengthened the case for aspirin use being causal [34].

In summary, there are two major types of matching. Frequency matching is used to produce approximately similar distributions of key confounding factors in the groups being compared. It should be considered simply as a method of improving study efficiency, and the matching factors and other confounders should be dealt with in the analysis by the usual stratification and multivariate methods. Specific individual matching is of particular value for complex confounders which cannot otherwise be dealt with, and situations where maximum efficiency is a priority. Such matching should only be carried out for factors which are true confounders. There should be good evidence that the matching factor is a strong risk factor for the outcome, with in addition an association with the exposure. Overmatching is produced if matching is carried out on a factor which is not a true confounder. Matching for a factor associated only with exposure will decrease efficiency and, if not appropriately analysed, will damage validity. It is important to avoid matching on a factor which is a component in the causal chain linking exposure and outcome, or on a factor which is affected by the exposure or the outcome, such as symptoms or signs.

## Multivariate methods

The final method of controlling confounding is to analyse the data using a mathematical model that has the outcome as the dependent variable, and includes both the postulated causal factor and confounding factors in the equation. Multivariate analysis is a major subject in itself, and the purpose of this section is to present the key principles which are important in interpreting the results of these analyses.

### Linear regression

While linear regression is not widely used in these studies, it is the simplest model from which the others are derived. For continuous variables, linear multiple regression is often appropriate, and is a standard technique included in most statistical texts and computer programs. For example, consider the assessment of whether maternal pre-pregnancy weight is related to the birth-weight of the baby, taking account of any relationship with the mother's height. A linear multiple regression model could be used, where the dependent variable is birthweight, and the model includes maternal pre-pregnancy weight as one independent (or 'predictor') variable and height as another. Standard multiple regression methods produce a coefficient for the maternal weight variable which shows the relationship between it and birthweight, independent of height.

The mathematical expression is:

$$y = a + b_1 x_1 + b_2 x_2$$

where $y$ is the outcome, birthweight, and is the dependent variable in the equation, $x_1$ is the mother's pre-pregnancy weight, $x_2$ is the mother's height, $a$ is a constant with no intuitive meaning (it is the birthweight if $x_1$ and $x_2$ are both zero), and $b_1$ and $b_2$ are the regression coefficients. These coefficients are calculated to be the values that give the best fit of the equation set out above to the observed data. (Terminology varies: $y$ can also be called the outcome variable or regressand the $x$ variables can be called predictor variables, covariates, or regressors).

This simple mathematical equation makes several assumptions. For example, it assumes that the change in birthweight with the change in the mother's pre-pregnancy weight is linear, and therefore the numerical value $b_1$ represents the amount of change in birthweight associated with a change in the mother's pre-pregnancy weight of one unit. A similar linear assumption holds for $b_2$. The equation also assumes that the change in birthweight with pre-pregnancy weight is the same irrespective of the value of the mothers' height, i.e. there is no *interaction* between these two variables. These are assumptions inherent in the mathematical form of the equation. If the variable $y$ represents 'risk', the coefficient $b_1$ with this linear model show the *difference* in risk associated with $x_1$, and independence of the effects of several variables means independence on a linear scale, i.e. the risk differences associated with each variable are additive. There are usually other assumptions involved in the ways in which the coefficients are calculated; for example, the usual method of calculation will make the assumption that the variable $y$ has a normal distribution.

## Log-linear models: Poisson regression

In many health situations the main variables are not continuous, or even if they are continuous, such as an incidence rate, they have limits; a rate cannot be negative. Outcomes are often dichotomous (binary): diseased or not diseased, cured or not cured. Exposures may be continuous, dichotomous, or have several categories (e.g. age, sex, stage of disease), and so standard linear regression will not be appropriate. Many other models have been developed and applied to these situations.

One model is to take the natural logarithm of the outcome variable, shown by ln $y$, and use the same equation as for linear regression but with ln $y$:

$$\ln y = a + b_1 x_1 + b_2 x_2$$

This transformation means that $y$ cannot be negative, as negative numbers do not have logarithms (ln $0 = 1$). This is a log-linear model; the right-hand side is linear, and the dependent variable has a logarithmic transformation. It is equivalent to an exponential model:

$$y = \exp(a + b_1 x_1 + b_2 x_2)$$

This model is widely used in the analysis of epidemiological cohort studies. The distribution of the dependent variable $y$ determines the best method of fitting the model to the data. In epidemiological cohort studies, where the frequency of positive outcomes is low, a model using a Poisson distribution is often suitable; this method is called *Poisson regression*. The interpretation of the results of any log-linear model is the same.

As these models use a logarithmic, or exponential, model, the interpretation of the coefficients is different from a linear model. Consider a simple model with only one independent variable $x_1$ on the right-hand side. The coefficient $b_1$, for variable $x_1$, estimates the change in ln $y$ for a change of one unit in $x_1$. If $x_1 = 1$ means that the subject is exposed, and $x_1 = 0$ means that they are unexposed, the change in outcome associated with $x_1$ is given by the following. Let $y_e$ be the risk in the exposed group and $y_u$ be the risk in the unexposed group. If $x_1 = 0$ (unexposed), ln $y_u = a$ (as $x_1 = 0$, $b_1 x_1 = 0$). If $x_1 = 1$ (exposed), ln $y_e = a + b_1$. Therefore the difference in the equations is $b_1$, which must equal ln $y_e - $ ln $y_u$, and this equals $\ln(y_e/y_u)$. Hence

$$b_1 = \ln(y_e/y_u)$$

and

$$\exp(b_1) = (y_e/y_u) = \text{risk in exposed/risk in unexposed}$$

Therefore in a log-linear model with a binary exposure variable, the exponential of a coefficient equals the *risk ratio (relative risk)* associated with that exposure. For a continuous exposure variable, the exponential of a coefficient represents the risk ratio associated with a one unit change in the exposure factor. This contrasts with the linear model described earlier, where the coefficient showed the risk difference associated with the factor. It follows that where we have two or more independent variables in a log-linear model, the definition of independent effects is that the risk ratio for each factor is constant, and so the joint effect of two 'independent' factors is additivity with regard to the log of disease risk, which is *multiplicity* in the effect on the absolute disease risk.

## Logistic regression

A further slightly different model is the most appropriate for case–control studies, although it can be used in any study design. It uses a further transformation of *y*. In the *logistic model* the logarithm of the odds, called the *logit* of disease risk, is used as the dependent variable in a linear regression equation. If *P* is the proportion of subjects in the study who have the outcome, or equivalently the probability that a randomly selected subject has the outcome, the logit of *P* is defined as $\ln[P/(1-P)]$ where ln means the natural logarithm (to base *e*).

The logistic regression equation has the form

$$\ln [P/(1-P)] = a + b_1x_1 + b_2x_2 + b_3x_3 + \ldots$$

where as before the *x* variables represent exposure factors and confounders, and the *b* terms are their coefficients. If an *x* variable is a numerical value (e.g. height), the *b* coefficient gives the change in logit *P* associated with a change of one unit of *x*, with the assumption of a linear relationship between the two. If *x* is binary, with the values of 0 or 1, the equation yields the odds ratio associated with *x*. For example, for sex we might define a variable so that $x_1 = 1$ for males and $x_1 = 0$ for females. For females, $x_1 = 0$, and so $b_1x_1$ is zero. For males, $x_1 = 1$, and so the equation for males differs from that for females by having the extra term $b_1x_1$, which is equal to $b_1$. The rest of the equation is the same. Therefore the difference in the logit *P* between males and females will be $b_1$:

$$\ln\left(\frac{P_m}{1-P_m}\right) - \ln\left(\frac{P_f}{1-P_f}\right) = b_1$$

where $P_m$ is the risk for males and $P_f$ is the risk for females. For two numbers *r* and *s*,

$$\ln r - \ln s = \ln (r/s)$$

Therefore

$$\ln\left[\frac{P_m/(1-P_m)}{P_f/(1-P_f)}\right] = b_1$$

where $P_m/(1 - P_m)$ is the odds of the outcome in males and $P_f/(1 - P_f)$ is the odds in females. Therefore the quantity in the brackets is the *odds ratio* comparing male and female subjects:

$$\ln(OR) = b_1$$

and

$$OR = \exp(b_1)$$

Thus with the logistic regression model, the exponential of a coefficient $b$ equals the odds ratio associated with the variable $x$, if this is a binary variable coded as 0 or 1. If $x$ is continuous, $b$ gives the odds ratio associated with a change in $x$ of one unit.

A simple example of this is given by the comparison between tolbutamide and placebo, using the data shown in Ex. 6.18. These data could be analysed by any log-linear model. We will apply a logistic model, as was done in the original analysis:

$$\ln [P/(1 - P)] = a + b_1 x_1$$

where $P$ is the probability of death, and $x_1$ is 1 for tolbutamide and zero for placebo. For the placebo group

$$P_p = 21/205 = 0.1024$$

(from Ex. 6.18, Subtable A). Therefore

$$\text{logit } P_p = \ln (0.1024/0.8976) = -2.171 = a.$$

For the tolbutamide group

$$P_t = 30/204 = 0.1471.$$

Therefore

$$\text{logit } P_1 = \ln(0.1471/0.8529) = -1.758 = a + b_1.$$

Thus

$$b_1 = -1.758 - (-2.171) = 0.413$$

and

$$\exp(b_1) = \exp(0.413) = 1.511.$$

Therefore the odds ratio is 1.511. We can also calculate the odds ratio from Ex. 6.18, Subtable A, by the usual method, with the same result: odds ratio = $(30 \times 184)/(21 \times 174) = 1.511$.

To account for other factors, the model becomes

$$\ln[P/(1-P)] = a + b_1 x_1 + b_2 x_2 + b_3 x_3 \ldots$$

where the other $x$ variables represent other factors. The value of multivariate analysis is that many other factors can be included in the equation. In the analysis of this study, a logistic model was used with 15 other factors (the nine factors shown in Ex. 6.12, plus sex, race, systolic blood pressure, diastolic blood pressure, visual acuity, and creatinine level). With all these other factors included, the value of $b_1$ in the presence of these other factors was 0.40, giving an odds ratio of 1.49 for tolbutamide. Thus although there were some considerable differences between the tolbutamide and placebo groups, as shown in Ex. 6.12, these did not in aggregate produce any great difference in the main result; the odds ratio for tolbutamide versus placebo only changed from 1.51 to 1.49. The results can also be expressed as the difference in mortality rates, as was done in the original paper [10].

## Use of dummy variables

Frequently, factors with several categories are relevant, and these are often best handled by using a number of 'dummy' binary variables to represent all the categories. **Exhibit 6.27** gives some results using this method. The data are from a case–control study comparing 83 patients with malignant melanoma with 83 controls chosen from the general population [35], and show the results for just two factors, the number of palpable moles (naevi) on the upper arm assessed by an interviewer (three categories) and the response to a question on whether the subject had ever had a severe sunburn (two categories). The results from cross-tabulations showed strong associations with both the number of moles and a history of sunburn. However, several other factors were associated with these two features and are also related to melanoma, which therefore are confounding factors. These included the severity of skin freckling (three categories), the usual reaction to sun exposure (four categories), and hair colour (three categories). Control for each of these confounders singly can be done fairly easily by cross-tabulations. However, to assess the relationship between moles and melanoma, with control for freckles, sun reaction, hair colour, and sunburn simultaneously by cross-tabulations, would mean that $3 \times 4 \times 3 \times 2 = 72$ separate tables showing the case–control distribution by numbers of moles would

MULTIVARIATE ANALYSIS

*A: Cross tabulations*

| | No. of moles on upper arm | | | History of sunburn | |
|---|---|---|---|---|---|
| | 0 | 1–2 | 3 + | No | Yes |
| Cases, number | 32 | 16 | 35 | 34 | 49 |
| Controls, number | 62 | 17 | 4 | 57 | 26 |
| Odds ratio | 1.0 (R) | 1.82 | 16.95 | 1.0 (R) | 3.16 |

*B: Logistic regression with one factor only*

| | | | | | |
|---|---|---|---|---|---|
| Coefficient *b* | | 0.6008 | 2.830 | | 1.150 |
| Exp(*b*) = odds ratio | | 1.82 | 16.95 | | 3.16 |

*C: Logistic regression with both factors, plus quantity of freckles (3 categories), reaction to sun exposure (4 categories), and hair colour (3 categories)*

| | | | | | |
|---|---|---|---|---|---|
| Coefficient *b* | | 0.3011 | 2.587 | | 0.4276 |
| Exp(*b*) = odds ratio | | 1.35 | 13.29 | | 1.53 |

**Ex. 6.27.** Multivariate analysis: results from a case–control study comparing 83 patients with malignant melanoma with 83 controls from the general population. Results are shown for two factors, number of moles on the upper arm and history of severe sunburn, derived by (A) cross-tabulation, (B) a logistic regression fitting only the one factor, and (C) a logistic regression fitting five factors, represented by 10 binary variables. From Elwood *et al.* [35]; fuller results are given in that paper

have to be generated, and in this small study many of these tables would have few or no observations.

Therefore it is more useful to include these five factors in a logistic regression equation, expressing each factor as a number of dummy variables, the number being 1 less than the number of categories. Thus for the number of moles, one binary variable was used with the value 1 for subjects who had one to two moles on the upper arm, and zero otherwise, and another with the value 1 was used for subjects with three or more moles, and zero otherwise. Where both these factors are zero the equation gives the risk in the referent category—subjects with no moles. If a logistic regression is fitted with just one factor, the results will be identical to a simple cross-tabulation, and the exponential of the coefficient *b* will be equal to the odds ratio obtained by the usual calculation on the simple table. These results are shown in Ex. 6.27, part B. Then if a model is fitted which includes the variables representing all the factors listed above, the coefficient *b* for each variable will give the odds ratio associated with that variable, controlled for the effects of all the other variables in the equation. Exhibit 6.27, part C, shows that with these coefficients, obtained from a model with 10 variables, the odds ratios for number of moles are still high, whereas the odds ratio for history of sunburn is 1.53, considerably lower than the crude odds ratio of 3.16. This shows that most of the association with sunburn seen in the simple analysis is not causal, but is produced by confounding by one or more of the other factors included in the equation. To determine which factor, analyses can be done fitting each confounding factor singly and seeing how the odds ratio for sunburn changes. The program used to calculate the coefficients will also allow the estimation of the statistical significance of these adjusted coefficients, and this aspect of multivariate analysis is considered further with the same example in Chapter 7 (Ex. 7. 12), p. 250.

The logistic model is the multivariate model most widely used in epidemiological studies and clinical trials, but many other models exist. To use such models the confounding factors must be recognized in advance, and quantitative information on them must be collected. Clearly, considerable care is necessary to use such models properly.

## Limitations of multivariate analysis

Multivariate analysis can deal with only a limited number of factors. Its scope is constrained by the number of study subjects, which should be much greater than the number of variables included. Most computer programs for such analyses have a limit to the number of factors they can deal with satisfactorily. Factors can be used in different ways. For example, a factor like age can be entered as one continuous variable or represented by a number of categories, each with a corresponding variable. If interactions are to be examined, extra interaction terms must be used. Thus for studies which include data on many factors, the most relevant must be selected before a multivariate model is applied. The next section on the use of the principles of confounding in analysis will be helpful in this regard.

## Multivariate analysis of matched data: conditional models

Multivariate analysis for individually matched studies uses methods that take account of the matching, i.e. they consider each case and its matched control(s) as a set. These methods are referred to as 'conditional' models. They require skilled application. The results are presented in the same way as has been shown, with the same interpretation of the coefficients. Further information is given in texts [36, 37].

Factors to be included in a multivariate model should be studied in detail, and issues such as the distribution of the observations, the need for transformations, and the appropriateness of assumptions such as a linear relationship to risk should be considered. Multivariate analysis is best regarded as a powerful but complex and demanding type of analysis, appropriate to the final stages of analysis of a study, rather than as a magical black box to provide a short cut to a result.

# Part 3. Other applications of confounding

## Use of the definition of confounding in designing a study

Now that we have discussed confounding and the methods available to control it, it is useful to go back to the definition of confounding and see how this can assist us in the *design* of studies. The definition of confounding provides an answer to the problem of feeling that because there are so many possible confounding factors, no satisfactory study can be designed.

In designing any study, we should make a list of the factors that are likely to be associated with the *exposure* under study, and another list of factors that are likely to be associated with the *outcome*. To do this, we may need to review the literature and consult reference works and people with specialized knowledge. Any factor that appears on both of these lists is a potential confounding factor, and we need to plan how to deal with it. Factors that appear on only one list, but which are likely to have a very strong association with either outcome or exposure, may be prudently included as potential confounding factors, as even a small difference in their distribution between the groups being compared may be sufficient to introduce confounding. The use of this approach will often reduce an apparently infinite number of potential confounders to a finite, and often fairly small, list of specific factors.

The options available for confounder control (Ex. 6.10) can then be considered. In practice, many potential confounders will not in fact be confounding, in that their associations with outcome and exposure in the study data are often weak and unimportant, but this will be known only if data on the confounders are collected. The most commonly used approach in non-randomized studies is to apply some restriction and to collect data on the potential confounders to allow stratification or multivariate methods to be used in the analysis. Individual matching should be used only when there are specific advantages to it.

In randomized studies only one list, of factors likely to be related to the outcome, is needed, and data on these should be collected, where possible, to assess whether the groups are in fact comparable on these factors. In large-scale randomized studies, for example of population interventions, samples of the groups may be selected for this purpose.

## Use of the definition of confounding in planning an analysis

Similarly, there are often a large number of potential confounding factors in the analysis. Initial data analysis can be used to decide if any of these factors are related to both the outcome and the exposure. This can be done by generating two sets of cross-tabulations: between each of the factors and outcome, and between each of the factors and exposure. The association between the potential confounding factor and the outcome should be examined within the non-exposed group, and the association between the potential confounding factor and exposure should be examined within the group without the outcome under consideration. Only those factors which show associations with both exposure and outcome need to be considered further as confounding factors. It is important to emphasize that it is the strength of the association, measured by the odds ratio or other measure, that matters, not its statistical significance. This type of initial analysis will often reduce a formidably large data set to a much simpler situation with only a few major confounding factors, and these can be analysed further by stratification or multivariate methods.

An alternative method of deciding which factors are confounding is often easier, and relies on the fact that confounding is demonstrated if a stratified or multivariate analysis is performed and the unconfounded relative risk or odds ratio estimate is different from the crude estimate. Therefore a practical approach to the analysis of a large data set is first to produce the basic table comparing exposure with outcome, and calculate the crude odds ratio or relative risk. Then each potential confounder is considered in a reasonable number of categories (five are usually sufficient), and stratified or multivariate analyses performed including the potential confounders, calculating the adjusted odds ratio or relative risk. If this adjusted ratio is similar to the crude ratio, there is no substantial confounding by that variable. In stratified analysis, the Mantel–Haenszel odds ratio or relative risk is usually used as the adjusted (unconfounded) estimate. Using multivariate methods, if a factor or a set of factors is confounding, the coefficient and therefore the odds ratio estimate for the exposure–outcome association will change when the confounding factors are added into the equation. Multivariate methods are very useful, as sets of potential confounding factors can easily be used and factors shown to have a confounding effect can be kept in the model while other factors are tested. The use of multivariate models to deal with confounding requires a close attention to the meaning of the various factors with regard to the causal hypothesis that is being assessed.

It is the size of the difference between the crude and adjusted risk ratio, not its statistical significance, which indicates confounding. This approach is different from the methods of selecting factors in multivariate models used in standard computer routines, such as forward and backward selection methods, as these are based on the statistical significance of each variable. In a large study with many variables, a strategy of setting a maximum accept-able change in the odds ratio or relative risk, such as 10 or 5 per cent, can be applied to potential confounders individually or in groups [38]. In pub-lished studies, a statement is sometimes given that many specified potential confounders were assessed, but that none of them changed the risk ratio estimate by more than a given percentage, and so they were not included in the final analysis. Models can be fitted including potential confounders cumulatively, or including all potential confounders and then excluding some; the critical change is the odds ratio for the main association being studied. Thus a large number of potential confounders can be reduced to a small number of actual confounders. Two or more potential confounders considered together may have a confounding effect, even if singly they do not; this is easily assessed using multivariate models. Therefore a reasonable approach is to proceed further with a reduced data set, keeping factors that have shown a confounding effect on simpler analysis plus those of major predetermined importance. This data set should then present a less forbid-ding challenge.

## Mendelian randomization: a special situation allowing control of confounding

The term 'Mendelian randomization' has been used for studies that exploit the random assortment of alleles at the time of gamete formation to give a method of avoiding confounding. The critical issue is that the random assort-ment of alleles should be independent of the distribution of behavioural and environmental factors in the population. Thus if a specific genetic allele is associated with a particular causal mechanism, the mechanism can be assessed on the basis of this allele, which is likely to be distributed independently of other factors. Thus an analysis based on Mendelian randomization may have advantages similar to a randomized clinical trial [39,40]. However, there are several limitations of this approach [41], and only a few examples as yet of its application.

What sparked interest in this issue was that an association was seen between low cholesterol levels and increased cancer rates in observational studies and in some trials of cholesterol-lowering agents. It was suggested that this could be either a causal effect, with a reduction in cholesterol causing an increase in cancer risk (which would require the treatment of high cholesterol to be reconsidered), or be due to presymptomatic cancers causing a reduction in cholesterol levels (protopathic bias). Conventional observational studies of this association will be limited by the many possible factors associated with cholesterol levels (such as other dietary factors). Katan [42,43] proposed comparing cancer risks in people with different polymorphisms of the apolipoprotein E gene. Individuals with the E2 allele have lower levels of cholesterol because their genotype gives them greater efficiency in removing cholesterol from plasma. Therefore if low cholesterol causes an increased risk of cancer, people with the E2 allele should have higher cancer risks, and a comparison of subjects with different gene types should be free of confounding as the gene type is distributed randomly.

In an example, many cohort and case–control studies have shown that people with a high intake of green cruciferous vegetables (such as broccoli and cabbage) show lower risks of lung cancer. This may be because these vegetables contain isothiocyanates, which may have a protective effect against cancer. Two genes, GSTM1 and GSTT1, are implicated in the production of the enzyme glutathione-S-transferase, which is thought to eliminate isothiocyanates. Subjects who have 'negative' alleles of these two genes do not produce glutathione-S-transferase, and so have a lesser ability to metabolize isothiocyanates. If this mechanism applies, these subjects should show a greater protective effect from a high intake of cruciferous vegetables than subjects with 'positive' alleles who do produce the enzyme. In a large case–control study of lung cancer in six East European countries, a dietary questionnaire was used and a blood sample was taken on which genotyping for the two genes was done. In subjects who were negative for one or both of the key alleles, a high consumption of cruciferous vegetables protected against lung cancer; the odds ratio for those who had both gene alleles negative was 0.28. No major protective effect was seen in people who were positive for the two genes: odds ratio 0.88 [44]. This gives support to the proposed mechanism. The advantage of using the logic of Mendelian randomization is that the presence of the relevant alleles should be independent of the many factors that could be confounding in a conventional dietary study. In this study it was shown that gene type was not associated with factors such as age, country, smoking, education, or dietary factors including cruciferous vegetable consumption.

# The limits of confounder control

A central issue in the interpretation of observational studies is whether the methods of control for confounding, which we have described in this chapter, can ever be good enough to give complete assurance that confounding has been controlled. On the one hand, studies such as the case–control studies and subsequently the prospective cohort studies of cigarette smoking and lung cancer have provided strong and consistent evidence demonstrating a causal relationship, and explaining it in quantitative terms, so that the strength of the available knowledge on that topic can be regarded as equivalent to the strength of evidence produced by randomized controlled trials in other contexts. Indeed, the aim of those carrying out epidemiological studies using observational methods is often stated in these terms—to be able to come to a similar level of confidence in the results as can be achieved by the randomized trial method. The counter-argument is that no observational study can control for a confounder that is not specifically included in the study, and even for those factors included, misclassification errors limit the ability to control their confounding effects.

The key advantage of the randomized trial method is its ability to reasonably exclude confounding, not only by factors that have been measured and assessed, but also by other factors. The real weakness of observational studies is that they provide no protection against the confounding effects of other factors that have not been measured, and may not be recognized or known. The methods described in this chapter can deal with confounding by factors that can be identified and measured, although even for these, confounding may not be completely controlled because of observational errors, limitations in how confounding factors are defined and measured, and statistical issues.

Several recent examples have been particularly influential in emphasizing the limitations of observational studies, even when well performed and analysed. These are situations where after extensive observational studies produced consistent results, large-scale randomized trials have produced quite different results. An example is the study of the potential protective effect of beta-carotene, contained in many vegetables. Extensive observational studies, both case–control studies and long-term prospective cohort studies, using the best available methods of dietary assessment and carried out by some of the world's leading research groups, produced generally consistent evidence that subjects with higher serum retinol or beta-carotene levels or with higher beta-carotene intake had substantially reduced cancer risks. This was supported by laboratory evidence that beta-carotene and its metabolites had an anti-carcinogenic action in animals. This evidence was collated over many years and a consensus formed that it was strong and consistent enough to justify intervention studies using beta-carotene dietary supplements to actively prevent many cancers [45]. Although the evidence for benefit was substantial, as Peto *et al.* [45] stated: 'Preventive measures, especially those which may be relevant over a long period to many million people, deserve particularly rigorous evaluation'. Large clinical trials were set up, but in contrast with all the previous evidence, these trials either showed no beneficial effect, or showed higher cancer rates in those receiving the beta-carotene supplements, and such trials had to be stopped promptly [46,47]. 'The cancer prevention community was stunned' by these results [48].

Another example relates to a reduction in the risk of coronary heart disease in women using oestrogen and/or progesterone hormones. Several observational studies showed that hormone users had a substantially reduced risk of coronary heart disease, with either no change in the risk of stroke or a slight reduction [49]. Therefore hormone therapies became widely recommended as a protection against heart disease in women. A trial involving over 16 000 post-menopausal women at 40 centres in the USA, the Women's Health Initiative (WHI) trial, was set up to validate this, but it showed an increased rate of heart disease and stroke in women randomized to hormone therapy (combined oestrogen–progesterone) [50]. As a result, this arm of the WHI trial was terminated early. Similar results were shown in other randomized trials. These clinical trials changed practice and destroyed the case for the benefits of hormone therapy that had been built up through observational studies. It has been pointed out that the confounding effects of socio-economic status had been inadequately dealt with in the observational studies and also that an analysis of observational studies taking account of the changes over time in the exposure (hormone use) changed the results, and these two influences together could explain the discrepancies between the observational studies and the clinical trials [51]; this commentary concluded by stating 'however, observational studies are not a substitute for clinical trials no matter how sophisticated the statistical adjustments may seem'.

Another example is that antioxidant vitamins such as vitamin C have shown protective effects against cardiovascular disease, cancer, and total mortality in many observational studies, but well-conducted randomized controlled trials of supplements with antioxidants do not show any beneficial effects. The largest observational study shows protective effects of high vitamin C plasma levels on coronary heart disease mortality, with odds ratios of 0.70 in men and 0.63 in women. This study controlled for age, systolic blood pressure, cholesterol, body mass index, smoking, diabetes, and vitamin supplement use. However, the largest randomized trial set up to verify this association showed a small increase in risk associated with vitamin C supplementation, with a relative risk of 1.06 [52]. This situation must be due to the influence of unmeasured confounding factors in the observational studies.

The challenge is the conflict between the desire to have the best quality scientific evidence and avoid premature action on the basis of apparently strong observational studies, and the reality that requiring a randomized trial may delay action for many years, or in some circumstances a randomized trial may never be done. For example, the definitive randomized trial of the preventive action of folic acid on birth defects is described in detail in Chapter 11. In this situation, an observational study completed 10 years before the randomized trial was completed in fact gave the correct answer, and public health action at that time would have prevented many birth defects which otherwise occurred. Another example is the current situation with screening by routine skin examinations with the aim of reducing deaths from melanoma, a dangerous skin cancer. Although authorities generally agree that a screening programme should only be instituted on the basis of randomized trial evidence, no randomized trial of skin screening has been done anywhere in the world, despite a successful pilot study [53], and none may ever be done because of the cost, the numbers of subjects, and the time required.

## Self-test questions (answers on p. 499)

**Q6.1** Suppose an as yet unidentified dietary constituent (X) greatly reduces the risk of cancer. It is distributed in foodstuffs in a similar way to an easily measured dietary constituent (D) which itself has no effect on cancer incidence. In a prospective cohort study, dietary intakes of D are measured, and subsequent cancer incidence recorded. What will be the result?

**Q6.2** In the same situation as in Q6.1, an intervention trial using pure compound D is carried out. What will the result be?

**Q6.3** An innovative pre-school reading programme is launched by asking teachers to volunteer to trial the programme, and the children in the programme are then compared with other children in the same school systems. What are the results likely to show?

**Q6.4** Exhibit 6.12 compares the characteristics of two groups in a randomized trial. Why are tests of the significance of the differences between the two groups not presented?

**Q6.5** The experience of treating a disease, which can present either early or late, is compared between two hospitals. In hospital A, the success rates are 40 per cent for early disease and 25 per cent for late disease, based on 500 and 100 patients in each category; in hospital B, the success rates are 60 per cent for early disease and 40 per cent for late disease, based on 100 and 200 patients, respectively. How does the performance of hospital B compare with hospital A for each stage of disease; and how does this compare with the crude comparison based on all patients treated in each hospital?

**Q6.6** Calculate the Mantel–Haenszel measure of relative risk for the data given in Q6.5.

**Q6.7** Again using the example given in Q6.5, assume that over the whole country 25 per cent of patients with this condition are early at presentation. Using a standard population of 25 per cent early and 75 per cent late disease, calculate the direct standardized success rates for each of hospitals A and B. What is the ratio of these direct standardized rates?

**Q6.8** In a case–control study, the role of previous injury in producing arthritis of the knee is assessed. In men, 300 of 900 men with arthritis of the knee reported previous injury, compared with 100 of 400 male controls. For women, four of 44 female cases reported previous injury, compared with 50 of 450 female controls. Calculate the overall crude odds ratio, the sex-specific odds ratios, and the Mantel–Haenszel odds ratio.

**Q6.9** In an individually pair-matched case–control study, 200 pairs are concordant for exposure and 100 pairs are concordant for lack of exposure; for 200 pairs, the case is exposed and the control is not; for 50 pairs, the control is exposed and the case is not. What is the odds ratio? What would the odds ratio be if an analysis ignoring the matching was performed?

**Q6.10** In a multivariate analysis, a binary variable represents oral contraceptive use, being coded 1 for ever use and zero for never use, in a prospective study assessing cardiovascular disease. On fitting ever use of oral contraceptives, plus age, the coefficient is 0.45. When the subject's weight is added to the equation, this coefficient changes to become –0.08. What is the odds ratio for the association with ever use of oral contraceptives, and what is the confounding effect of weight?

# References

1.  **Charig CR, Webb DR, Payne SR, Wickham JEA.** Comparison of treatment of renal calculi by open surgery, percutaneous nephrolithotomy, and extracorporeal shockwave lithotripsy. *BMJ* 1986; **292**: 879–882.

2. **Charig CR.** Confounding and Simpson's paradox: multiple regression would confound the clinicians. *BMJ* 1995; **310**: 329.

3. **Simpson EH.** The interpretation of interaction in contingency tables. *J R Statist Soc* 1951; **2**: 238–241.

4. **Paffenbarger RS, Hale WE.** Work activity and coronary heart mortality. *N Engl J Med* 1975; **292**: 545–550.

5. **Adish AA, Esrey SA, Gyorkos TW, Jean-Baptiste J, Rojhani A.** Effect of consumption of food cooked in iron pots on iron status and growth of young children: a randomised trial. *Lancet* 1999; **353**: 712–716.

6. **Altman DG, Schulz KF, Moher D,** *et al.* The revised CONSORT statement for reporting randomized trials: explanation and elaboration. *Ann Intern Med* 2001; **134**: 663–694.

7. **Dodd JM, Hedayati H, Pearce E, Hotham N, Crowther CA.** Rectal analgesia for the relief of perineal pain after childbirth: a randomised controlled trial of diclofenac suppositories. *BJOG* 2004; **111**: 1059–1064.

8. **Cook CC, Scannell TD, Lipsedge MS.** Another trial that failed. *Lancet* 1988; **i**: 524–525.

9. **English DR, Burton RC, Del Mar CB, Donovan RJ, Ireland PD, Emery G.** Evaluation of aid to diagnosis of pigmented skin lesions in general practice: controlled trial randomised by practice. *BMJ* 2003; **327**: 375–380.

10. **University Group Diabetes Program.** A study of the effects of hypoglycemic agents on vascular complications in patients with adult-onset diabetes. II: mortality results. *Diabetes* 1970; **19**(Suppl.2): 785–830.

11. **Coronary Drug Project Research Group.** Influence of adherence to treatment and response of cholesterol on mortality in the Coronary Drug Project. *N Engl J Med* 1980; **303**: 1038–1041.

12. **Shapiro S, Venet W, Strax P, Venet L, Roeser R.** Ten- to fourteen- year effect of screening on breast cancer mortality. *J Natl Cancer Inst* 1982; **69**: 349–355.

13. **Bruner AB, Joffe A, Duggan AK, Casella JF, Brandt J.** Randomised study of cognitive effects of iron supplementation in non anaemic iron deficient adolescent girls. *Lancet* 1996; **348**: 992–996.

14. **Ashby D.** Can iron supplementation improve cognitive functioning? *Lancet* 1996; **348**: 973.

15. **Tunis SR, Stryer DB, Clancy CM.** Practical clinical trials: increasing the value of clinical research for decision making in clinical and health policy. *JAMA* 2003; **290**: 1624–1632.

16. **Labrie F, Candas B, DuPont A,** *et al.* Screening decreases prostate cancer death: first analysis of the 1988 Quebec prospective randomized controlled trial. *Prostate* 1999; **38**: 83–91.

17. **Labrie F, Candas B, Cusan L,** *et al.* Screening decreases prostate cancer mortality: 11-year follow-up of the 1988 Quebec prospective randomized controlled trial. *Prostate* 2004; **59**: 311–318.

18. **Boer R, Schroder FH.** Quebec randomized controlled trial on prostate cancer screening shows no evidence for mortality reduction. *Prostate* 1999; **40**: 130–134.

19. **Elwood M.** A misleading paper on prostate cancer screening. *Prostate* 2004; **61**: 372.

20. **Mantel N, Haenszel W.** Statistical aspects of the analysis of data from retrospective studies of disease. *J Natl Cancer Inst* 1959; **22**: 719–748.

21. International Agency for Research on Cancer. *Cancer Incidence in Five Continents*, Vol. VIII. Lyon, France: International Agency for Research on Cancer, 2002.

22. Elwood JM, Gallagher RP, Davison J, Hill GB. Sunburn, suntan and the risk of cutaneous malignant melanoma: the Western Canada Melanoma Study. *Br J Cancer* 1985; **51**: 543–549.

23. Lyon JL, Gardner JW, West DW, Stanish WM, Hebertson RM. Smoking and carcinoma *in situ* of the uterine cervix. *Am J Public Health* 1983; **73**: 558–562.

24. Karlberg J, Chong DS, Lai WY. Do men have a higher case fatality rate of severe acute respiratory syndrome than women do? *Am J Epidemiol* 2004; **159**: 229–231.

25. Elwood JM. Wood exposure and smoking: association with cancer of the nasal cavity and paranasal sinuses in British Columbia. *Can Med Assoc J* 1981; **124**: 1573–1577.

26. Daly E, Vessey MP, Hawkins MM, Carson JL, Gough P, Marsh S. Risk of venous thromboembolism in users of hormone replacement therapy. *Lancet* 1996; **348**: 977–980.

27. Halvorsen I, Andersen A, Heyerdahl S. Girls with anorexia nervosa as young adults. Self-reported and parent-reported emotional and behavioural problems compared with siblings. *Eur Child Adolesc Psychiatry* 2005; **14**: 397–406.

28. Scott WK, Zhang F, Stajich JM, Scott BL, Stacy MA, Vance JM. Family-based case–control study of cigarette smoking and Parkinson disease. *Neurology* 2005; **64**: 442–447.

29. Swerdlow AJ, De Stavola BL, Floderus B, *et al.* Risk factors for breast cancer at young ages in twins: an international population-based study. *J Natl Cancer Inst* 2002; **94**: 1238–1246.

30. Carlsson S, Hammar N, Grill V, Kaprio J. Alcohol consumption and the incidence of type 2 diabetes: a 20-year follow-up of the Finnish twin cohort study. *Diabetes Care* 2003; **26**: 2785–2790.

31. Cederlöf R, Jonsson E, Kaij L. Respiratory symptoms and 'angina pectoris' in twins with reference to smoking habits: an epidemiological study with mailed questionnaire. *Arch Environ Health* 1966; **13**: 726–737.

32. Herbst AL, Ulfelder H, Poskanzer DC. Adenocarcinoma of the vagina: Association of maternal stilbestrol therapy with tumor appearance in young women. *N Engl J Med* 1971; **284**: 878–881.

33. Hulten K, Van Kappel AL, Winkvist A, *et al.* Carotenoids, alpha-tocopherols, and retinol in plasma and breast cancer risk in northern Sweden. *Cancer Causes Control* 2001; **12**: 529–537.

34. Forsyth BW, Horwitz RI, Acampora D, *et al.* New epidemiologic evidence confirming that bias does not explain the aspirin/Reye's syndrome association. *JAMA* 1989; **261**: 2517–2524.

35. Elwood JM, Williamson C, Stapleton PJ. Malignant melanoma in relation to moles, pigmentation, and exposure to fluorescent and other lighting sources. *Br J Cancer* 1986; **53**: 65–74.

36. Rothman KJ, Greenland S. *Modern Epidemiology* (2nd edn). Philadelphia, PA: Lippincott–Raven, 1998.

37. Clayton D, Hills M. *Statistical Models in Epidemiology*. Oxford: Oxford Scientific Publications, 1993.

38. Maldonado G, Greenland S. Simulation study of confounder-selection strategies. *Am J Epidemiol* 1993; **138**: 923–936.

39. Hingorani A, Humphries S. Nature's randomised trials. *Lancet* 2005; **366**: 1906–1908.
40. Davey Smith G, Ebrahim S. 'Mendelian randomization': can genetic epidemiology contribute to understanding environmental determinants of disease? *Int J Epidemiol* 2003; **32**: 1–22.
41. Brennan P. Commentary: Mendelian randomization and gene-environment interaction. *Int J Epidemiol* 2004; **33**: 17–21.
42. Katan MB. Apolipoprotein E isoforms, serum cholesterol, and cancer. *Lancet* 1986; **i**: 507–508.
43. Katan MB. Apolipoprotein E isoforms, serum cholesterol, and cancer. *Int J Epidemiol* 1986; **33**: 9 (reprinted from *Lancet* 1986; **i**: 507–508).
44. Brennan P, Hsu CC, Moullan N, *et al.* Effect of cruciferous vegetables on lung cancer in patients stratified by genetic status: a Mendelian randomisation approach. *Lancet* 2005; **366**: 1558–1560.
45. Peto R, Doll R, Buckley JD, Sporn MB. Can dietary beta carotene materially reduce human cancer rates? *Nature* 1981; **290**: 201–208.
46. The Alpha-Tocopherol Beta Carotene Cancer Prevention Study Group. The effect of vitamin E and beta carotene on the incidence of lung cancer and other cancers in male smokers. *N Engl J Med* 1994; **330**: 1029–1035.
47. Omenn GS, Goodman GE, Thornquist MD, *et al.* Effects of a combination of beta carotene and vitamin A on lung cancer and cardiovascular disease. *N Engl J Med* 1996; **334**: 1150–1155.
48. Duffield-Lillico AJ, Begg CB. Reflections on the landmark studies of beta-carotene supplementation. *J Natl Cancer Inst* 2004; **96**: 1729–1731.
49. Stampfer MJ, Colditz GA. Estrogen replacement therapy and coronary heart disease: a quantitative assessment of the epidemiologic evidence. *Prev Med* 1991; **20**: 47–63.
50. Rossouw JE, Anderson GL, Prentice RL, *et al.* Risks and benefits of estrogen plus progestin in healthy postmenopausal women: principal results from the Women's Health Initiative randomized controlled trial. *JAMA* 2002; **288**: 321–333.
51. Petitti DB, Freedman DA. Invited commentary: how far can epidemiologists get with statistical adjustment? *Am J Epidemiol* 2005; **162**: 415–418.
52. Lawlor DA, Davey SG, Kundu D, Bruckdorfer KR, Ebrahim S. Those confounded vitamins: what can we learn from the differences between observational versus randomised trial evidence? *Lancet* 2004; **363**: 1724–1727.
53. Aitken JF, Elwood JM, Lowe JB, Firman DW, Balanda KP, Ring IT. A randomised trial of population screening for melanoma. *J Med Screen* 2002; **9**: 33–37.

# Chapter 7

# Chance variation

*Although men flatter themselves with their great actions, they are not so often the result of a great design as of chance.*

—La Rochefoucauld: Maxims; 1665

In this chapter, we will discuss the effects of chance variation that can be assessed by applying statistical tests. The chapter falls into three parts: the application of statistical tests and confidence limits to a simple 2 × 2 table; applications to stratified and matched studies, and to multivariate analysis; and life table methods for the consideration of the timing of outcome events in a cohort study or intervention study. Reference will be made to the Appendix, in which summaries of the statistical methods presented in this book are given. Appendix Table 15 shows the relationships between the value of a statistic and the probability or *P*-value. The conversion between statistical results and probability values can also be done using a Microsoft Excel spreadsheet, and useful commands are listed in Appendix Table 16.

## Part 1. Statistical tests and confidence limits in a simple table

The third non-causal explanation for an association is that it is due to chance variation, or random number variation, the fall of the dice, bad luck, or whatever synonym you prefer. The science of statistics is concerned with measuring the *likelihood* (or *probability*) that a given set of results has been produced by this mechanism. In this chapter we shall look at the probability of chance variation being responsible for an observed association. This chapter is designed to act as a bridge between the rest of the text and a conventional basic course or text in biostatistics.

A range of statistical techniques will be presented and discussed. For reference purposes, the tests most widely used for each type of study are summarized in the Appendix.

The main objective of this section is to see how the results of statistical tests fit in with other considerations in assessing causality. These principles can be appreciated using simple examples, but also apply to results which use much more complex statistics. Many important papers now published use complex statistical methods that will not be familiar to the general reader. However, working through some simpler and widely used statistical methods can clarify most of the general principles of interpretation of statistical tests. Often, application of the simpler methods can greatly help understanding.

We shall also present in more detail some relatively simple statistical methods, particularly a test for variation in a 2 × 2 table (the Mantel–Haenszel statistic) and variations of it that can deal with cohort data using person-time denominators, life-table methods, and matched studies. Because of the wide application and the excellent performance of these statistics, even in comparison with much more complex types, we will present these in sufficient detail for readers to be able to apply such statistics to their own work and to the key results from published papers.

## The role of statistics

So far in this text we have discussed the *measurement* of the association between an exposure and an outcome, in terms of the relative risk, odds ratio, or attributable risk. We have discussed how to judge whether the estimate of association is acceptable, as being reasonably free of bias and confounding. The order of consideration of non-causal explanations, observation bias, confounding, and chance, is important. If there is substantial observation bias, there is no point in adding a statistical analysis to a biased result. The assessment of bias depends on consideration of the design and conduct of the study. Some analysis methods may help to deal with bias, for example by restricting the study to certain subgroups, using a particular comparison group, and so on. Once observation bias has been dealt with, it is appropriate to consider confounding. We may have a situation in which there could be severe confounding by a factor not included in the study design, in which case further data manipulation is not helpful. More frequently, there may be confounding which can be dealt with by stratification or multivariate analysis, or has been dealt with by randomization, matching, or restriction in the study design. These steps reviewed so far take us to the point of having an estimate of the association, which is, in our best judgement, not compromised by bias and is adjusted as far as possible for confounding. It is this estimate of the association on which we now concentrate and to which we can now apply statistical tests.

## Discrete versus continuous measures

The statistical methods described here are limited to those applicable to discrete measures of exposure and of outcome, i.e. two or a small number of categories. This is for two main reasons. We are concerned mainly with disease causation and with the evaluation of interventions. In most applications, the outcome measures are qualitative: the onset of disease, death, recurrence, recovery, return to work, and so on. Even where the biological issues are quantitative, the practical issues are often qualitative, and it may be appropriate to convert continuous data to a discrete form. For example, in a comparison of agents used to control high blood sugar, the analysis may be based on a comparison of the change in blood glucose levels in each group of subjects, using methods appropriate for this quantitative outcome. However, it may be more relevant clinically to assess the value of the agents by the proportion of treated subjects who move from having clinically unacceptable blood sugar levels to being 'well controlled', as defined by preset clinically relevant criteria.

The second reason is that introductory statistics courses and texts emphasize methods of dealing with continuous data: the normal distribution, $t$-tests, regression, analysis of variance, and so on. Thus methods applicable to discrete variables may be less familiar. Standard statistical texts should be consulted with regard to the analysis of data using continuous variables.

## The concept of significance

The statistical method the reader is most likely to be familiar with is that of significance testing. The question is: is the difference in outcome between the two groups of subjects larger than we would expect to occur purely by chance? Consider a simple intervention study (**Ex. 7.1**).

This study gives the success rate of the new treatment as 20 per cent. Even accepting the study design as being perfect with no bias, we would not interpret this as meaning that for all similar groups of subjects exposed to this intervention, the success rate would be 20.00 per cent. The 200 subjects chosen are a sample from the uncounted total of all possible subjects who could be given that intervention, and 20 per cent is the estimate of the success rate in that total group of potential subjects. On the basis of pure chance, we should understand that the next sample of 200 subjects would be likely to give a slightly different result. However, 20 per cent is our best estimate of the true success rate. Similarly, in the comparison group, our best estimate is 10 per cent. The significance testing technique tests how likely it is that a difference as

| A SIMPLE COMPARATIVE STUDY | | | | |
|---|---|---|---|---|
| Treatment group | Outcome | | | Incidence of |
| | Success | No success | Total patients | success (%) |
| New therapy | 40 | 160 | 200 | 20 |
| Conventional therapy | 20 | 180 | 200 | 10 |
| Total | 60 | 340 | 400 | 15 |

**Ex. 7.1.** A simple comparative study: hypothetical data

large as the one we have seen (or larger) could occur purely by chance, if the true situation is that both the intervention and the comparison groups have the same true success rate. This would occur on the *null hypothesis* that the effect of the intervention is no different from that of the comparison therapy. This is sometimes referred to as the concept that the two groups of subjects are independent samples drawn from the same population. Therefore statistical tests test the hypothesis that the true success rate in the two groups is the same, and that the observed differences are produced purely by chance variation around that common value. Our best estimate of the common value of the success rate is based on all the subjects in the study, and therefore is 15 per cent in this example.

## Simple statistical tests for a 2 × 2 table

One commonly used test in this situation is the *chi-squared statistic*, written $\chi^2$, applied to the 2 × 2 table formed from the study results, which gives a value of 7.84 (**Ex. 7.2a**). To interpret this we need to know the number of *degrees of freedom* of the statistic. The number of 'degrees of freedom' is the number of cells in the body of the table that can vary independently, given the marginal totals (i.e. the totals which appear at the margins of the table). For the table in Ex. 7.2, if the marginal totals are known, only one number within the table needs to be known—all the rest are then derived from it—and so the table has one degree of freedom (*d.f.*). An $n \times n$ table has $(n-1) \times (n-1)$ degrees of freedom. Looking up 7.84 in a table of the chi-squared distribution on one degree of freedom (Appendix Table 15, p. 552) shows that the probability or *P*-value is between 0.01 and 0.001; alternatively, using an Excel spreadsheet and entering =chidist(7.84,1) gives 0.005. Thus the test shows that, *if* the true success rate is the same in the two groups, the probability of a difference as large as or larger than the one we have observed occurring purely by chance variation is between 1 in 100 (0.01) and 1 in 1000 (0.001). It is considerably

STATISTICAL TESTS OF A NULL HYPOTHESIS

| Exposure | Outcome | | Total no. patients | Success rate (%) |
|---|---|---|---|---|
| | Positive (success) | Negative | | |
| New treatment | a (40) | b (160) | $N_1$ (200) | $S_1$ (20%) |
| Comparison | c (20) | d (180) | $N_0$ (200) | $S_0$ (10%) |
| Total | $M_1$ (60) | $M_0$ (340) | $T$ (400) | $S$ (15%) |

Appropriate statistical tests for departures from the null hypothesis:

(a) Chi-square statistic $\chi^2 = \dfrac{(ad-bc)^2 T}{N_1 N_0 M_1 M_0} = 7.84$

Equivalently $\chi^2 = \sum \dfrac{(\text{obs}-\text{exp})^2}{\text{exp}}$ for each of the four cells

$$= \frac{(a-N_1 M_1/T)^2}{N_1 M_1/T} + \frac{(b-N_1 M_0/T)^2}{N_1 M_0/T} + \frac{(c-N_0 M_1/T)^2}{N_0 M_1/T} + \frac{(d-N_0 M_0/T)^2}{N_0 M_0/T}$$

$= 7.84$

From the table of the $\chi^2$ distribution on 1 d.f., the probability $P$ of this or a larger value occurring on the null hypothesis lies between 0.01 and 0.001 (from Appendix Table 15), or using Appendix Table 16, $P = 0.005$.

(b) Comparison of two proportions

Standardized normal deviate $= \dfrac{S_1 - S_0}{\sqrt{\left\{ S(1-S)\left(\dfrac{1}{N_1} + \dfrac{1}{N_0}\right)\right\}}}$

$= 2.80$

From a table of the normal distribution (Appendix Table 15), the two-sided probability corresponding to 2.80 lies between 0.01 and 0.001, or using Appendix Table 16, $P = 0.005$.

(c) For a continuity corrected version of the $\chi^2$ statistic, the formulae are:

$$\chi^2_c = \frac{(|ad-bc|-\frac{1}{2}T)^2 T}{N_1 N_0 M_1 M_0}$$

and

$$\chi^2_c = \frac{(|a-N_1 M_1/T|-\frac{1}{2})^2}{N_1 M_1/T} + \text{etc.}$$

Hence $\chi^2_c = 7.08$
From Appendix Table 15, $P$ is between 0.01 and 0.001, or using Appendix Table 16, $P = 0.008$.

**Ex. 7.2.** Two appropriate statistical tests applied to a 2 × 2 table: arithmetic examples use the data shown in Ex. 7.1

less than 5 per cent (0.05), and so is conventionally accepted as 'statistically significant'.

Another commonly used test is a test of *difference in proportions*, testing whether the 20 per cent success rate in the intervention group is different from the 10 per cent success rate in the control group **(Ex. 7.2b).** This formulation yields a *standardized normal deviate* of 2.80. This also corresponds to a two-sided *P*-value of between 0.01 and 0.001 (Appendix Table 15, p. 000), or using Excel we can enter =2*(1-normsdist(2.8)) and this yields 0.005 (Appendix Table 16).

We have applied two statistical tests to the same data. They should give the same results. In fact, the chi-squared statistic on one degree of freedom is the square of the normal deviate: $2.8^2 = 7.84$. The cut-off point at 5 per cent significance for $\chi^2$ on one degree of freedom is 3.84, which is the square of 1.96, the cut-off for the normal deviate. As an alternative to calculating the chi-squared statistic from the formula shown in Ex. 7.2, its square root, the *chi statistic*, can be calculated and looked up in tables of the normal deviate, which are often more detailed than tables of the chi-squared statistic. This relationship between $\chi^2$ and a standardized normal deviate holds only for the situation where $\chi^2$ has one degree of freedom.

Studies which produce results that can be simplified to the $2 \times 2$ format exemplified here can be dealt with using either of these techniques, and the statistical methods apply to both cohort and case–control designs. The statistic tests the departure of the data from the null hypothesis of no association; therefore it can be regarded as a test of the significance of a risk difference (attributable risk) from the null value of 0, or of the difference of the risk ratio (relative risk or odds ratio) from the null value of 1.

## One-sided and two-sided tests

The tests used above are *two-sided* tests; that is, they estimate the probability that if the null hypothesis were true, a difference would occur which would be as large as or larger than that observed in either direction, i.e. the intervention group having either the higher or the lower success rate. A *one-sided* test estimates only the probability of occurrence, on the null hypothesis, of the observed result or results that are more different from the null hypothesis in the same direction. A one-sided test is appropriate in situations where the direction of the effect is established before the data are collected. Thus if Ex. 7.1 was drawn from a study designed specifically to assess whether the new therapy was better than the conventional treatment, discounting any possibility that it could be worse, a one-sided test could be used. This will estimate the probability of occurrence, on the null hypothesis, of the difference observed (the success rate being 10 per cent higher in the new therapy group) or a larger difference in the predetermined direction. Except with very small numbers, the two-sided probability is simply twice the one-sided probability, and therefore a one-sided test with a probability given as 5 per cent (0.05) is equivalent to a two-sided test with a probability value of 10 per cent (0.1) (see Appendix Table 15, p. 552). Note that chi-squared statistics, because they square the deviations between observed and expected values, directly give two-sided tests, while many tables of the distribution of the standardized normal deviate directly give a one-sided probability value, which is then doubled if a two-sided test is required. In Excel, the command =(1-normsdist(z)) gives the one-sided $P$-value for a normal deviate $z$, and =2*(1-normsdist(z)) gives the two-sided probability.

## Small numbers, continuity corrections, and exact tests

The expected value in each cell in a 2 × 2 table need not be a whole number; it has a continuous distribution. However, the observed values must be whole numbers. In calculating the chi-squared statistic or normal deviate, a 'continuity correction' which allows for this can be used (see **Ex. 7.2c**); it is sometimes called a Yates' correction after the statistician Frank Yates who introduced it. Its effect is to reduce the calculated statistic somewhat; this reduction is greater when the number of observations in the table is small. However, its use is controversial; some statisticians argue that the use of a continuity correction gives a more accurate estimation of the $P$-value [1], while others disagree [2]. With reasonably large numbers, the continuity correction will make very little difference. For the data in Ex 7.2, the continuity corrected $\chi^2$ statistic is 7.08, compared with the uncorrected value of 7.84, corresponding to $P$-values of 0.0078 and 0.0051, respectively (Appendix Table 16). The test of comparison of proportions makes an assumption of having reasonable numbers of subjects and gives the square root of the uncorrected $\chi^2$ value.

Thus the issue of whether to use a continuity correction is related to how $P$-values are interpreted. If we reduce the stress on particular cut-off values of the $P$-value, such as 0.05, the problem is put into perspective. If the use of a continuity correction changes a result from being less than to being greater than 0.05, this merely shows that the true probability value is very close to 0.05 and should be interpreted accordingly. Also, if the difference is substantial, it means the number of observations is small, and a better solution is to use an *exact* probability test. One of these, the Fisher test for 2 × 2 tables, is described in Appendix Table 4, but others are available for other situations and statistical advice should be sought. Many computer programs provide exact tests. An approximate rule is that $\chi^2$ statistics become unreliable where any expected numbers in the tables are less than 5. This often occurs if tables with many cells are generated, and the solution may be to combine some categories. The same consideration applies where different results arise from different, but applicable, statistical tests, or even from the same test performed using a different calculator or computer program. All these serve to emphasize that we should guard against over-interpreting the precise value of the $P$-value, using it instead as a general measure of probability.

## The Mantel–Haenszel test

Although the usual $\chi^2$ tests are appropriate for simple tables, more generally applicable methods that can be extended to deal with stratified data are very useful in epidemiological and clinical studies.

Many statistical tests are derived from the principle that if we calculate the difference between an observed value $a$ and its expected value on the null hypothesis $E$, square that, and divide it by the variance $V$ of the observed value, the quantity (the statistic) resulting will follow a $\chi^2$ distribution on one degree of freedom (1 d.f.), i.e.

$$\chi^2 = (a - E)^2/V.$$

As we shall see, this general formula can be applied to many different situations, using appropriate calculations to obtain $E$ and $V$.

The $\chi^2$ distribution on 1 d.f. is simply related to the normal distribution. If a variable $\chi$ follows a normal distribution, its square $\chi^2$ will follow a $\chi^2$ distribution on 1 d.f. Thus an equivalent formula to that given above is

$$\chi = \sqrt{\chi^2} = (a - E)/\sqrt{V}.$$

That is, the difference between the observed value $a$ and its expected value $E$, divided by the standard deviation of $a$ (i.e. the square root of the variance) gives a normal deviate, often referred to as chi, $\chi$, or $Z$.

A most useful test, the Mantel–Haenszel test, for a $2 \times 2$ table is shown in **Ex. 7.3** [3]. It is of the above form, with the $\chi^2$ statistic being given by the squared difference between one value in the table and its expected value, divided by the variance of the observed value. The value $a$ is usually taken as the number of exposed cases; the expected number is derived simply from the totals in the margins of the table as $N_1M_1/T$. The variance is calculated from a formula based on the 'hypergeometric' distribution, also shown in Ex. 7.3. Further explanation is not essential here; it applies to a table where the 'marginal totals' are fixed, and this assumption is also made in the Fisher test and the usual $\chi^2$ tests. From this, we can calculate $\chi^2$ or $\chi$ using the formulae

---

## GENERAL TEST FOR A 2 × 2 TABLE

Table showing fixed marginal totals

|                | Success | No success | Total |
|----------------|---------|------------|-------|
| New treatment  | $a$     | $b$        | $N_1$ |
| Old treatment  | $c$     | $d$        | $N_0$ |
| Total          | $M_1$   | $M_0$      | $T$   |

*General formulae*

Observed number of 'exposed cases' = $a$
Expected value of $a$ on null hypothesis = $E = N_1 M_1 / T$

Variance of $a$ under hypergeometric distribution $= V = \left( \dfrac{N_1 N_0 M_0 M_1}{T^2(T-1)} \right)$

Chi-squared statistic, 1 degree of freedom $= \dfrac{(a-E)^2}{V} = \dfrac{(a - N_1 M_1 / T)^2}{N_1 N_0 M_0 M_1 / T^2(T-1)}$

Normal deviate, $\chi$ $= \sqrt{\chi^2} = \dfrac{(a-E)}{\sqrt{V}}$

Continuity corrected versions: $\chi^2_c = \dfrac{(|a-E|-0.5)^2}{V}$

$\chi_c = \dfrac{|a-E|-0.5}{\sqrt{V}}$

---

**Ex. 7.3.** The Mantel–Haenszel test for a 2 × 2 table with reasonable numbers. This is applicable to both cohort and case–control data

given above. For a continuity correction, we reduce the absolute value $|a - E|$ by 0.5, before squaring. For the table in Ex. 7.1,

observed value of $a = 40$

expected value of $a = N_1 M_1 / T = 200 \times 60/400 = 30$

variance of $a = N_1 N_0 M_1 M_0 / T^2 (T - 1) = 200 \times 200 \times 60 \times 340/$
$$(400 \times 400 \times 399) = 12.78.$$

Then

$$\chi^2 = (a - E)^2 / V = (40 - 30)^2 / 12.78 = 7.82$$

and from Appendix Table 15, $P$ lies between 0.01 and 0.001, and

$$\chi = 2.80$$

---

### TEST FOR COHORT STUDY WITH PERSON-TIME DATA

|  | Outcome positive | Person-time |
|---|---|---|
| Exposed | $a$ | $N_1$ |
| Unexposed | $b$ | $N_0$ |
| Total | $M_1$ | $T$ |

*Statistical test*

Observed no. of 'exposed cases' $\quad = a$

$\quad$ expected value of $a \qquad E = N_1 M_1 / T$

$\quad$ variance of $a \qquad\qquad V = N_1 N_0 M_1 / T^2$

Chi-squared statistic $\chi^2$, 1 degree of freedom $= \dfrac{(a-E)^2}{V} = \dfrac{(a - N_1 M_1 T)^2}{N_1 N_0 M_1 / T^2}$

---

**Ex. 7.4.** Person-time data: for cohort data using person-time denominators, formulae very similar to those shown in Ex. 7.3 are applicable. For a continuity correction, subtract 0.5 from the absolute value of $|a - E|$

and from Appendix Table 15 or 16, $P = 0.005$ (two-sided). These values are almost identical to those given by the tests used in Ex. 7.2. If a continuity correction is used, $\chi^2 = 7.06$, $P = 0.008$.

This test, as shown in Ex 7.3, was first applied to case–control studies [3], and is also applicable to cohort studies and surveys using count data. A very similar formula, shown in **Ex. 7.4**, is used for cohort data with a person-time denominator. Later in this chapter we will discuss how this basic test, with some variations, can be applied to stratified data, to matched studies, and to cohort studies taking into account follow-up time.

These formulae are 'asymptotic', i.e. they are derived by making assumptions which are valid only where reasonable numbers of observations are available; a guide to 'reasonable' would be that the smallest expected number in the $2 \times 2$ table on which the result is based should be greater than five. This limitation does not apply to stratified subtables, which can be smaller if only the summary estimates are to be used. Where numbers of observations are smaller, 'exact' tests should be used, such as Fisher's test for a simple $2 \times 2$ table; there are several other exact tests for different situations [1,4].

## The concept of precision; confidence limits

These tests of significance yield a single value, which is the probability of a difference the same as or larger than that observed in the study occurring purely

| | TWO COMPARATIVE STUDIES | | | |
| | Numbers of subjects | | | |
| | Success | No success | Total | Success rate (%) |
|---|---|---|---|---|
| Study A | | | | |
| New therapy | 40 | 160 | 200 | 20 |
| Old therapy | 20 | 180 | 200 | 10 |
| | | | | |
| Study B | | | | |
| New therapy | 10 | 26 | 36 | 28 |
| Old therapy | 5 | 31 | 36 | 14 |

Study A: relative risk = 2.0 $\chi^2$ = 7.84 $P$ = 0.005

Study B: relative risk = 2.0 $\chi^2$ = 2.11 $P$ = 0.14

**Ex. 7.5.** Two simple comparative studies: hypothetical data. Statistics calculated without continuity corrections. With a continuity correction they are 7.08 and 1.35, respectively

by chance, on the null hypothesis that the outcome is the same in each of the groups being compared. Two sets of data representing trials of therapy are shown in **Ex. 7.5**; in both, the success rate is twice as high with the new therapy. In study A, the difference seen would have occurred purely by chance about once in 200 occasions ($P$= 0.005). In study B, it would occur purely by chance on about 14 per cent of occasions ($P$= 0.14). Using the conventional $P$ = 0.05 cut-off, the result in A is significant, whereas that in B is non-significant.

Reporting results by concentrating only on significance tests and $P$ values at best makes poor use of the data, and at worst can be misleading. A superficial review of these two studies might conclude that they are inconsistent, as study A shows a significant benefit while study B shows no significant difference. In fact, the two studies are consistent, showing exactly the same advantage for the new therapy. It is the precision of the studies, not the estimate of effect, which differs.

The way to avoid this dependency on an arbitrary cut-off, and to use the information in the study more fully, is to calculate *confidence limits* for the result rather than the $P$-value. The concept is as follows. Any one study provides one estimate of the association, for example the relative risk shown in the study is an estimate of the true relative risk. This estimate has variability; another study of the same design would give a different estimate of this relative risk. What we are interested in is the true relative risk in the population from which these samples of participants have been drawn. **Ex. 7.6** shows a

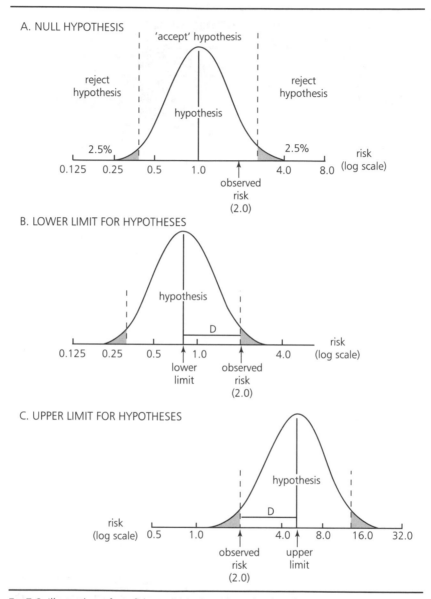

A. NULL HYPOTHESIS

'accept' hypothesis

reject
hypothesis

reject
hypothesis

hypothesis

2.5%

2.5%

risk
(log scale)

0.125    0.25    0.5    1.0    4.0    8.0

observed
risk
(2.0)

B. LOWER LIMIT FOR HYPOTHESES

hypothesis

D

risk
(log scale)

0.125    0.25    0.5    1.0    4.0

lower
limit

observed
risk
(2.0)

C. UPPER LIMIT FOR HYPOTHESES

hypothesis

D

risk
(log scale)    0.5    1.0    4.0    8.0    16.0    32.0

observed
risk
(2.0)

upper
limit

**Ex. 7.6.** Illustration of confidence limits based on the data in Ex. 7.5, study B. The limits shown are 95 per cent, two-sided limits, i.e. the unacceptable values of relative risk are those corresponding to the highest 2.5 per cent and the lowest 2.5 per cent of the distribution

diagrammatic representation of the statistical test applied to the data from study B in Ex. 7.5. In hypothesis testing, a specific value is stated as the prior hypothesis, usually as here a relative risk of 1, representing the null hypothesis of no association. The statistical test then assesses if the observed value of the relative risk is consistent or inconsistent with this prior value, using a preset level of probability. To be able to do this we must hypothesize what the true relative risk in the underlying population is, and how the risks observed in a multitude of small samples will be distributed.

Exhibit 7.6, part A, shows the expected distribution of the observed relative risk in a multitude of samples of the same size as the one we have used, on the assumption that the null hypothesis applies and the true relative risk is 1.0. Therefore the distribution is centred on the null hypothesis value of 1.0. It has a normal distribution, but the scale of relative risk is logarithmic. This is because relative risk is a ratio measurement; relative risk values of 2.0 and 0.5 are different from the null value of 1.0 by different amounts on an arithmetic scale, but by the same amount on a logarithmic scale. The width of the normal curve is determined by the standard deviation of these estimates, which is estimated by the standard deviation of the observed relative risk value. We shall come to the issue of how we can calculate that in due course. Note that in the diagram the observed value of relative risk, 2.0, lies within the central part of the distribution and therefore is a value quite 'likely' to occur in taking a sample from such a distribution centred on 1.0. An arbitrary value of 5 per cent probability has been used as a definition of 'likely'. We conclude that although a relative risk of 2.0 has been observed, the relative risk in the population from which the sample was drawn is quite likely to be 1; this is what we mean when we say that the result is not statistically significant.

However, it is clear that the distribution could be moved and centred on many other values, while still keeping our observed value in the central 'acceptable' region. If we take successively lower values for the population relative risk as the hypothesis, this is equivalent to moving the distribution to the left. The standard deviation does not change, since it does not depend on the central value. We can move the distribution to the left until it reaches the point shown in Ex. 7.6, part B. If we moved it any further, the observed value would be moved into the region defining values with a probability less than 0.05, such that we should reject the hypothesis that the observed relative risk is consistent with the hypothesized value of the relative risk in the population. The value of the centre of the distribution, when the observed relative risk is at this cut-off point, is then the lowest 'acceptable' value for the population relative risk; it is referred to as the lower 95 per cent confidence limit. Similarly, moving the distribution to the right gives successively higher values of the population relative risk, until we reach a value such that the observed relative risk reaches the critical point in the lower tail of the distribution (Ex. 7.6, part C). This gives the upper limit of the 'acceptable' population relative risk—the upper 95 per cent confidence limit. Any value between the two limits defined in this way is 'acceptable' as a value for the relative risk in the population from which our sample is drawn. In this way we can define limits for the relative risk, and we can be 95 per cent confident that these limits will include the true value.

While the use of these diagrams can aid in the understanding of confidence limits, it does not provide a practical method for calculating them. However, the basic formulae can be derived from the diagram. Given reasonable numbers in the samples studied, these distributions are normal, and therefore the points which define the 5 per cent rejection region are located 1.96 standard deviations from the mean. This standard deviation is equal to the standard deviation of the logarithm of the estimated relative risk. We use natural (base e) logarithms. Thus, if we know the logarithm of the observed relative risk (ln $RR$) and its standard deviation (dev ln $RR$), we can calculate the 95 per cent confidence limits as follows:

$$\text{95 per cent confidence limits of ln } RR = (\text{ln } RR - 1.96 \text{ dev ln } RR) \text{ and}$$
$$(\text{ln } RR + 1.96 \text{ dev ln } RR)$$

$$\text{95 per cent confidence limits of } RR = \text{exponential (ln } RR - 1.96$$
$$\text{dev ln } RR) \text{ and exponential}$$
$$(\text{ln } RR + 1.96 \text{ dev ln } RR).$$

Of course limits other than 95 per cent can be calculated using different values of the normal deviate corresponding to that proportion, which can be obtained from a table of the normal distribution such as that given later in Ex. 7.15 or Appendix Tables 15 or 16. Thus, for 99 per cent two-sided confidence limits, we use a value of 2.58 instead of 1.96. Just as we have discussed one-sided and two-sided statistical tests, we can use one-sided or two-sided confidence limits, with the same issues being involved. The above example is based on two-sided limits.

The calculation of dev ln $RR$, the standard deviation of the logarithm of the relative risk, is not always simple. Formulae for the calculation of standard deviations for various study designs are given in Appendix Tables 1–3.

In presenting study results, confidence limits are much more informative than $P$-values. Many leading clinical and epidemiological journals will no longer accept papers using only $P$-values. Confidence limits are particularly useful when the result of the study is non-significant. The presentation of confidence limits may guard against the common fallacy of interpreting studies like study B as showing 'no difference' between the intervention and control group. While the overall result is consistent with the null hypothesis, the confidence limits show that the study is also consistent with a relative risk of 5.0, a considerable effect. A better interpretation of study B is that, while it has demonstrated a relative risk of 2.0, the 95 per cent confidence limits show that the result is consistent with anything from a small detrimental effect of the intervention to a large beneficial effect, and therefore the study is inconclusive rather than demonstrating that the intervention has no effect.

## Approximate test-based limits

In addition to the above procedures, a simple method which allows the standard deviation, and therefore confidence limits, to be calculated from a test statistic is sometimes useful [5], but it should be seen only as an approximate method (**Ex. 7.7**). It is derived from the logic that, for a normally distributed

---

### APPROXIMATE TEST-BASED CONFIDENCE LIMITS

Given that the logarithm of the relative risk, ln $RR$, is normally distributed, and on the null hypothesis the expected value of ln $RR$ is zero, a standardized normal deviate will be given by

$$\chi = \frac{\text{observed (ln } RR) - \text{expected (ln } RR)}{\text{standard deviation of (ln } RR)} = \frac{\ln RR}{\text{dev ln } RR}$$

This is equal to $\chi$, calculated by the formulae in Ex. 7.3 and Ex. 7.4, or by other appropriate methods. Hence standard deviation of ln $RR$ = dev ln $RR$ = ln $RR/\chi$
The $y\%$ confidence limits of ln $RR$ are

ln $RR$ - $Z_y$ (dev ln $RR$) and ln $RR$ + $Z_y$ (dev ln $RR$)

where $Z_y$ is the normal deviate corresponding to $y\%$, e.g. 1.96 for 95% two-sided limits.
Hence $y\%$ confidence limits for ln $RR$ = ln $RR$ ± $Z_y$ (dev ln $RR$)
= ln $RR$ ± $Z_y$ (ln $RR/\chi$)
= ln $RR$ $(1\pm Z_y/\chi)$
and the 95% confidence limits for $RR$ = exp {ln $RR(1\pm Z_y/\chi)$}

---

**Ex. 7.7.** Calculation of approximate 'test-based' confidence limits

variable, the difference between the observed value and the expected value, divided by the standard deviation (the square root of the variance $V$) gives a normal deviate. This normal deviate is calculated as the test statistic $\chi$ or $\sqrt{\chi^2}$ from any of the tests we have described; the $\chi$ statistic without a continuity correction should be used.

Thus the Mantel–Haenszel analysis will give us ln $RR$, the logarithm of the $RR$ (or $OR$), and $\chi$. The expected value of $RR$ or $OR$ is 1, and so the expected value of its logarithm is zero. Therefore dev ln $RR$ can be calculated as follows:

$$\text{dev ln } RR = (\ln RR - 0)/\chi = \ln RR/\chi.$$

Thus for the data shown in Ex. 7.5, study A, the standard deviation is

$$\text{dev ln } RR = \ln RR/\chi = \ln 2.0/\sqrt{7.84} = 0.248,$$

The 95 per cent two-sided confidence limits for ln $RR$ are

$$\ln RR - (1.96 \times \ln RR/\chi) \text{ and } \ln RR + (1.96 \times \ln RR/\chi),$$

and the limits for the relative risk itself are

$$\text{exponential } [\ln RR \pm (1.96 \times \ln RR/\chi)]$$

which gives limits of 1.23 and 3.25. As we already know from the $P$-value, these limits for study A do not include the value 1.0. For study B the limits are 0.79 and 5.10, and these are shown in Ex. 7.6; they do include the null hypothesis value.

The test-based method is reasonably accurate for relative risks and odds ratios close to 1 (but not exactly 1, where it gives no result), which are based on fairly large numbers of observations. It can be applied both to a single table and to a stratified data set, as it is based on the Mantel–Haenszel estimates of odds ratio or relative risk, and the summary chi statistic. These confidence limits are derived from exactly the same information as went into the $P$-values, and are only approximations. The calculation uses an assumption of equivalence of two different statistics, which only applies under the null hypothesis and gives reasonable results only when the odds ratio or relative risks are reasonably close to the null, between 0.2 and 5.0. The method is even less reliable with risk difference measures [6]. It is better to use the formulae for standard deviation of ln $RR$ and the confidence limits that are given in Appendix Tables 1–3, and such calculations are available in many computer programs.

# Part 2. Statistical methods in more complex situations

## Analyses with stratification

The use of stratification to control for a confounding variable was discussed in Chapter 6. The Mantel–Haenszel test is easily applied to stratified data from any type of study. The test can be regarded as a test of the summary relative risk or odds ratio estimate.

We recall that the Mantel–Haenszel $\chi^2$ test for a $2 \times 2$ table is calculated as (Ex. 7.3)

$$\chi^2 = (a - E)^2/V$$

where $a$ is one of the values in the table, such as the number of exposed cases, $E$ is its expected value, and $V$ is its variance. If the data are stratified into several $2 \times 2$ tables, a $\chi^2$ test for the association after stratification is given by

$$\chi^2 = (\Sigma_i a_i - \Sigma_i E_i)^2/\Sigma_i V_i$$

where $\Sigma_i a_i$ means 'the sum of the values $a$ in each table, represented by $a_1$, $a_2$, $a_3$, ... over $I$ tables, where $I$ is the number of tables', i.e. the values of $a$, $E$, and $V$ are calculated in each table and summed, and $\chi^2$ is calculated using the three summations; it still has one degree of freedom irrespective of the number of subtables.

An application to a simple case–control study is shown in **Ex. 7.8**; these data were shown previously in Ex. 6.23 and relate to the association between melanoma and sunburn history. The single-factor table shows an odds ratio of 1.40, which is statistically significant: $\chi^2 = 4.94$, $P = 0.03$ (Appendix Table 15, p. 552). However, part of the association is produced by confounding by tendency to sunburn. Adjustment for this by stratification gives an odds ratio of 1.19, which is not statistically significant; the summary $\chi^2 = 1.16$, $P = 0.3$, indicating that this or a more extreme result would occur in nearly one of three studies of this size if the null hypothesis were true.

The same formula is applicable to cohort or intervention studies with observations on individuals, as shown in Appendix Table 2. For person-time data from a cohort study, the values of $E_i$ and $V_i$ are calculated using a formula adapted from that in Ex. 7.4, which is shown in Appendix Table 3.

## Assumptions in stratification: interaction

The calculation of a summary measure of odds ratio or relative risk implies that this single estimate applies to all the different strata. This is usually a

---

### MANTEL-HAENSZEL ANALYSIS OF STRATIFIED DATA

*Table A. All subjects*

|  | Cases | Controls | Total |
|---|---|---|---|
| Severe sunburn | 136 | 98 | 234 |
| Mild sunburn | 343 | 347 | 690 |
|  | 479 | 445 | 924 |

$OR = 1.40$

$a = 136$   $E = 121.31$   $V = 43.67$

$\chi^2 = 4.94$   $P = 0.03$

*Subtable $B_1$. Subjects who sunburn easily*

|  | Cases | Controls | Total |
|---|---|---|---|
| Severe sunburn | 119 | 76 | 195 |
| Mild sunburn | 227 | 173 | 400 |
|  | 346 | 249 | 595 |

$OR = 1.19$

$a = 119$   $E = 113.39$   $V = 31.96$

*Subtable $B_2$. Subjects who do not sunburn easily*

|  | Cases | Controls | Total |
|---|---|---|---|
| Severe sunburn | 17 | 22 | 39 |
| Mild sunburn | 116 | 174 | 290 |
|  | 133 | 196 | 329 |

$OR = 1.16$

$a = 17$   $E = 15.77$   $V = 8.30$

*Stratified analysis, adjusting for tendency to sunburn*
Summary $OR = 1.19$ (see Ex. 6.23 for calculation)

$$\text{Summary } \chi^2 = \frac{\left(\sum_i a_i - \sum_i E_i\right)^2}{\sum_i V_i} = \frac{\{(119+17)-(113.39+15.77)\}^2}{(31.96+8.30)}$$

$$= 1.16 \ P = 0.3 \text{ (Appendix Table 15 or 16)}$$

---

**Ex. 7.8.** Calculation of the Mantel-Haenszel $\chi^2$ statistic from the case–control data shown in Ex. 6.23, p. 194.

reasonable a priori assumption, but it should be checked by examining the stratum-specific ratios. While substantial variation in stratum-specific odds ratios may be due only to small numbers, a summary estimate may disguise important real variation. With an ordered confounder, such as age, there may be a regular trend in the odds ratio estimates over strata of the confounder.

Methods are available which compare the stratum-specific values with the summary odds ratio, and test the hypothesis that the summary estimate applies to all strata. A simple test is based on the familiar logic of squaring the difference between an observed value and its expected value, and dividing by the variance to give a chi-squared statistic. For each stratum, we calculate the difference between the observed log odds ratio (or relative risk) $L_i$ and the summary log odds ratio $L_s$ (which is its expected value), square it, and divide by the variance of the observed log odds ratio $V_i$. This gives a measure of the 'goodness of fit' of the model applying the summary odds ratio in each stratum to the observed data. Summing over all subtables gives

$$\chi^2_{(I-1)} = \sum_i \frac{(L_i - L_s)}{V_i}$$

where $L_i$ and $V_i$ are the log odds ratio and its variance for each subtable, and $L_s$ is the log of the summary odds ratio (e.g. the Mantel–Haenszel odds ratio). Given $I$ subtables, $\chi^2$ has $I - 1$ degrees of freedom. The formulae for the variances in the different study designs are given in the Appendix. This is a test of the hypothesis that the odds ratios are homogeneous. Other tests can assess a linear trend in the odds ratios over the strata, which may sometimes be more relevant. However, substantial numbers of observations are required to detect heterogeneity in stratum-specific relative risks.

**Exhibit 7.9** shows an example of variation of the odds ratio estimate. In this study 217 patients with *in situ* carcinoma of the cervix were compared with 243 population-based controls [7]. A significant association between the disease and smoking was seen, with an odds ratio of 6.6, which is highly significant (Table A). After subdivision into three categories by age, the Mantel–Haenszel age-adjusted odds ratio is 6.3, only slightly reduced compared with the crude odds ratio, and has 95 per cent confidence limits of 4.1 to 9.5. Thus age is not a major confounder, as is expected because frequency matching on age has been done. However, the odds ratios in each of the three strata of age are considerably different, being 27.9, 5.9, and 2.8 in successively older age groups; all these odds ratios are significantly different from 1, but the confidence limits show that the odds ratio in the youngest age group is significantly different from the overall Mantel–Haenszel estimate, and also significantly different from the other odds ratios. The chi-squared statistic testing for heterogeneity of the odds ratio, calculated as above, is 12.1 on 2 d.f., $P < 0.01$, and so there is statistically significant variation in the stratum-specific odds ratios. The summary odds ratio of 6.3 is not an adequate description of the relationship of smoking with disease, and so in this study the results for the different age groups should be shown and discussed. Further stratification to control for religious affiliation and number of sexual partners reduced all the odds ratios, but the significant variation in odds ratios in different age groups remained.

---

INTERACTION IN A STRATIFIED ANALYSIS

| A. *Full table* | | Cases | Controls | |
|---|---|---|---|---|
| All ages: | smokers | 130 | 45 | |
| | non-smokers | 87 | 198 | Odds ratio = 6.6 |
| | | 217 | 243 | $\chi^2 = 83.1$; 95% confidence limits = 4.3, 10.0 |

*B. Subtables by age*

| Age 20–29: | smokers | 41 | 6 | *OR* = 27.9 |
|---|---|---|---|---|
| | non-smokers | 13 | 53 | $\chi^2 = 49.7$; 95% C.L. = 9.8, 79.6 |
| Age 30–39: | smokers | 66 | 25 | *OR* = 5.9 |
| | non-smokers | 37 | 83 | $\chi^2 = 35.8$; 95% C.L. = 3.2, 10.8 |
| Age 40 + | smokers | 23 | 14 | *OR* = 2.8; |
| | non-smokers | 37 | 62 | $\chi^2 = 6.7$; 95% C.L. = 1.3, 6.0 |

Odds ratio after adjustment for age, Mantel-Haenszel method = 6.3
$\chi^2$ statistic after adjustment for age, 1 d.f. = 82.3
95 per cent confidence limits of adjusted *OR* = 4.1, 9.5

$\chi^2$ for heterogeneity on the three subtables = 12.1  d.f. = 2  P<0.01

---

**Ex. 7.9.** An example of interaction defined here as non-homogeneity of the odds ratio in different categories of a third modifying variable. In this case-control study comparing 217 patients with *in situ* carcinoma of the cervix with 243 population-based female controls, a significant association with smoking is seen (Table A); adjustment for confounding by age makes little difference to this result. However, the odds ratios in the three age categories are substantially different, as shown by their confidence limits (C.L.) and by the $\chi^2$ test for homogeneity over the three subtables. Data from Lyon *et al.* [7], also shown in Ex. 6.24. Calculations shown in Appendix Table 1. The heterogeneity statistic uses the variance formula in 4A of this table

   This analysis assumes a multiplicative model, as discussed in Chapter 3; the relative risk estimates are assumed to be constant. This multiplicative model is assumed in techniques such as the Mantel–Haenszel estimate of odds ratio, and in many multivariate analyses, such as those using the logistic regression model. The attractiveness of this model arises from both its mathematical advantages, as it is a relatively simple model, and the empirical evidence that it appears to apply to a wide range of biomedical applications.
   The situations where such a model can be tested are those in which there are two or more strong risk factors, and enough subjects with the various combinations of categories of these risk factors can be identified and their risks assessed directly. Important examples in medicine which have shown that a

multiplicative model appears to be an appropriate description of the natural state of affairs include the interactions between several major risk factors for coronary heart disease, as shown in the Framingham Study and other major prospective studies [8,9], and the interactions between factors relating to several cancers, such as smoking and asbestos exposure in relation to lung cancer [10] and several others.

There are also some examples where this model does not seem to be appropriate. One relatively simple alternative, also described in Chapter 3, is an additive model in which the risk of disease in subjects exposed to more than one factor is the sum of the excess risks conferred by each of the factors. Such a model implies that the absolute excess risk associated with one factor will be constant in different categories of other factors. This means that the relative risk or odds ratio must vary. For example, in Ex. 7.9 the odds ratio varies with age. However, we know that the baseline risk of *in situ* carcinoma of the cervix increases with age over the age range given in non-smokers; therefore it is possible that the decrease in odds ratio with increase in age may reflect a relatively constant attributable risk associated with smoking in different age groups. We cannot directly test this hypothesis from this case–control study alone, although it could be assessed by using information on the absolute risk in different age categories relevant to the same population. The appropriateness of these different models, and their relevance in both public health and biological terms, has been much discussed. The terms 'interaction', 'synergism', or 'antagonism' can all be used in these contexts, but they are meaningful only if the underlying model regarded as the non-interaction situation is described. Caution in the acceptance and interpretation of interaction is desirable, as it is difficult to detect unless the risk factors concerned have large effects and subjects representing a wide range of categories of the joint distribution of the factors involved are available. In the analysis, it is appropriate not only to show whether a model such as a multiplicative model fits the data, but also that alternative models do not.

## Ordered exposure variables and tests of trend

Frequently the outcome variable has only two categories, while the exposure or intervention variable may have a number of ordered categories. For example, the incidence of lung cancer, a yes/no outcome variable, may be compared in a number of groups of individuals categorized by different levels of smoking, or the survival of a group of patients, a yes/no outcome variable, may be described in terms of a graded measure of the severity of the disease.

To compute relative risks or odds ratios with several exposure categories, an arbitrary category is chosen as the reference category. This is usually the unexposed or minimally exposed category of subjects, although another choice may be made if, for example, that category is extremely small. The relative risks for each of the other categories of exposure are calculated by comparing each category with this constant reference group. If the categories of exposure represent a logically ordered variable, a reasonable a priori hypothesis may be that the association will show a regular dose–response effect, with increasing (or decreasing) relative risks with increasing levels of exposure. An appropriate statistical method in those circumstances is to use the whole data set and test for a linear dose–response effect. A commonly used test is the trend test developed by Mantel [11] as an extension of the Mantel–Haenszel test, which in essence comprises a regression test of the odds ratio against a numeric variable representing the ordered categories of exposure (Appendix Table 7). Where the exposure categories are defined numerically, such as different measured amounts of smoking, they may be represented by numbers taken as the midpoint of the exposure category, or some variation of it such as its logarithm; otherwise arbitrary values such as 0, 1, 2, etc. are chosen to represent categories which, although ordered, are not defined in precise quantitative terms. An example would be stage of disease, the ordering reflecting increasing extent of disease on a qualitative scale. This test yields a chi-squared statistic on 1 d.f. which tests a linear trend in odds ratio over the ordered categories of the exposure variable, and also a chi-squared statistic on $k - 2$ d.f., where $k$ is the number of exposure categories, which tests the deviation of the data from the linear trend. The sum of these two statistics will yield approximately the standard chi-squared statistic for homogeneity, which has $k - 1$ d.f.

Data from a case–control study assessing risk factors for twin births [12] are shown in **Ex. 7.10.** The data show the numbers of cases (twin births) and controls (single births) by maternal parity, in four groups. An ordinary or global chi-squared statistic can be calculated for this 2 × 4 table; it has three degrees of freedom and tests the hypothesis of homogeneity, i.e. that the ratio of cases to controls and therefore the odds ratio is the same in each category. The result is $\chi^2 = 91.2$, $P < 0.001$ (Appendix Table 15 or 16). This statistic would be the same if the same data were in a different order, for example if the odds ratios with increasing parity were 1.0, 1.84, 1.36, and 1.17, although such an irregular pattern would make a direct effect of parity less plausible. It is more informative to apply a linear trend test. Using the formula given in Appendix Table 7, with scores of 0, 1, 2, and 3 for parity, the trend test yields $\chi^2 = 88.0$, d.f. = 1, $P < 0.0001$. The deviation from the linear trend is given by the difference between these, giving $\chi^2 = 3.2$, d.f. = 2, $P = 0.2$; this is non-significant.

TEST FOR TREND IN AN ORDERED VARIABLE

| | Degree of exposure (parity of mother) | | | |
|---|---|---|---|---|
| | 0 | 1 | 2 | 3 + |
| Cases (twins) | 716 | 582 | 454 | 720 |
| Controls (singletons) | 1833 | 1269 | 853 | 1003 |
| Odds ratio | 1.0 (R) | 1.17 | 1.36 | 1.84 |

| | | | |
|---|---|---|---|
| Global $\chi^2$ statistic, test for homogeneity | = 91.2 | d.f. = 3 | $P < 0.001$ |
| Trend $\chi^2$ statistic, test for linear trend | = 88.0 | d.f. = 1 | $P < 0.001$ |
| Residual $\chi^2$ statistic, test for deviations from trend | = 3.2 | d.f. = 2 | $P = 0.2$ |

Thus the data are consistent with a linear increase in twinning by parity
However, this analysis takes no account of confounding

**Ex. 7.10.** Application of a test for trend to an ordered variable. Data from Elwood [12]. Formulae given in Appendix Table 7, p. 530.

The interpretation is that there is a positive association between the frequency of twin births and greater parity of the mother, which is consistent with a linear trend.

Such trend tests should be used with caution. Particularly where there are only a few categories of the exposure variable, a trend can be fitted and may be significant even if inspection of the data shows no regular pattern over the ordered exposure categories. The tests are appropriate primarily where there is an a priori hypothesis of an approximately linear relationship between odds ratio or relative risk and the ordered exposure variable. In such circumstances, the test can be more powerful than the standard chi-squared test for homogeneity in an $n \times 2$ table.

The Mantel trend test can deal easily with stratified data, so that the Mantel–Haenszel estimator of the odds ratio for each category can be calculated after stratification, and the test then assesses a linear trend in these adjusted odds ratios. For example, the analysis in Ex. 7.10 was repeated after stratification for maternal age.

## Statistical tests for data with individual matching

As shown in Chapter 6, in a case–control study controls can be chosen to be matched to the cases on certain confounding factors, and this technique will control matching if and only if the appropriate matched analysis is used, based on the matched sets of cases and controls. For matched case–control data with

---

MATCHED PAIR ANALYSIS

|  |  | Controls | |
| --- | --- | --- | --- |
|  |  | Outcome positive | Outcome negative |
| Cases | Outcome positive | 31 | 30 s |
|  | Outcome negative | 7t | 52 |

Odds ratio = $s/t$ = 30/7 = 4.3

$$\chi^2 \text{ on 1 d.f. } = \frac{(s-t)^2}{s+t} = \frac{23^2}{37} = 14.3 \quad P < 0.001$$

Continuity corrected $\chi^2 = \dfrac{(|s-t|-1)^2}{s+t} = 13.1 \quad P < 0.001$

---

**Ex. 7.11.** Statistical test for 1:1 matched case–control studies: note that both the odds ratio and $\chi^2$ depend only on the numbers of discordant pairs. Data from Ex. 6.26, p. 199.

one control per case, the resultant analysis is simple, and the appropriate statistical test is McNemar's chi-squared test [13], which is shown in **Ex. 7.11.** This test is a special application of the Mantel–Haenszel test for subtables each representing one matched pair. Note that for the calculation of both the odds ratio and the statistic, the only contributors are the pairs which are disparate in exposure, i.e. the pairs where the case was exposed but the control was not, and those where the control was exposed and the case was not. On the null hypothesis the numbers of each of these will be the same.

For a matched case–control study in which a fixed ratio other than one to one is used, such as two or three controls per case, formulae for the calculation of odds ratio estimates and statistical tests are given in Appendix Table 6. Matched cohort studies will not be discussed in detail, as they are less common. The measures of association (relative and attributable risk) are calculated in the same way as for an unmatched cohort study. For statistical tests, the methods for matched case–control data are applicable, although usually very similar results are given by analysing the data in the unmatched format.

## Statistical tests in multivariate analysis

An introduction to multivariate analysis in the control of confounding was given in Chapter 6, and the multiple logistic model was described. In this model, each dependent variable represents an exposure factor. For binary factors (those with only two categories), the odds ratio is estimated as the exponential of the coefficient for that variable, if appropriate coding has been used. There are two main ways in which statistical tests are applied to such models. One is to estimate the significance of each coefficient by taking the ratio of its value to that of its standard error as a standardized normal deviate. The other is to assess the goodness of fit of an entire model to the data set, comparing models by calculating a statistic representing the difference in the log likelihood (a measure of the 'fit' of the model to the data) produced by adding or deleting variables. The log likelihood statistic, or deviance, is a numerical value that indicates the deviation of the fitted model from the data, and the better the model fits the data, the smaller is the statistic. If an exposure variable is added to the model, and that exposure is related to the outcome variable, the value of the log likelihood statistic will decrease. The value of the change in the log likelihood statistic is distributed approximately as a chi-squared statistic, and if $K$ extra variables are entered into the model, the change in the log likelihood can be considered as a chi-squared statistic on $K$ degrees of freedom. This method can be used to assess not only if one extra variable is significant, but if a set of variables, which may represent a number of factors or different categories of one factor, has a significant effect on the fit of the model.

The statistical aspects of the multivariate analysis that was previously presented in Chapter 6 (Ex. 6.27) are shown in **Ex. 7.12**. In this case–control study involving 83 cases and 83 controls [14], the overall model with no independent variables fitted has $n - 1 = 165$ d.f. and a deviance of 230.1. The results of fitting variables singly into the model are equivalent to those from cross-tabulations. Fitting the two binary variables, which together represent the number of moles, gives a change in deviance of 38.1 on 2 d.f. $P < 0.001$. Similarly, for sunburn, coded as one binary variable, the chi-squared statistic is 13.0 on 1 d.f., $P < 0.001$. Therefore both factors show significant associations in single-factor analyses. These chi-squared statistics are the same as those obtained from cross-tabulations (with no continuity correction). The coefficient from the model where only one factor is fitted gives the crude odds ratio associated with that variable, and most computer programs for this analysis produce a standard error estimate of this coefficient, which can be used to calculate confidence limits.

In this analysis there were three other relevant factors (number of freckles in three categories, hair colour in three categories, and usual skin reaction to sun exposure in four categories). Therefore the full model fitted had 10 variables representing the number of moles, sunburn history, and the three other

## MULTIVARIATE ANALYSIS

*Coefficients and standard errors*

| Factor | Model with only one factor | | | | Model with 10 variables representing 5 factors | | | |
|---|---|---|---|---|---|---|---|---|
| | Coeff | Std error | OR | 95% limits | Coeff | Std error | OR | 95% limits |
| No. of moles (reference = 0) | | | | | | | | |
| 1–2 | 0.6008 | 0.4107 | 1.82 | 0.82–4.08 | 0.3011 | 0.4697 | 1.35 | 0.54–3.39 |
| 3+ | 2.830 | 0.5705 | 16.95 | 5.54–51.84 | 2.5870 | 0.6095 | 13.29 | 4.02–43.89 |
| Sunburn history (reference = none) | | | | | | | | |
| yes | 1.150 | 0.3246 | 3.16 | 1.67–5.97 | 0.4276 | 0.4207 | 1.53 | 0.67–3.50 |

*Deviance statistics*

| Model | Deviance | d.f. | Change in deviance | d.f. | |
|---|---|---|---|---|---|
| No variables | 230.1 | 165 | — | — | |
| Moles only | 192.1 | 163 | 38.1 | 2 | $P < 0.001$ |
| Sunburn only | 217.1 | 164 | 13.0 | 1 | $P < 0.001$ |
| Full model | 157.7 | 155 | — | — | |
| Full model less moles | 183.4 | 157 | 25.7 | 2 | $P < 0.001$ |
| Full model less sunburn | 158.9 | 156 | 1.2 | 1 | $P < 0.25$ |

**Ex. 7.12.** Multivariate analysis: the analysis previously shown in Ex. 6.27, fitting a multiple logistic model to data from a case-control study of 83 patients with melanoma and 83 controls. Coeff, fitted coefficient; Std error, Standard error of coefficient; OR, Odds ratio = exponential (coefficient); Limits, exp(coeff ± 1.96 × std error); deviance, log likelihood statistic

factors, and this full model had a deviance of 157.7 with $n - 10 - 1 = 155$ d.f. The results from this full model give coefficients whose exponentials give the odds ratio of each variable, controlled for the presence of all the other variables in the model. The overall effect of a factor represented by a number of variables is best judged by comparing the deviance of the full model, with all factors fitted, with that of the model with that one variable removed. This change in deviance shows the effect of that single factor given that all the other factors are included. Thus, as shown in Ex. 7.12, the factor of number of moles remains highly significant in the presence of all other factors, as removing it from the full model gives a significant increase in the deviance. However, if the sunburn is removed from the full model, the increase in deviance is not statistically significant. The interpretation is that the effect of number of moles on melanoma risk is reduced slightly by control for confounding by the other variables included in this analysis, but remains as a strong and statistically significant association, while the association seen with sunburn history in crude data is greatly reduced by controlling for confounding by the other variables, and is no longer statistically significant.

Multivariate analysis for *individually matched studies* uses 'conditional' models which take account of the matching, i.e. they consider matched sets of cases and controls as sets. They require skilled application. The results are presented in the same way as has been shown, with the same interpretation of the coefficients. Further information is given in the literature [4,15].

## Problems of multiple testing

Some general points about the interpretation of published results can be emphasized. First, let us consider the situation where the results are reported as 'statistically significant'. To interpret this, we must first consider whether the results reported are free from problems of observation bias and confounding. The statistical significance of the result is in itself no protection against these problems. Indeed, an easy way to produce highly significant results is to use a design which is open to severe observation bias; for example biased recall between cases and controls in a retrospective study, or an intervention study using a subjective outcome measure made by someone involved in the intervention being assessed. When these issues have been dealt with, the next step is to know whether the statistical methods used are appropriate and correctly applied.

The issue of multiple testing poses a particular problem in interpretation. The familiar statistical tests such as those that have been described above are designed for hypothesis testing, to be applied to one particular result that has arisen in the course of a study designed to test that association. Where a study produces a large number of associations, such as a study of patient prognosis which assesses 20 factors and uses conventional 5 per cent significance level tests, we expect at least one of these factors to appear as statistically significant even if none of them in truth is related to the outcome. Greater problems arise in observational studies where very large numbers of factors can be assessed, or in explorations of very large data sets. For example, comparisons of all causes of mortality with occupational categories using death registrations and census data may involve comparisons of perhaps 100 categories of causes of death with several hundred possible occupations. Genetic and proteonomic studies may assess fairly small numbers of subjects, applying very large banks of markers, which will produce many associations by chance alone. Special statistical methods, some of which are quite complex, have been developed for these situations. In intervention trials, repeated testing may be planned, as discussed below.

The issue of to what extent the existence of other comparisons should be taken into account when assessing a particular result is one of considerable dispute. It is valuable to distinguish between results from *hypothesis testing studies* that have been specifically set up to test a particular hypothesis, and those from studies in which a large number of associations have been examined. The latter studies may be considered as having a *hypothesis generation* function, and the validity of particular results from the study will be uncertain until confirmatory evidence is available from further work. A further issue in the interpretation of positive results is publication bias, which is discussed in the next chapter.

## Appropriate and inappropriate subgroup analyses

In most clinical trials and observational studies, the studies will usually be designed and have adequate statistical power to test the main comparisons specified in the protocol. However, there will be a great tendency to test for many other differences, for example in subgroups. **Exhibit 7.13** shows some results of an important randomized trial which assessed the use of both streptokinase and aspirin in reducing the death rate in patients who had a suspected acute myocardial infarction [16]. Some of the results for aspirin are shown. In the whole trial, over 8500 patients were randomized to receive aspirin starting as soon as possible after the onset of symptoms, and a similar number were randomized to placebo. The overall result shows a reduced death rate in the aspirin group, with an odds ratio of 0.77 and 95 per cent confidence limits of 0.70 to 0.85. These confidence limits are calculated by the methods shown in Appendix Table 2, and are identical to those reported in the paper.

DANGERS OF SUBGROUP ANALYSIS

| | | Aspirin | | | Placebo | | | Odds ratio | 95% confidence limits | | MH odds ratio | Heterogeneity test | |
|---|---|---|---|---|---|---|---|---|---|---|---|---|---|
| | | deaths | total number | death rate % | deaths | total number | death rate % | | | | | Chi sq | P value |
| All patients | | 804 | 8587 | 9.36 | 1016 | 8600 | 11.81 | 0.77 | 0.70 | 0.85 | | | |
| Prior myocardial infarct | Yes | 219 | 1454 | 15.08 | 219 | 1484 | 14.76 | 1.02 | 0.84 | 1.25 | | | |
| | No | 576 | 7038 | 8.18 | 778 | 7005 | 11.11 | 0.71 | 0.64 | 0.80 | 0.78 | 9.30 | 0.0023 |
| Astrological birth sign | Gemini / Libra | 150 | 1357 | 11.05 | 147 | 1442 | 10.19 | 1.09 | 0.86 | 1.39 | | | |
| | Other | 654 | 7228 | 9.05 | 868 | 7157 | 12.13 | 0.72 | 0.65 | 0.80 | 0.77 | 9.67 | 0.0019 |

**Ex. 7.13.** Dangers of subgroup analysis: data from a large randomized trial of aspirin in treatment of a suspected acute myocardial infarction, showing total results, and a subgroup analysis by prior myocardial infarction, one of 26 subgroup analyses done. Also shown is an analysis of astrological birth sign. From ISIS-1 (Second International Study of Infarct Survival) Collaborative Group [16]

This 23 per cent reduction in deaths is obviously clinically important, and is statistically significant. With these data, relative risks could equally easily be used.

A small number of subgroup analyses were planned in the protocol to the study, but many others were carried out, comparing groups subdivided by sex, age groups, different levels of blood pressure and heart rate, with or without cardiograph abnormalities, and so on. One result was that no beneficial effect of aspirin was seen in patients who had had a previous myocardial infarction (odds ratio 1.02), and the effect was correspondingly greater in those who had not had a previous infarction (odds ratio 0.71). This difference is substantial, the confidence limits do not overlap, and a statistical test of heterogeneity shows that the difference in effects is highly significant ($P = 0.002$). This would seem to be clinically important, as it suggests that this aspirin is a useful therapy only for patients who have no previous history of myocardial infarction. However, this subgroup analysis was unplanned and was one of 26 such analyses, of which this was the only one which showed a statistically significant variation. Thus, despite its statistical significance, this is likely to be a chance finding, and in the discussion in the paper the investigators suggest that it is implausible, given other knowledge of the effects of aspirin on heart disease. To demonstrate the dangers of unplanned subgroup analyses, the investigators also published the results from a subdivision of patients by astrological birth sign. As shown in Ex.7.13, this showed that patients with Gemini or Libra birth signs showed no benefit of aspirin (odds ratio 1.09), and the benefit was confined to those with other birth signs (odds ratio 0.72). This difference is also statistically significant with a similar $P$ value for heterogeneity as was found in the other subdivision ($P = 0.002$).

Therefore, to be reliable, a subgroup analysis should be defined in advance, before the data are examined, giving a specific hypothesis that can be tested. In contrast, the subgroup analysis by birth sign used one of many possible ways of grouping birth signs, and this choice was influenced by the data. Such analyses have been referred to as *post hoc*, after the fact, data-driven, or the result of data dredging or fishing.

## Repeated testing in trials: stopping rules and data-monitoring groups

In intervention trials, it is often desirable to monitor the results at regular intervals, or continuously, so that the trial can be stopped as soon as a definitive result is obtained, or when it is clear that no significant difference will be seen. This introduces a problem of multiple testing, and specific statistical methods have been developed, such as sequential trial designs [17]. An example of these is shown in the trial discussed in Chapter 11. It also requires an *independent data-monitoring group*, as the investigators themselves should not know the ongoing results of the trial. Most major trials have an independent data-monitoring group, which will assess interim results and decide if the trial should be continued or stopped earlier than anticipated. This is only one of their functions; they act as an independent assessment group on all aspects of the trial design, and particularly the collection, coding, input, and interpretation of the data. They contribute to statistical and clinical decision-making, and to quality control including ethical safeguards. The statistical methods used take into account the fact that the data are being examined on many occasions. For example, during the randomized trial of clofibrate in the treatment of heart disease, referred to in Chapter 6 (Ex. 6.14), on three occasions during the monitoring of the trial the death rate was lower in the treatment than in the placebo group, and would have been significantly lower if tested by the routine statistical test using a 5 per cent cut-off. However, the difference was not significant when assessed by methods appropriate for repeated monitoring of a trial, and so the trial was continued; the final results showed no significant difference between the group randomized to clofibrate and the comparison group.

Several major randomized trials have been stopped early or modified after such monitoring. In the trial of prevention of neural tube defects discussed in detail in Chapter 11, the results passed the level of significance demanded by a sequential test when only about two-thirds of the original planned number of participants had been enrolled, and the trial was terminated early. The recent studies of beta-carotene are another good example. As was discussed in Chapter 6, case–control and cohort studies had shown associations between high intakes or high blood levels of beta-carotene and lower cancer and heart disease rates, and these results were supported by the antioxidant properties of beta-carotene, protecting against DNA damage and inhibiting carcinogens in experimental situations. A trial of various nutritional interventions, including beta-carotene, was carried out in almost 30 000 subjects in rural China, and demonstrated a 13 per cent reduction in total cancer mortality [18]. However, a randomized trial in a well-nourished lower risk group, 22 000 American doctors, showed no effect [19], and a trial on 29 000 male smokers in Finland showed an 18 per cent *increase* in lung cancer incidence and an 8 per cent increase in total mortality in those randomized to beta-carotene [20]. Then in a large trial in the USA involving 18 000 subjects who were smokers or ex-asbestos workers, interim results assessed by the monitoring committee showed a 28 per cent increase in lung cancer incidence and a 17 per cent increase in total mortality [21]. The trial was terminated 20 months early, and the use of beta-carotene supplementation as one part of a further trial involving female health professionals in the USA was also stopped.

## Interpreting non-significant results

The interpretation of the results that are reported as not showing statistical significance also raises several issues. Again, we must consider first the issues of observation bias and confounding, assessing whether there are problems that could make the observed result smaller than the true result; these include the problem of random error. Again, we must assess if the statistical methods used are appropriate and correctly applied, although the issue of multiple testing is not important here. The main issue in interpreting non-significant results is to what extent we can accept that there is no true difference between the groups being compared. A *type 2*, or *beta*, error is made if the result is non-significant when there is a true difference. The computation of confidence limits is very useful, as these show the range of values of the association with which the results are compatible. Where limits are not shown in the original material, it is often possible to calculate approximate limits from the statistical test data, as shown in Ex. 7.7. If the non-significant result is based upon a small study, the confidence limits will be wide, making it clear that we cannot conclude that there is no appreciable difference between the groups being compared. The consideration of confidence limits calculated for two or more studies of the same topic will often show that the studies are not inconsistent, despite the fact that in one the result may be statistically significantly different from the null hypothesis value and in the other study it might not; indeed, that was shown in Ex. 7.5.

## Statistical power and the size of a study

Go back to Ex. 7.5 (p. 235) and look again at study B. This result is rather unsatisfactory. From 72 subjects, there is a higher success rate in the intervention compared with the comparison group, but this effect is not statistically significant, and the confidence limits show that we cannot confidently decide whether the intervention is beneficial or not. The basic problem is that the study is too small. It does not provide a definite answer. In technical terms, the study lacks *power*. To avoid committing ourselves to performing studies like study B, it would be helpful to be able to predict the power of a study. We shall now present some fairly simple mathematical aspects of this; but readers who wish to avoid these may go on to the section on dealing with a statistician (p. 264).

## Factors affecting the power of a study

Several factors affect the power of a study (**Ex. 7.14**). The first is the *strength of the association*, for example the difference in outcome rates between the two groups, or the relative risk or odds ratio. The larger the true difference, the easier it will be to detect.

The second is the *frequency of the outcome*. The effective size of a cohort or intervention study is not the total number of subjects in the study, but depends mainly on the number of subjects who experience the outcome events. Similarly, the effective size of a case–control study depends mainly on the number of cases and controls who have the exposure under consideration. In study B in Ex. 7.5, the number of subjects experiencing outcome events is considerably less than the total number of subjects (15 rather than 72). If this number were increased, for example by doing the study on patients with a higher frequency of success, or by extending the follow-up time, the study would have more power even though the same number of patients were entered initially. The maximum power for a fixed total number of subjects and a particular relative risk will be when about half the subjects have the outcome, or in a case–control design where half have the exposure under consideration.

---

FACTORS INFLUENCING THE NECESSARY SIZE OF A STUDY

| | |
|---|---|
| Strength of the association | Size decreases as the difference in frequency increases; size depends approximately on the square of the difference |
| Frequency of the outcome (cohort and intervention studies) or of the exposure (case–control studies) | Size minimum when frequency close to 50 per cent |
| Significance level | Size increases as significance level decreases, i.e. a more stringent test is used; higher for a two-sided than for a one-sided test |
| Power | Size increases as power increases |
| Confounding | Size increases if confounder control, by stratification or multivariate methods, is required; may decrease in individually matched study |
| Error | Size increases if non-differential misclassification of either exposure or outcome |

**Ex. 7.14.** Factors influencing the necessary size of a comparative study

The next factors to be considered are the significance level and the power. The *significance level* is the cut-off point that will be used to determine whether the association found is regarded as statistically significant. It is most frequently at the $P = 0.05$ level, using a two-sided test. The significance level, or alpha ($\alpha$), is the frequency with which a 'significant' result occurs when in truth there is no difference; this type of error is called an *alpha*, $\alpha$, or *type 1* error. In setting a significance level, we are deciding what risk we will accept that the study will show an (incorrect) significant result when the true situation is that there is no difference. In some circumstances the direction of the effect may be regarded as fixed and tests used which assess only effects in one direction, and a one-sided test may be used. If we are to apply a 5 per cent one-sided test rather than a 5 per cent two-sided test, fewer subjects will be required.

The *power* of a study is its ability to demonstrate an association, given that the association exists. The frequency with which we will see no significant difference, if in truth there is a difference, is referred to as beta ($\beta$); this is a beta, or type 2, error. A more powerful study is one that is less likely to miss an effect; the power of the study is $1 - \beta$. If in reality a true association is present, our ability to recognize it will be greater with a larger sample, a stronger association, and a higher frequency of outcome. A typical value of power is 80 per cent; the study is designed so that the chance of detecting a true difference is 80 per cent, and we accept that we will miss the true difference in 20 per cent of instances. For an exploratory study we may decide that missing a true difference (i.e. obtaining a false-negative result) is unimportant, and we may be content with a lower power, requiring fewer subjects. If we need to be confident that we will not miss a true effect, we may need a power of 90 per cent or more, which will require many more subjects.

For both significance level ($\alpha$) and power ($\beta = 1 -$ power), the corresponding normal deviates $Z_\alpha$ and $Z_\beta$, go into the formula, usually in a term $(Z_\alpha + Z_\beta)^2$, which we call $K$ for convenience. The deviates for commonly used values of $\alpha$ and $\beta$, and the corresponding values of $K$, are given in **Ex. 7.15**.

These four factors are the components of the formulae generally used for sample size determination, which will be described below. Two other factors also affect the necessary size. If confounder control by stratification or multivariate methods is to be used, the study size required is increased. However, an individually matched study, where the analysis will use the matched sets, may need a smaller sample size for the same power. Non-differential misclassification, as described in Chapter 5, will lead to a larger sample size being needed. This effect can be assessed by calculating the observable odds ratio or risk difference after allowing for misclassification, as shown in Chapter 5, and using it

CONSTANTS FOR USE IN SAMPLE SIZE FORMULAE

A. *Table relating normal deviates to power and to significance level*

| Power $(1-\beta)$ (%) | Z-value (Normal deviate) | Significance level $(\alpha)$ | |
|---|---|---|---|
| | | One-sided | Two-sided |
| 99.5 | 2.58 | 0.005 | 0.01 |
| 99 | 2.33 | 0.01 | 0.02 |
| 98 | 1.96 | 0.025 | 0.05 |
| 95 | 1.64 | 0.05 | 0.1 |
| 90 | 1.28 | 0.1 | 0.2 |
| 80 | 0.84 | 0.2 | 0.4 |
| 70 | 0.52 | 0.3 | 0.6 |
| 50 | 0.0 | 0.5 | |

B. *Values of $K = (Z_\alpha + Z_\beta)^2$, for commonly used values of $\alpha$ and $\beta$*

| | | Power | | | | | |
|---|---|---|---|---|---|---|---|
| | | 50% | 80% | 90% | 95% | | |
| Sigificance level | | | | | | Sigificance level | |
| Two-sided | 0.1 | 2.7 | 6.2 | 8.6 | 10.8 | 0.05 | One-sided |
| value | 0.05 | 3.8 | 7.9 | 10.5 | 13.0 | 0.025 | value |
| | 0.02 | 5.4 | 10.0 | 13.0 | 15.8 | 0.01 | |
| | 0.01 | 6.6 | 11.7 | 14.9 | 17.8 | 0.005 | |

**Ex. 7.15.** Normal deviates corresponding to frequently used values for significance levels $(Z_\alpha)$ and power $(Z_\beta)$; and table of $K$ where $K = (Z_\alpha + Z_\beta)^2$. The value of $Z_\beta$ is the normal deviate corresponding to the one-sided test for (1 − power)

for the determination of the size of the study needed. Methods of determining study size with allowance for these various factors are available, which is why the formulae given below should be used only as a guide, and expert advice should be sought for any major study. Finally, the study size given in the formulae refers to the number of study participants in *each* group being compared who complete the study and provide full data for analysis. In designing a study, allowance has to be made for non-response and possible incompleteness of data.

The power of a study is increased by increasing the number of subjects in the study, in the intervention or case group, or in the comparison group, or in both. When a similar effort is required to enrol a test or a comparison subject, studies with equal numbers in each group are optimal. A slight variation of this may be made on the basis of the projected effects, as the information in the study depends on the number of subjects with the outcome in a cohort study, or the number with the exposure in a case–control study, and slight modifications of the ratio may be made to design a study where the number of outcome events or exposed subjects is likely to be the same. For example, more than half the patients in a trial may be allocated to the new therapy, on the basis of the anticipated benefit yielding equal numbers of deaths in each group. It may be easier to increase the size of the comparison group than of the intervention or case group because more potential subjects are available, data on them has already been collected, or the number of exposed subjects or cases is fixed. The power of the study is increased by increasing the number of controls, but this is less effective than increasing both groups.

## Estimating the size of study which is needed

From the four parameters of the expected frequency of the outcome in the control group, the difference in outcome rates, the significance level, and the power, a calculation of the sample size to satisfy those criteria can be made. Some appropriate formulae are illustrated in **Ex. 7.16.** The formulae can obviously be used in other ways. It is often useful to calculate the power of the study from the sample size readily available, to show if a proposed investigation is worthwhile or if more ambitious methods need to be used. The following examples will show the application of these formulae.

(1)  For a clinical trial. Suppose that the mortality rate in 2 years from conventional therapy is 40 per cent, and a new therapy would be useful if the rate fell to 30 per cent. How many patients do we need? Setting a significance level of 0.05 one-sided, and a power of 80 per cent, yields $K = 6.2$ and $n = 279$, i.e. 279 subjects in each group. If we were content to detect a larger difference, such as 20 per cent mortality with the new therapy, then $n = 62$; note the large change in $n$ for a substantial change in $(p_1 - p_2)$.

(2)  For an epidemiological cohort study. We wish to test whether the breast cancer rate is increased in oral contraceptive users, and estimate a 10-year cumulative incidence in unexposed women of 0.01 (1 per cent). We set significance at 0.05 two-sided and power at 90 per cent, and wish to be able to detect a doubling of risk to 0.02; hence $K = 10.5$ and $n = 3098$.

(3)  A colleague hopes that a new therapy will increase the proportion of patients recovering from his current 40 per cent to 60 per cent. He sees 100 patients each year whom he would like to enter into a trial. Is it worth it?

Set significance at 0.05 one-sided. Hence $Z_\alpha = 1.64$; $p_1 = 0.4$, $p_2 = 0.6$, $n = 50$; therefore $Z_\beta = 2.04 - 1.64 = 0.40$. From Ex. 7.15, the power is less

## FORMULAE FOR SAMPLE SIZE ESTIMATION

*For cohort or trial design, with equal groups*

$$n = \frac{(p_1 q_1 + p_2 q_2) \cdot K}{(p_1 - p_2)^2}$$

$n$ = number of subjects in each group

where $p_1$ = frequency of outcome in group 1 $\qquad q_1 = 1 - p_1$
$\qquad p_2$ = frequency of outcome in group 2 $\qquad q_2 = 1 - p_2$
$K = (Z_\alpha + Z_\beta)^2$ where $Z_\alpha$ and $Z_\beta$ are normal deviates corresponding to significance level $\alpha$ and power $(1 - \beta)$.

To calculate power

$$Z_\beta = \frac{(p_1 - p_2) \cdot \sqrt{n}}{\sqrt{(p_1 q_1 + p_2 q_2)}} - Z_\alpha$$

*For case–control study*

Same formulae, where
$\quad p_1$ = frequency of exposure in cases
$\quad p_2$ = frequency of exposure in controls

Use of odds ratio

Given the proportion of controls exposed, $p_2$, and the odds ratio predicted, $OR$, the proportion of cases exposed, $p_1$, is given by:

$$p_1 = \frac{p_2 \cdot OR}{1 + p_2(OR - 1)}$$

*Unequal groups*

If there are $c$ comparison subjects for each exposed subject or case

$$n = \frac{(1 + 1/c) \cdot \bar{p}\,\bar{q} \cdot K}{(p_1 - p_2)^2} \quad \text{where } \bar{p} = \left(\frac{p_1 + p_2}{2}\right) \text{and } \bar{q} = 1 - \bar{p}$$

$$Z_\beta = \frac{(p_1 - p_2) \cdot \sqrt{n}}{\sqrt{((1 + 1/c)\bar{p}\,\bar{q})}} - Z_\alpha$$

where $n$ = number of exposed subjects or cases

**Ex. 7.16.** Formulae for calculating the size of a study: for the meaning and values of $Z_\alpha$, $Z_\beta$ and $K$, see Ex. 7.15. A formula for 1:1 matched studies is given in Appendix Table 8, p. 534.

than 70 per cent; for more accuracy, use Excel to give the one-sided probability of this value of 0.40 in the normal distribution (Appendix Table 16). This yields 0.35, i.e. a power of $1 - 0.35$ or 65 per cent. His study would miss a difference of the size given on one occasion out of three, and is too weak. For adequate power (e.g. 80 per cent), he would need 74 patients in each group; for 90 per cent, 103 patients. Thus a 2-year accrual period would be likely to be satisfactory if all subjects seen could be entered into the study.

(4) In a case–control study, we wish to be able to detect a doubling of risk (odds ratio = 2) associated with a factor which is present in 10 per cent of the normal population from which the control series will be drawn. Hence $p_2 = 0.1$ and $p_1$ is given by Ex. 7.16 as 0.182; if power = 80 per cent, and significance level = 0.05 two-sided, $K = 7.9$ and $n = 280$. We need approximately 300 cases and 300 controls. If controls are easily found, we might wish to try a study with, say, three controls per case. Keeping the other parameters the same, $p = 0.14$, $q = 0.86$, and $n = 190$; a study design with 200 cases and 600 controls would give similar power to one with 300 cases and 300 controls.

The formulae given here are fairly simple. More complex sample size calculations are available in standard texts, websites, and computer programs [22–24]. The justification for presenting only a simple formulation here is that the general reader should use such formulae only as a broad guide. In practice, many quantities are unknown when a study is being contemplated; not only the likely difference between the outcomes, but the extent of loss of information by drop-outs or missing data and the extent to which stratification or other techniques will have to be used which will reduce the power of the study. The main usefulness of these sample size formulae is to indicate a minimum value for the number of subjects necessary for a particular study, or conversely the approximate power that is achievable with the numbers available. Such calculations may show that the numbers of subjects needed far exceed those readily available, or conversely that the power of the study is very low, perhaps 50 per cent or less. Such results should be taken to indicate that the study as envisaged is not a worthwhile endeavour and a different approach is necessary, such as moving from a single-centre to a multi-centre study, or addressing the question on a different set of subjects or in a different way. We need to emphasize that these calculations take only statistical sampling variation into account. There is no allowance for incomplete records, drop-outs, or errors in ascertainment, and no allowance for the requirements of more detailed analysis to adjust for confounding or assess results in subgroups.

It is often helpful to compare the power produced by studies with different numbers of subjects, and to calculate a 'power curve', i.e. a graph showing the relationship between sample size and power within the other constraints of the study. This will help to choose the most efficient design, which is the one that gives the most information for least cost in subjects, time, and finances.

The major properties of the formulae are useful guides (Ex. 7.16). The number of patients required is inversely proportional to the square of the difference in outcome rates; in other words, if the difference to be detected is halved, the number of subjects required will be four times as large. The biological effect of a factor will be expected to give a certain ratio of outcome events; the difference in numbers corresponding to a fixed ratio will be greater if the frequency of the outcome is higher, up to 50 per cent. Given that a new intervention reduces mortality by a third, it is easier to detect a difference between 45 and 30 per cent mortality than between 15 and 10 per cent; often a study design can be made more efficient by selecting subjects who have a high risk of the outcome under investigation. There is little room to manoeuvre in terms of significance levels, and one should not be overly tempted to use one-sided significance levels unless these are clearly indicated. The remaining factor is the relationship between the number of subjects and power. A study with 80 per cent power requires about twice as many subjects as one with 50 per cent power, and a very powerful study with 95 per cent power requires about 60 per cent more subjects than one of 80 per cent power.

As mentioned earlier, when a similar effort is required to enrol a test or a comparison subject, studies with equal numbers in each group are optimal, but otherwise studies with more controls and cases can be used. Exhibit 7.16 shows that the power of a study with $n$ subjects in each group is equalled by one with $c$ controls per test subject, and $n[1 + (1/c)]/2$ test subjects; therefore an alternative to finding 100 cases and 100 controls is to use, say, two controls per case and find 75 cases and 150 controls. A little arithmetic will show the decreasing benefit of increasing the ratio of controls to cases; unless data for controls are very easy to obtain, for example by being available on a computer file, it is rarely worth using ratios greater than 5:1.

It is a requirement of the scientific review process for research funding that investigators show that their proposed study will have sufficient statistical power to give an adequately precise result. Increasingly ethical committees are also examining this aspect, as a study with inadequate power is unethical because it will not provide scientific value. Reports of completed studies should describe the initial planned study size and its rationale, particularly if the final study includes fewer or more subjects.

## Dealing with a statistician about study design

When designing a major study, statistical help should be requested in regard with sample size. However, the non-statistical reader should be prepared for the questions which the statistician will ask, which amount in principle to a prediction of the results of the study. In cohort studies and trials, we need to predict the *frequency of the outcome in the control group* and *the size of the difference* between control and exposed groups which we regard as worth detecting. To arrive at this judgement it is worth thinking in operational terms; if the frequency of the outcome in the comparison series, such as patients treated on conventional therapy, is a certain percentage, to what would this have to change before we would wish to employ the new therapy? For a case–control design, the statistician will want to know the likely *frequency of exposure* in the comparison group, which may be obtained from literature or a pilot study, and the *size of the association* to be detected, best expressed as the odds ratio. The remaining questions are to define the *significance level* and the desired *power* of the study. For the first, there is rarely a good reason to stray from the convention of the 5 per cent level. The question of one-sided and two-sided tests has been alluded to. As to power, a frequently used starting point is 80 per cent in an exploratory study; in a study to reassess a finding or in other circumstances where it is important not to miss a true association, higher power is desirable.

## Part 3. Lifetable methods: the analysis of cohort and intervention studies taking the timing of the outcome events into consideration.

So far in this text we have presented the results of cohort and intervention studies in terms of the numbers of subjects with and without the outcome in question ('count data'), or the numbers of subjects experiencing the outcome divided by the total person-years of observation ('person-time data'). These methods are valid only if the outcome can be adequately expressed in this simple form, which is true only if the follow-up time period is the same for the different groups of subjects being compared, or if the risk of the outcome is constant over the time course of the study. Lifetable methods of analysis were developed to overcome these difficulties. They are used in intervention trials and cohort studies where the risk of the outcome events varies with the time interval since the intervention or exposure, and where the period of follow-up varies for different individuals in the study. All aspects of the scheme for critical appraisal described in this text are applicable to these studies.

# Survival curves

In cohort studies where the period of follow-up of individuals varies, the number of outcome events must be related to the person-time experience during which an event could occur. In the person-time type of analysis shown in Chapter 3 we assumed that the risk of the outcome was constant over time, and therefore groups of subjects could be adequately compared by looking only at their total person-time experience and the number of events occurring. In many situations this is manifestly not true. For example, after an acute myocardial infarction, the risk of death is initially high and then decreases rapidly. If we compare 50 patients who have each been followed up for 1 year with 600 patients who have each been followed up for 1 month, the total person-time experience of each group is the same, but we would expect the death rates, as deaths per unit person-time, to be much higher in the second group. To reduce this problem we divide the follow-up period into small sections, and assess the probability of an outcome event happening in each small section of the follow-up period. Because these methods have been most widely used in assessing survival after diagnosis or treatment, they are often referred to as *survival* analyses. However, the methods can be applied to any non-recurrent outcome event, such as death, recovery, onset of a complication, return to work, or discharge from hospital. The results can be expressed either as the proportion of subjects at different times who have not undergone the event, as is seen in a survival curve, or as a proportion of subjects who have undergone the event, which gives a *cumulative incidence* curve. **Exhibit 7.17** shows a survival curve for a group of patients with breast cancer, showing the proportion of the original group who are still alive at various points from the date of diagnosis; at 3 years after diagnosis, 68 per cent of patients are still alive. The same data could be plotted to show the cumulative incidence of death; at 3 years, 32 per cent have died.

To construct such a curve, we need to know for each individual in the study the *starting date* of the period of observation, the *finishing date* of this period, and the *outcome* for that individual. The starting date in a clinical situation may be defined as the date of diagnosis, the date of first treatment, or in a randomized study the date of randomization. In an epidemiological cohort study the starting date may be the date of first exposure to the exposure under investigation, such as working in a particular job or using a drug.

In a simple example assessing survival in a group of patients, the survival curve is simply the proportion surviving at various points in time. The 'curve' has, in fact, a step-type pattern; if we start with 10 patients the survival rate is 100 per cent until one dies, then it remains at 90 per cent until another dies,

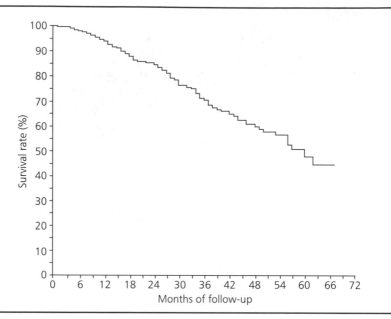

**Ex. 7.17.** Survival of 596 patients with breast cancer from date of confirmed diagnosis, calculated by the product limit method. For this graph, only deaths from breast cancer were counted; the few other deaths were not, the observations being censored at that point

and so on. As the number of patients enrolled in the study increases, each step becomes smaller and the curve appears smoother. Usually we do not know all the dates of death, as some patients will still be alive at the time of analysis and others may have been lost to follow-up, so that their current status will be unknown. The observations on these patients are *censored*. Censoring also occurs if the particular endpoint under study is precluded by another event; for example, if we wish to count only deaths from a certain cause, other deaths produce censored observations. We shall describe two commonly used methods for constructing a survival curve: the product-limit method (also known as the Kaplan–Meier estimate) and the actuarial or life-table method.

## The product-limit method

Consider the data in **Ex. 7.18,** which shows survival times for 20 subjects, and at this point ignore the treatment designation. The data show survival time in months, calculated from the date of diagnosis to the date of death, arranged with the subjects in order of increasing survival time. Eight subjects are still alive or have been lost to follow-up. For them, we use the date of the last

SURVIVAL DATA

| Patient no. | Survival time, (months)* | Treatment group |
|---|---|---|
| 14 | 1 | A |
| 12 | 1 | A |
| 13 | 3 + | A |
| 4 | 4 | A |
| 7 | 6 | A |
| 2 | 9 + | B |
| 9 | 11 + | A |
| 8 | 11 + | B |
| 19 | 12 | A |
| 20 | 13 | B |
| 1 | 15 | A |
| 3 | 16 | B |
| 15 | 22 | B |
| 5 | 22 + | A |
| 10 | 23 | A |
| 6 | 23 | B |
| 16 | 25 + | B |
| 11 | 32 + | B |
| 17 | 32 + | B |
| 18 | 41 | B |

* + indicates a censored observation

**Ex. 7.18.** Hypothetical survival data arranged in order of increasing survival time for a clinical trial with 10 patients in each of two treatment groups. Note: Trials of this size are not recommended; this is for explanation only

follow-up assessment, but indicate that their survival times are censored. The product-limit method is based on two simple concepts. First, subjects with censored observations are included in the total number of subjects at risk of death only up to the time of their censoring. Secondly, we use a simple application of probability logic in calculating that the chance of surviving 2 months equals the probability of surviving the first month multiplied by the probability of surviving the second, and so on with subsequent months.

The calculations are shown in **Ex. 7.19.** Two deaths occurred in the first month, so that the probability of surviving that month was 18/20 or 0.9, and the survival at 1 month, i.e. at the end of the first month, was 0.9. No deaths occurred during the second month and during the third month there was one censored observation but still no deaths, so that the cumulative survival by the

### SURVIVAL CURVE CALCULATION

| Interval $i$ | Interval between deaths (months) | No. of deaths at end of interval $d_i$ | No. of patients alive immediately prior to end of interval $n_i$ | Probability of surviving interval $P_i = 1 - (d_i/n_i)$ | Value of survival curve subsequent to interval $S_i = S_{i-1} \times P_i$ | Standard error of survival curve |
|---|---|---|---|---|---|---|
| 0 | 0 | — | — | 1.0000 | 1.0000 | — |
| 1 | 0–1 | 2 | 20 | 0.9000 | 0.9000 | 0.0671 |
| 2 | 1–4 | 1 | 17 | 0.9412 | 0.8471 | 0.0814 |
| 3 | 4–6 | 1 | 16 | 0.9375 | 0.7941 | 0.0919 |
| 4 | 6–12 | 1 | 12 | 0.9167 | 0.7279 | 0.1054 |
| 5 | 12–13 | 1 | 11 | 0.9091 | 0.6618 | 0.1147 |
| 6 | 13–15 | 1 | 10 | 0.9000 | 0.5956 | 0.1209 |
| 7 | 15–16 | 1 | 9 | 0.8889 | 0.5294 | 0.1242 |
| 8 | 16–22 | 1 | 8 | 0.8750 | 0.4632 | 0.1251 |
| 9 | 22–23 | 2 | 6 | 0.6667 | 0.3088 | 0.1221 |
| 10 | 23–41 | 1 | 1 | 0.0000 | 0.0000 | |

**Ex. 7.19.** Calculation of product limit estimate of survival curve from data in Ex. 7.18. Formula for standard error given in text

end of the third month was $0.9 \times 1 \times 1 = 0.9$. During the fourth month one death occurred; because only 17 subjects were under follow-up at the time the probability of survival was 16/17 or 0.94, and the cumulative survival at the end of the fourth month was $0.94 \times 0.9 = 0.85$. The survival curve changes only when a death occurs; hence a calculation need be made only when this happens. Therefore each relevant interval ends when one or more deaths occur. The resultant step-type curve is shown in **Ex. 7.20.**

The estimation of survival by this method not only allows for censoring, but gives an efficient estimate since in each section of the follow-up period the information available on all subjects observed during that interval is used. The adjustment made for censored observations assumes that they are censored randomly, i.e. we assume that the subjects whose data are censored at a certain time have a subsequent course similar to that of the subjects remaining under follow-up. If this is not so, bias will result; for example, if those lost to follow-up do worse than those followed, perhaps because very ill subjects no longer attend for treatment, the calculated survival curve will overestimate the actual survival which would be correctly calculated if full information were available. The product-limit method gives the survival curve that is the most likely estimate, in statistical terminology the 'maximum likelihood' estimate of the true survival curve.

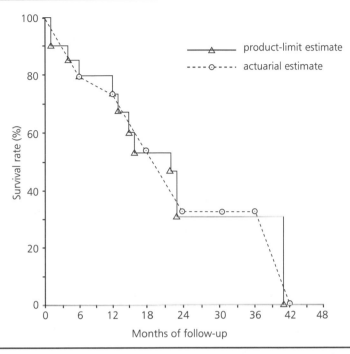

**Ex. 7.20.** Survival curves for the data shown in Ex. 7.18. The step pattern is the product-limit survival curve calculated in Ex. 7.19. The dotted line is the actuarial curve calculated in Ex. 7.21

## The actuarial or life-table method

Because hand calculation of the product-limit estimate is tedious with a large set of data, the actuarial or life-table method can be used. This gives an approximation to the product-limit estimate, with the number of calculations being reduced by grouping the data into suitable intervals of follow-up, such as 1 year or 3 months. Calculations for the data used in Ex. 7.18, with a 6-month interval, are shown in **Ex. 7.21.** For each time interval we calculate the probability of surviving that interval, which is given as 1 minus the probability of dying during that time interval. The probability of dying is given by the number of deaths during the interval divided by the number of subjects under follow-up during that interval. This denominator is estimated as the number of subjects alive at the beginning of the interval minus half the number whose data are censored during the interval. We are making the assumption that if subjects are censored during an interval, their follow-up experience is

ACTUARIAL SURVIVAL

| Interval (months) | Patients alive at start $r_i$ | Patients censored $c_i$ | Patients 'at risk' $n_i = r_i - \frac{1}{2}c_i$ | Deaths during interval $d_i$ | Probability of surviving interval $P_i = 1-(d_i/n_i)$ | Survival curve estimate $S_i = S_{i-1} \times P_i$ |
|---|---|---|---|---|---|---|
| 0–6 | 20 | 1 | 19.5 | 4 | 0.7949 | 0.7949 |
| 7–12 | 15 | 3 | 13.5 | 1 | 0.9259 | 0.7360 |
| 13–18 | 11 | 0 | 11.0 | 3 | 0.7273 | 0.5353 |
| 19–24 | 8 | 1 | 7.5 | 3 | 0.6000 | 0.3212 |
| 25–30 | 4 | 1 | 3.5 | 0 | 1.0 | 0.3212 |
| 30–36 | 3 | 2 | 2.0 | 0 | 1.0 | 0.3212 |
| 37–42 | 1 | 0 | 1.0 | 1 | 0.0 | 0.0 |

**Ex. 7.21.** Calculation of actuarial estimate of survival curve from the data in Ex. 7.18. using 6-month intervals. This example is to show the method; the actuarial method is not advisable with such small numbers, but is useful with large sets of data

approximately half that interval. The cumulative probability of survival is calculated, as with the product-limit method, as the product of the probability of survival over each of the intervals up to that point. The resultant survival curve is shown in Ex. 7.20.

Survival curves are usually shown with an arithmetic horizontal scale, and either an arithmetic or a logarithmic vertical scale. If the risk of death during each section of the follow-up period is in fact the same, a survival curve with an arithmetic vertical scale will show an exponential decreasing curve, while one with a logarithmic scale will show a straight line. Product-limit estimates, being actual calculations of survival rate at every event, are best shown by stepped patterns, while actuarial estimates are an approximation and can reasonably be shown as a series of points connected by straight lines. The intervals chosen for actuarial calculation need not be of equal length and are often chosen on a convenient arbitrary basis, such as annual intervals; but they should be short enough to keep the number of censored observations in any interval relatively small.

## Accuracy of estimates

The standard error of the survival rate $S_i$ at the end of a given interval is given by

$$SE = S_i \sqrt{\left( \sum_i \frac{1-P_i}{n_i P_i} \right)}$$

using the notation shown in Ex. 7.19. The summation $\Sigma_i$ is over all the intervals up to and including the last interval $i$. This formula is applicable to both product-limit and actuarial calculations and, although approximate, is adequate for most purposes. In the usual way, the 95 per cent two-sided confidence limits are given as the estimate $S_i \pm 1.96 \times$ standard error.

## Relative survival rates and disease-specific survival rates

Analyses of survival for groups of patients are often reported in terms of *relative survival*, which is total survival divided by the survival expected in a group of subjects of the same age and gender composition in that country and at that time. The expected values are derived from life tables routinely produced from vital statistics data. This is a way of taking account of the proportion of deaths that will be due to causes other than the disease of interest.

For example, suppose that the survival at 5 years after diagnosis for a group of men diagnosed with prostate cancer at age 70 is calculated by the product-limit method shown in this chapter, and is 72 per cent. This estimate has variation depending on the number of men assessed, and so the 95 per cent confidence limits might be from 68 to 76 per cent. From life tables, the expected survival of a group of 70-year-old men over 5 years is 83 per cent. We can regard this as being without sampling variation because it is based on the whole community and on large numbers. Thus the relative survival for the group is 0.72/0.83, i.e. 87 per cent, with confidence limits obtained by dividing the upper and lower limits by the same factor of 0.83, giving limits of 82 to 92 per cent. Similarly, the overall 5-year survival for a group of women with breast cancer diagnosed at age 60 might be 79 per cent, and the expected survival of a group of women of this age is 96 per cent, giving a relative survival of 82 per cent. Although the total survival of the men with prostate cancer was lower than that of the women with breast cancer (72 per cent compared with 79 per cent), their relative survival was higher (87 per cent compared with 82 per cent) as a greater proportion of their total mortality was due to the expected mortality in a group of that age and sex. The relative survival is taken as an indicator of the disease-specific survival, i.e. the survival and corresponding mortality specifically due to prostate cancer or breast cancer, respectively.

Alternatively, disease-specific survival can be calculated by the methods already shown. Using the product-limit method, each death from a specific disease such as prostate cancer or breast cancer is counted as an event, and deaths from any other cause are regarded as censoring. The danger with this analysis is that it is open to biases in the allocation of deaths; there is always the suspicion that subjects who have a diagnosis of a severe disease will tend to be certified as dying from that disease, even if their cause of death is in fact independent of it.

In clinical trials and cohort studies with much smaller numbers of individuals, disease-specific analyses may be appropriate, as attention can be paid to possible biases in outcome assessment and steps taken to ensure that the attribution of the cause of death is not biased by the exposure or intervention of the subject. Thus an independent panel, blind to the treatment allocation in a trial, may review the clinical and pathological information to classify causes of death. Where disease-specific survival is regarded as the prime endpoint, it is always useful to do an analysis of total survival in addition.

## Differences between groups

To compare the survival experiences of two (or more) groups of subjects we could select an arbitrary point in time and compare the survival at that point using a simple $2 \times 2$ table of deaths versus survivors at that point, or using the formula given above for the standard error of the actuarial estimate at that point. Such a comparison is unsatisfactory as the results will depend on the particular time point used. One alternative is to find a mathematical formula which will describe the form of the survival curve adequately and compare the relevant parameters of the formula. These methods are called parametric, as the shape of the curve is assumed; for example, in some situations there may be a simple linear relationship between the logarithm of the survival rate and time. Such methods are clearly dependent on the validity of the parametric model chosen.

To avoid both these difficulties, a non-parametric test is often used. Such a test compares the order in which the outcome events occur in each group of subjects, without reference to the precise timing. Thus the tests evaluate the whole curve, but make no assumptions about its shape.

### The log-rank test

Although there are several different non-parametric tests, one method is simple and at the same time powerful and appropriate over a wide range of circumstances [25,26]. This is the log-rank test, and it will come as no surprise to the reader that this is an application of the Mantel–Haenszel test that has been discussed earlier. At each point in time at which a death occurs, a $2 \times 2$ table showing the number of deaths and the total number of subjects under follow-up is created, as shown in **Ex. 7.22.** For each such table, the observed deaths in one group, the expected deaths, and the variance of the expected number are

---

LOG-RANK STATISTIC

For each time interval $i$:

| | Deaths at end of interval $i$ | Subjects still alive at end of interval $i$ | Subjects alive immediately prior to end of interval $i$ |
|---|---|---|---|
| 'Exposed' | $a_i$ | $b_i$ | $N_{1i}$ |
| 'Unexposed' | $c_i$ | $d_i$ | $N_{0i}$ |
| Total | $M_{1i}$ | $M_{0i}$ | $T_i$ |

$$\text{Log-rank statistic} = \frac{\left(\sum_i a_i - \sum_i E_i\right)^2}{\sum_i V_i}$$

where $E_i = N_{1i}M_{1i}/T_i$
and $V_i = N_{1i}N_{0i}M_{1i}M_{0i}/T_i^2(T_i-1)$

---

**Ex. 7.22.** The log-rank statistic: for each time interval, ending when one or more deaths occurs, a 2 × 2 table is created which has usual format (compare Ex. 7.3). The log-rank statistic is calculated as the stratified Mantel–Haenszel statistic, summing over all time intervals, and yields a $\chi^2$ statistic on one degree of freedom

calculated in the same way as was shown in Ex. 7.3. These quantities are summed over all tables, and the Mantel–Haenszel statistic is derived from the summations. The calculation for the data given in Ex. 7.18, comparing the two treatment groups, is shown in **Ex. 7.23.**

The log-rank test calculations produce the observed to expected ratio for each group, which relates the number of deaths observed during the follow-up period to the number expected on the null hypothesis that the survival curve for that group would be the same as that for the combined data. A subgroup of subjects with a mortality rate higher than the whole group will have an observed to expected ratio greater than 1. Therefore, in the data used in Ex. 7.23, in group A more deaths are observed (7) then expected (3.49). Examination of the survival curves, calculated for each group by the method shown in Ex.7.19, shows that there are more early deaths in group A.

## Several exposure categories

The log-rank method can be expanded to look at a number of different categories of subjects, which might correspond to graded severities of disease, stages of disease, dose regimens of treatment, and so on. Comparison between

CALCULATION OF LOG-RANK STATISTIC

| Interval $i$ | Interval between deaths (months) | No. of deaths at end of interval | | No. of patients alive immediately prior to end of interval | | Expected deaths $E_i$ | Variance $V_i$ |
|---|---|---|---|---|---|---|---|
| | | Group A $a_i$ | Both groups $M_{1i}$ | Group A $N_{1i}$ | Both groups $T_i$ | | |
| 1 | 0–1 | 2 | 2 | 10 | 20 | 1.0000 | 0.4737 |
| 2 | 1–4 | 1 | 1 | 7 | 17 | 0.4118 | 0.2422 |
| 3 | 4–6 | 1 | 1 | 6 | 16 | 0.3750 | 0.2344 |
| 4 | 6–12 | 1 | 1 | 4 | 12 | 0.3333 | 0.2222 |
| 5 | 12–13 | 0 | 1 | 3 | 11 | 0.2727 | 0.1983 |
| 6 | 13–15 | 1 | 1 | 3 | 10 | 0.3000 | 0.2100 |
| 7 | 15–16 | 0 | 1 | 2 | 9 | 0.2222 | 0.1728 |
| 8 | 16–22 | 0 | 1 | 2 | 8 | 0.2500 | 0.1875 |
| 9 | 22–23 | 1 | 2 | 1 | 6 | 0.3333 | 0.2222 |
| 10 | 23–41 | 0 | 1 | 0 | 1 | 0.0000 | 0.0000 |

$$\sum a_i = 7 \qquad \sum E_i = 3.4983 \qquad \sum_i V_i = 2.16347$$

Log-rank statistic = $(7–3.4983)^2/2.1634 = 5.67$
This is a chi-square statistic on 1 d.f., so $P = 0.018$

**Ex. 7.23.** Calculation of log-rank statistic from the data in Ex. 7.18: the quantities $a_i$, $E_i$, and $V_i$ are calculated for each time period $I$; a time period ends when a death occurs, or two or more deaths occur together. The formula is shown in Ex. 7.22

the curves can be based on either an overall chi-squared statistic with $(n-1)$ degrees of freedom, where $n$ is the number of groups compared, which assesses the total variation from the null hypothesis that survival is the same in each group, or by a trend statistic on one degree of freedom which assesses the linear component of a trend in difference in survival experience over the ordered groups.

Thus, **Ex. 7.24** shows a further analysis of the survival of the breast cancer patients whose overall survival was shown earlier in Ex. 7.17. The patients have been divided into four groups in terms of the measurement of oestrogen receptor (ER) concentration in the tumour [27]. The graph shows that survival is better for those with a higher concentration of oestrogen receptors. The log-rank analysis for the four groups gives an overall $\chi^2$ of 60.4 on 3 d.f. ($P < 0.0001$), and the trend statistic, assessing whether survival changes in a linear fashion with a change in receptor concentration, gives a $\chi^2$ of 48.6 on 1 d.f. ($P < 0.0001$).

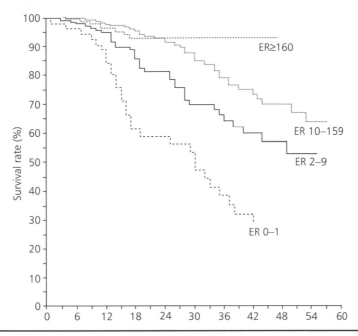

**Ex 7.24.** Survival curves for 583 breast cancer patients (those shown in Ex. 7.17, less 13 with incomplete data) divided into four groups on the quantity of oestrogen receptor (ER) in the breast tumour, measured in femtomoles per milligram. Derived from Godolphin *et al.* [27]

## Control for confounding

Since the log-rank method of analysis is derived from the Mantel–Haenszel statistical method, it can easily be adapted to the consideration of confounding variables. The logic is the same as that with the simpler types of data analysis already discussed, in that the experience of the groups to be compared is examined within categories of the confounding factor by generating survival curves for the groups to be compared for each subcategory of the confounder. The log-rank statistic allows the data to be summarized over levels of the confounding factor, giving an overall observed to expected ratio, and an overall chi-squared statistic which assesses the difference between the groups being compared after control for the confounder. For example, the data shown in Ex. 7.24 show that survival in breast cancer patients is related to oestrogen receptor concentration. It is important to know whether this effect is independent of the effect of other prognostic factors such as staging. Therefore a stratified analysis in which the effect of oestrogen receptor status was assessed within clinical stage categories, and the log-rank statistic was calculated over the strata, was done. This showed that the observed to expected ratios were little changed; the ratio for subjects with the highest receptor concentration was 0.44 before control for clinical stage and 0.45 after such control, and the trend statistic was 48.6 before controlling for stage and 47.3 afterwards. This shows that the prognostic effect of oestrogen receptor quantity is independent of clinical stage [27].

## Multivariate analysis

Beyond this type of analysis, multivariate methods can be applied to survival data. Such methods are similar in principle to the logistic regression model described earlier in this chapter. A powerful method with wide applicability is the proportional hazards model developed by Cox [28]. This model allows the survival curve to take any form, i.e. the *hazard function*, or instantaneous mortality rate, is allowed to vary with the time from the start of follow-up. However, it is assumed that the relative effect of any factor on the hazard function will be constant over time. Thus, if the hazard function at time $t$ in the referent group of subjects is expressed as $\lambda_{0,t}$, the function for subjects with a factor $x_1$ is given by

$$\lambda_{1,t} = \lambda_{0,t} \cdot \exp(b_1 x_1)$$

or

$$\ln \lambda_{1,t} = \ln \lambda_{0,t} + b_1 x_1$$

where $b_1$ is the coefficient related to $x_1$. If $x_1$ has the values 0 or 1, the exponential of $b_1$ will be the ratio $\lambda_{1,t} / \lambda_{0,t}$, i.e. the ratio of the hazard function, which is a relative risk. With multiple factors, the model becomes

$$\lambda_{k,t} = \lambda_{0,t} \cdot \exp(b_1 x_2 + \dots b_k x_k)$$

Of course, methods that can deal with a multivariate analysis and the complexity of censored survival data are complex, and specialist statistical and programming advice is required.

As stated at the beginning of the chapter, this review of key statistical methods emphasizes that statistical methods are one component of the process of assessing causation, along with the consideration of observation bias and confounding. In subsequent chapters, we will consolidate and develop this theme.

## Self-test questions (answers on p. 501)

**Q7.1** Two studies of the effects of a new treatment on recovery from a disease are available. The first study gives a relative risk of 2.2, with a chi-square statistic on one degree of freedom of 9.6. The second study gives a relative risk of 4.6, with a chi-square statistic of 1.8. How would you interpret these results? (Use Appendix Table 15, or the Excel functions shown in Appendix Table 16).

**Q7.2** In a study of injury in different work groups, there were 16 injuries in 1 year in a group of 1000 employees working on special processes, while for a larger group of 10 000 workers there were 40 injuries in a year. What is the relative risk of injury and the associated chi-square statistic (use Ex. 7.4). What are the 95 per cent two-sided confidence limits for the relative risk? (Use Appendix Table 2, section 4A).

**Q7.3** In a case–control study, 52 of 400 controls are exposed to the agent in question compared with 34 of 100 cases. Calculate the odds ratio, the Mantel–Haenszel chi-square statistic, and the 95 per cent two-sided confidence limits. Use Ex. 7.3 and Appendix Table 1.

**Q7.4** A cohort study gives a result showing a relative risk of 2.25 with 95 per cent two-sided confidence limits of 0.88 to 5.75. How do you interpret this?

**Q7.5** The background rate of smoking cessation over 1 year is assumed to be 10 per cent. A specific programme is thought worthwhile if it would double this to 20 per cent. It is assumed that the cessation programme could not reduce the cessation rate. You want to design a study which has high confidence (90 per cent) that you can detect an effect of this magnitude. How many subjects do you need? Use Exs 7.15 and 7.16.

**Q7.6** If the answer from the last question suggests a number beyond your resources, how could you design the study to use a smaller number?

**Q7.7** You want to set up a case–control study to assess a factor that you expect to be present in 10 per cent of the control sample. You want to be able to detect a relative risk of 2, with 80 per cent power and using a two-sided 0.05 significance level. Cases and controls are equally difficult to recruit. What is the minimum number of subjects you require?

**Q7.8** If in the case–control study described in Q7.7, controls are much easier to recruit than cases, how many cases are needed if four controls per case are recruited?

**Q7.9** In an individually matched case–control study there are 200 pairs in which the case is exposed and the control is not, and 50 where the control is exposed and the case is not. What is the odds ratio, the chi-square statistic, and the approximate 99 per cent two-sided confidence limits? Use Exs 7.11 and 7.7, (p. 248 and 239).

**Q7.10** In a case–control study, 50 of 100 cases and 20 of 100 controls in men have the exposure of interest. In women, 60 of 100 cases and 10 of 100 controls are exposed. What are the results? Are the results different for men and women?

**Q7.11** From the data in Ex. 7.18, calculate the survival curve for each of groups A and B. What is the survival rate and 95 per cent confidence limits for each group at 18 months? Do these results agree with the log-rank statistic calculated in Ex. 7.23?

# References

1. **Armitage P, Berry G, Matthews JNS.** *Statistical Methods in Medical Research.* (4th edn). Oxford: Blackwell Scientific, 2002.
2. **Kleinbaum DG, Kupper LL, Morgenstern H.** *Epidemiologic Research: Principles and Quantitative Methods.* Belmont, CA: Lifetime Learning Publications, 1982.
3. **Mantel N, Haenszel W.** Statistical aspects of the analysis of data from retrospective studies of disease. *J Natl Cancer Inst* 1959; **22**: 719–748.
4. **Rothman KJ, Greenland S.** *Modern Epidemiology* (2nd edn). Philadelphia, PA: Lippincott–Raven, 1998.
5. **Miettinen O.** Estimability and estimation in case-referent studies. *Am J Epidemiol* 1976; **103**: 226–235.
6. **Greenland S.** A counterexample to the test-based principle of setting confidence limits. *Am J Epidemiol* 1984; **120**: 4–7.
7. **Lyon JL, Gardner JW, West DW, Stanish WM, Hebertson RM.** Smoking and carcinoma *in situ* of the uterine cervix. *Am J Public Health* 1983; **73**: 558–562.
8. **Truett J, Cornfield J, Kannel W.** A multivariate analysis of the risk of coronary heart disease in Framingham. *J Chronic Dis* 1967; **20**: 511–524.
9. **Pooling Project Research Group.** Relationship of blood pressure, serum cholesterol, smoking habit, relative weight and ECG. abnormalities to incidence of major coronary events: final report of the Pooling Project. *J Chronic Dis* 1978; **31**: 201–306.
10. **Saracci R.** Asbestos and lung cancer: an analysis of the epidemiological evidence on the asbestos-smoking interaction. *Int J Cancer* 1977; **20**: 323–331.
11. **Mantel N.** Chi-square tests with one degree of freedom; extensions of the Mantel–Haenszel procedure. *Am Stat Assoc J* 1963; **58**: 690–700.
12. **Elwood JM.** Maternal and environmental factors affecting twin births in Canadian cities. *Br J Obstet Gynaecol* 1978; **85**: 351–358.
13. **McNemar Q.** Note on the sampling of the difference between corrected proportions or percentages. *Psychometrika* 1947; **12**: 153–157.

14. **Elwood JM, Williamson C, Stapleton PJ.** Malignant melanoma in relation to moles, pigmentation, and exposure to fluorescent and other lighting sources. *Br J Cancer* 1986; **53**: 65–74.

15. **Clayton D, Hills M.** *Statistical Models in Epidemiology.* Oxford: Oxford Scientific Publications, 1993.

16. **ISIS-2 (Second International Study of Infarct Survival) Collaborative Group).** Randomised trial of intravenous streptokinase, oral aspirin, both, or neither among 17,187 cases of suspected acute myocardial infarction: ISIS-2. *Lancet* 1988; **332**: 349–360.

17. **Armitage P.** *Sequential Medical Trials* (2nd edn). Oxford: Blackwell Scientific, 1975.

18. **Blot WJ, Li J-Y, Taylor PR,** *et al.* Nutrition intervention trials in Linxian, China: supplementation with specific vitamin/mineral combinations, cancer incidence, and disease-specific mortality in the general population. *J Natl Cancer Inst* 1993; **85**: 1483–1492.

19. **Hennekens CH, Buring JE, Manson JE,** *et al.* Lack of effect of long-term supplementation with beta carotene on the incidence of malignant neoplasms and cardiovascular disease. *N Engl J Med* 1996; **334**: 1145–1149.

20. **The Alpha-Tocopherol Beta Carotene Cancer Prevention Study Group.** The effect of vitamin E and beta carotene on the incidence of lung cancer and other cancers in male smokers. *N Engl J Med* 1994; **330**: 1029–1035.

21. **Omenn GS, Goodman GE, Thornquist MD,** *et al.* Effects of a combination of beta carotene and vitamin A on lung cancer and cardiovascular disease. *N Engl J Med* 1996; **334**: 1150–1155.

22. **Pocock SJ.** *Clinical Trials: A Practical Approach.* Chichester: John Wiley, 1983.

23. **Machin D, Day S, Green SB.** *Textbook of Clinical Trials* (2nd edn). Chichester: John Wiley, 2006.

24. **Fleiss JL, Levin B, Paik MC.** *Statistical Methods for Rates AND Proportions* (3rd edn). New York: John Wiley, 2003.

25. **Mantel N.** Evaluation of survival data and two new rank order statistics arising in its consideration. *Cancer Chemother Rep* 1966; **50**: 163–170.

26. **Peto R, Pike MC, Armitage P,** *et al.* Design and analysis of randomized clinical trials requiring prolonged observation of each patient. II: analysis and examples. *Br J Cancer* 1977; **35**: 1–39.

27. **Godolphin W, Elwood JM, Spinelli JJ.** Estrogen receptor quantitation and staging as complementary prognostic indicators in breast cancer; a study of 583 patients. *Int J Cancer* 1981; **28**: 667–683.

28. **Cox DR.** Regression models and life-tables. *J R Statist Soc Series B* 1972; **34**: 187–220.

Chapter 8

# Combining results from several studies: systematic review and meta-analysis

*And differing judgements serve but to declare.*

*That truth lies somewhere, if we knew but where.*

—William Cowper: Hope, 1782

In the first part of this chapter, we discuss systematic reviews and the role of meta-analysis. In the second part, we present the most widely used statistical methods for meta-analysis and related issues such as exploring differences between studies.

## Part 1. Systematic reviews and meta-analysis

So far in this book, we have concentrated on the assessment of the methods and results of a single study. For most topics many studies will be available, which need to be assessed, compared, and summarized. Traditionally, there was no particular method of doing this. Authors of reviews and textbooks would identify relevant studies through ad hoc methods, comment on selected studies in a narrative fashion, and come to conclusions. These conclusions would be strongly influenced by the importance given to each study, but the criteria used to judge studies would not be stated, and often was not recognized by the author. The criteria might include the type of study, the size of the study, and the reputation of the investigators and the journal publishing the study. Such criteria may have certain validity, but the key issue is that the criteria were not explicitly defined. As a result different experts reviewing the same material could come to very different conclusions.

In contrast to this traditional review, now referred to as a *narrative* review, the emphasis over the last two decades has been on improving *systematic reviews*. The key feature of these is that the methods of doing the review are explicitly documented, just as the methods of any other study are described, so that in principle they can be reproduced by others. It is now accepted good practice that the methods by which studies are identified, the criteria determining whether a study is included in the review or excluded, the factors used to give different importance to different studies, and the methods used to consolidate the results and come to conclusions are all explicitly described. Such systematic reviews are at the centre of developments in *evidence-based medicine* and *evidence-based health care*.

Within this overall process of systematic review, *meta-analysis* refers to statistical methods using the data from numerous studies to produce an estimate of an overall association and to explore variations between the studies. A systematic review need not include a meta-analysis, as meta-analysis is only relevant if several studies provide data that can be sensibly combined. Thus only a few years after the first randomized trial of tuberculosis treatment was published (described in Chapter 1, Ex. 1.8), Daniels and Bradford Hill [1] reported a comparative review of the three studies on the topic then available. The first published meta-analysis may be a pooled data analysis by Goldberg in 1906 from a review of 44 studies of urinary infections in typhoid [2]. Systematic reviews and meta-analysis have developed very rapidly since the 1980s as a result of the development of good statistical methods for combining study results, the recognition of the value of using all available information to avoid publication bias, the greater power and accessibility of computer based systems for retrieving literature, and the development of the Cochrane Collaboration. All of these influences will be discussed in this chapter.

Two examples will show the power and relevance of meta-analysis, both with regard to breast cancer. In 1992, a major meta-analysis of the treatment of early breast cancer was published, which gave a much clearer assessment of the effects of hormonal, cytotoxic, and immune therapy than had been given by the many trial results and reviews up to that time [3]. The work involved identifying and obtaining the raw data from 133 randomized trials, estimated to include 79 per cent of all trials of these therapies; information was obtained for some 90 per cent of the patients randomized, giving data on 75 000 women treated, with 24 000 deaths and 31 000 recurrences. This international collaborative analysis is continuing to produce more and more information, now with information on recurrences and deaths over 15 years since treatment [4,5]. The definitive information on the treatment of breast cancer now comes from these analyses, rather than from a reviewer's choice of the 'best' trial or from the most 'authoritative' textbook.

A similar effort with regard to aetiology resulted in a meta-analysis of observational studies on the relationship between oral contraceptive use and the incidence of breast cancer. The data from 54 case–control and cohort studies, including 53 000 breast cancer cases and 100 000 controls, were newly analysed, a major effort involving the chief investigators of all these studies [6]. This analysis included about 90 per cent of the known worldwide information on the question. Among other findings, this meta-analysis showed a small but important increased risk of breast cancer in current users of oral contraceptives, which decreased after cessation of use. This association had not been shown previously in any of the individual studies. Several other analyses of other aetiological factors have been produced from the same data set, including the assessment of abortion which was mentioned in Chapter 5 [7].

## Meta-analyses based on individual subject data, or on results of each study

There are two major types of meta-analysis. A meta-analysis may be based on the results of each study, published or unpublished, or it may be a new analysis using the original data for each participant in each of the studies. The use of study results only is obviously much easier; however, there is little ability to deal with limitations or biases in these results. There is no clearly accepted terminol ogy for these two approaches. Some authors refer to the combined analysis of individual subject data as *pooled analysis* [8], reserving the term meta-analysis for the more restricted analysis of results from each study. Others use the term meta-analysis to include both these approaches, and refer to analyses of *individual patient data* (IPD) as opposed to aggregate data [9]. In this chapter we will use *meta-analysis* to refer to all combined analyses, and use the term *pooled analysis* specifically to refer to analyses using individual subject data.

A meta-analysis which involves access to the original individual subject data can not only summarize the main results, but can also produce new analyses on issues which could not be covered within any one study, such as the assessment of effects within subgroups, the interactions between two or more factors, or the more adequate control of confounding. The meta-analyses of aetiological and treatment issues of breast cancer just mentioned used individual subject data. Such pooled analyses are particularly valuable where the major limitations of individual studies are not only in sample size, but in the adequacy of confounder control and the limited analysis of subgroups. Such meta-analyses require the active support of the investigators of each original study, and a great deal of work in editing, perhaps recoding, and checking the original data to produce consistently formatted data for analysis. The most successful efforts have had substantial funding for these central functions, and support for meetings of investigators who are involved throughout the process. The analysis of these pooled data sets is in principle the same as the analysis of one large study, with the individual studies being treated as strata in the analysis.

However, most meta-analyses are simpler, being based on the results of previous studies, and these are also very valuable. The great majority of systematic reviews in the Cochrane database include only meta-analyses of published results. The methods available for the analyses of the results of many studies to produce summary estimates of the overall effect and measures of the precision of that summary measure, and to explore issues of variation between studies, will be discussed in part 2 of this chapter.

## The Cochrane Collaboration

In 1992 in Britain, the Cochrane Centre was founded with support from the Research and Development Programme of the National Health Service. It is named in honour of Professor Archie Cochrane, who in a long career in epidemiology and health care research argued strongly that all health care interventions should be demonstrated to be effective, where possible by randomized trials [10,11]. This developed into the international Cochrane Collaboration, launched in 1993. This international network prepares and disseminates systematic reviews of health care interventions, using meta-analysis methods. Most of these are restricted to randomized controlled trials, but the work also extends to meta-analyses of observational studies [12,13]. The Cochrane Collaboration website (www.cochrane.org) provides freely accessible information on the extensive databases available (which will be described later in this chapter), and on methodological issues in systematic reviews and meta-analysis. The *Cochrane Handbook for Systematic Reviews of Interventions* [9] is a valuable reference source relating to much of the material included in this chapter, and also discussing methods of accessing literature and formatting systematic reviews, which will not be covered in detail here. The website also provides access to the *RevMan* computer software, which supports Cochrane format reviews, and includes meta-analysis. There is a good user guide and a glossary of terms [14,15]. Databases linked to the Cochrane site will be described later in this chapter.

## Format of reports of systematic reviews

A recommended process for the reporting of systematic reviews originated from a conference on the Quality of Reporting of Meta-analyses (QUOROM), which has produced a checklist of headings which should be addressed in a systematic review, and a flowsheet detailing the identification, extraction, and selection of studies for review [16]. This arose from the CONSORT statement for randomized trials, discussed in Chapter 5, and is available from the CONSORT website (www.consort-statement.org/QUOROM.pdf). The Cochrane review process has a fixed protocol including these points [9], and the Cochrane RevMan software (to be discussed later) encourages reviewers to produce reports in a consistent format. An example will be given (Ex. 8.3).

## Systematic review and meta-analysis: the process

The term 'systematic review' describes a process with several important steps, one of which is meta-analysis (**Ex. 8.1**). These steps are to define the objective and the question, to set the criteria for studies to be included in the review, to identify, retrieve, and review these studies, to abstract the data required for the review and analysis, to perform a meta-analysis when appropriate, to report and interpret the results, and finally to plan for the review of new evidence as it arises.

### Objectives of systematic reviews and meta-analyses

The objectives of any systematic review and any meta-analysis within that review need to be clear and explicit, just as the objectives of any other scientific study should be. So far in this book we have discussed the assessment of the results of a single study in terms of the conclusions we can reach about the interpretation of the association being assessed. We have discussed issues of internal validity, i.e. how far we can interpret the association in terms of a causal relationship, and external validity, i.e. how widely the conclusions can be applied. In systematic reviews and meta-analysis, the same key issues of internal and external validity need to be assessed in terms of the totality of evidence provided by the studies included in the review. The general objective is

---

STEPS IN A SYSTEMATIC REVIEW

1. Define the objective and the question
2. Define the criteria for inclusion of studies
3. Find all eligible studies
4. Review the methods and results of each study
5. Summarize the results of each study in a standard format
6. Apply statistical methods to produce a summary result
7. Assess variation between studies (heterogeneity)
8. Review and interpret findings, and report them
9. Set up plan for monitoring new evidence and revising the review

**Ex. 8.1.** Steps in a systematic review

to define the key association which is addressed, and assess the interpretation of this association in terms of a cause and effect relationship, with attention to both internal and extra validity.

The review should answer a relevant question, and care in defining the question is crucial. For example, for a review of the effects of one drug in treating a certain illness, we would need to define the clinical endpoints used and decide whether to include studies which assess the drug used alone, studies of its use combined with other therapies, or studies based only on certain types of patients, certain dosages, and routes of administration, or with a defined extent of follow-up. Some of the most productive meta-analyses have taken broad questions. The reviews of breast cancer treatment referred to above assessed major comparisons, for example patients randomized to treatment with tamoxifen with those not offered it, including trials in which the other treatments received and the selection of the patients varied greatly. One of the values of meta-analysis is that it may indicate variation between studies that show the importance of other factors.

Within that overall objective for the systematic review, a meta-analysis will have certain objectives which come from the strengths of this method. The first objective is to increase the statistical power and therefore the precision of the estimate of effect. Meta-analysis was originally designed to counteract the prime weakness of individual randomized trials, which was small size and therefore imprecision of the results. Meta-analysis, by combining data from a number of studies, increases statistical power and increases the precision of the estimate of association. For example, a recent report from the breast cancer treatment pooled analysis referred to earlier shows an improvement in 15-year mortality from 60 to 55 per cent in patients with advanced breast cancer with the use of radiotherapy: a clinically important but, in absolute terms, small benefit that would not be apparent in a single study, but was clear and highly significant statistically in the combined analysis [5]. Clearly this objective is only met if it can be accepted that a single estimate of the overall association is compatible with the results of the individual studies.

A further objective is to provide information on questions that are inadequately addressed by individual studies. This applies mainly where there are a large number of available studies, and is particularly applicable to meta-analyses using individual patient data. Such pooled analyses have the ability to explore relationships within the data, for instance variations in the key association by characteristics of subjects such as age or sex and disease-related characteristics, and may lead to conclusions which an individual study cannot assess. Thus, for example, the pooled analysis of data from many studies of breast cancer and oral contraceptive use showed a relationship between current use and increased risk, which decreased rapidly after cessation of use. This had not been recognized in any of the previous studies, although it was apparent in several studies once the meta-analysis was done [6].

A related objective is to provide further assessment of hypotheses that may have arisen from individual studies. For example, in the same example as above, earlier studies of breast cancer and oral contraceptive use had led to specific hypotheses that risk was increased with use at young ages, or use before a first pregnancy, and some interesting biological hypotheses had been produced to match these epidemiological associations. Meta-analysis, particularly using pooled individual patient data, has the power to test such hypotheses on the larger set of data; in this example, neither of these specific hypotheses was sustained.

A further objective, or unanticipated result, of many meta-analyses has been to simplify the questions. Empirically, many meta-analyses have shown that the results of related but different interventions or exposures have been fairly consistent. Meta-analyses of clinical trials were often criticized for combining trials that had, for example, different combinations of drugs or different dosages, yet often these meta-analyses have shown that the differences in major effects have been small. For example, with regard to the effects of blood-pressure-lowering agents, meta-analyses have revealed differences between classes of drugs, but few important differences between individual drugs or dosages have been shown [17]. Similarly, the meta-analysis of oral contraceptive use and breast cancer showed consistent results for studies of women in different countries and ethnic groups and differing risks of breast cancer [6].

## Publication bias

One of the key concepts stimulating the development of systematic reviews and meta-analysis has been the recognition of the problem of publication bias. Just as a particular association may be one of a number tested in a study, one study is merely one member of the universe of all studies that have been done. We will have incomplete knowledge about these studies. If the subset which we know about differs from the others, because the results of the study influence whether we know about it or not, publication bias exists. In particular, positive and statistically significant results are generally more likely to lead to publications and scientific presentations. Publication bias was described in 1979 as the *file drawer* problem by Rosenthal [18], who summarized it by saying that 'journals are filled with the 5 per cent of studies which show type 1 errors, while the file drawers back at the lab are filled with the 95 per cent of the studies that show non-significant results'.

Peto *et al.* [19] considered what may happen in one situation, that of clinical trials of new therapies for cancer. Suppose that over a given period there are 120 large clinical trials with several hundred patients involved in each, and 1200 small clinical trials with perhaps 50 subjects involved in each (**Ex. 8.2**). Let us further suppose that the large trials test therapies that have survived preliminary evaluation, and so, of the 120 new therapies tested, 20 are actually beneficial. If the power of these large trials is 90 per cent, 18 of the 20 will be correctly reported as beneficial. Of the 100 therapies that are not beneficial and are assessed by large trials, five will be expected to show significant results because of the use of a significance level of 5 per cent. Further, because large trials are major undertakings, even those with negative results are likely to be reported. Therefore the published literature should give a fair representation of the total results from large trials. Of the 1200 small trials, representing therapies for which less previous work has been done, let us assume that 100 of the interventions tested are in fact beneficial. As the power of a small study to detect these benefits may only be 50 per cent, there will be 50 correct reports of benefit and 50 false–negative results. Of the 1100 non-beneficial new interventions assessed by small trials, some 55 may have erroneously positive results. Suppose further that all these 105 positive reports, showing a significant effect of the new intervention, are published, whereas the 1095 results of small trials that show no significant difference are not published. The implications of this scenario are several. First, perhaps half of the *statistically significant* benefits reported for new therapies on the basis of *small* trials may be incorrect; therefore a consideration of the size and the power of the study is important even when the results of that study are statistically significant. From this we could argue that all results from small studies should be ignored, but that leads to the difficulty that many of the large studies would not be done if it were not for the encouraging results from previous small studies. A wise counsel might be to regard only the results of large studies as definitive. A useful test is to ask whether the study would have been published if it had shown no benefit of the new intervention.

Several processes leading to publication bias have been identified [20]. As well as the non-publication of research results, there are issues of *delayed publication* in that some results are reported much later than others, and *multiple publication* with some studies being reported in more than one primary source. Studies with results regarded as favourable or interesting will tend to be cited more frequently in other sources, and so will be easier to find (*citation bias*). Studies published in different languages will be accessed differently, with

## PUBLICATION BIAS

| Type of trial | True situation | No. of trials in progress | Numbers with results which show | | |
| --- | --- | --- | --- | --- | --- |
| | | | No significant difference | New therapy better | |
| Large (Several hundred patients) | No difference | 100 | 95 | 5 | Significance level 0.05 |
| | New therapy better | 20 | 2 | 18 | Power 90% (optimistic) |
| Small (Several dozen patients) | No difference | 1100 | 1045 | 55 | Significance level 0.05 |
| | New therapy better | 100 | 50 | 50 | Power 50% |

| Proportion of trial results which are correct (no adjustment for publication bias) | |
| --- | --- |
| large trials showing no difference | 98% |
| large trials showing a significant difference | 78% |
| small trials showing no difference | 95% |
| small trials showing a significant difference | 48% |

**Ex. 8.2.** Publication bias: the problem of judging one result in terms of others, and the issue of publication bias, in that small trials with no significant difference will often not be published. Adapted from Peto et al. [19]

English-language studies easiest to find (*language bias*). Within publications, there may be selection in terms of which outcomes are reported or emphasized in the publications (*outcome reporting bias*). Most literature-searching processes depend on words identified as keywords, or words in the title or the abstract of an article; results only noted in the body of the article will be harder to access.

Publication bias arises through research studies that produce less 'exciting' results not being accessible. Not all research studies are completed, not all are submitted for publication, not all are accepted, particularly by high-profile journals where the acceptance rate of submissions may be very low, and not all published papers will be included in computerized databases. Some surveys of researchers have shown that non-submission of research results is the largest factor, but the importance of different factors will vary by the type of study and the subject matter [20]. Publication bias is inevitable (and even desirable) as while researchers and particularly those who conduct meta-analyses want to obtain access to the complete spectrum of research on each topic, most users of research results rely on scientific journals to filter the information and present them with a selection which is of high quality, relevant, digestible, and even interesting. Scientific journals are commercial enterprises which have to be read to stay in business, whether owned by commercial companies or by professional societies. Probably every experienced researcher has the experience of having done a research study that does not seem to justify the effort required to prepare it for publication, and papers with non-significant or expected results require much greater effort on the part of the authors to make them acceptable for publication. While journals may not have explicit policies of favouring positive or new and exciting results, this is likely still to apply even if not explicit; most editors ask reviewers not only for comments on scientific quality, but also on 'Will this be new and interesting to our readers?' Some editorial decisions can clearly produce publication bias; the present author has seen a paper rejected by a major journal with the stated reason that the journal had previously published a study with different results, and therefore they would not publish this new study although it was considerably larger and used stronger methods.

Of particular concern is the deliberate prevention or delay of publication of research by commercial or other interests. Melander *et al.* [21] reviewed 42 controlled trials of selective serotonin-reuptake inhibitor (SSRI) antidepressant drugs submitted to the Swedish drug regulatory authority for marketing approval, and accessed all published reports based on those trials. Sixty per cent of the studies done resulted in full stand-alone publications, but the studies showing significant differences were three times more likely to appear as stand-alone publications and were more likely to lead to multiple publications than were the studies with non-significant results. Although both intention to treat analyses and per protocol analyses (only subjects who were compliant with the protocol) were available, the intention to treat results were usually less favourable and were reported in only 24 per cent of the stand-alone publications. The conclusion was that if only published information were reviewed, rather than all the studies that had been done, 'any attempt to recommend a specific drug is likely to be based on biased evidence'.

This issue has been raised again with the use of these drugs in the treatment of childhood depression. In 2003 the UK Committee on Safety of Medicines prohibited the use of any SSRI drugs except one, fluoxetine, for the treatment of childhood depression. This was after a meta-analysis had found that the published data suggested beneficial effects for several SSRIs, particularly paroxetine, but a review including unpublished information suggested that the risks outweighed the benefits [22]. The review gave evidence that trials with unfavourable results tended not to be reported. An accompanying editorial noted evidence from an internal drug company memorandum suggesting that negative results were being withheld, and stated that the selective reporting of research was a serious abuse of patients and doctors involved in the trials [23].

## Finding the relevant studies

Some studies are much easier to locate than others. A search for all available published information on a topic is a major undertaking, may never be complete, and much of the information obtained may be of dubious quality. If unpublished information is to be included, the difficulties are greatly increased. While a complete search is the ideal, more limited searches of published literature identified through major databases will be a considerable improvement on a casual search of a few textbooks and journals.

Studies published in the major medical and scientific literature, which is abstracted on to easily available databases such as Medline, will be the most easily found. However, even here, the number of relevant studies found will depend on the search technique and how thoroughly it is applied. Many studies are not included in computerized databases because they appear as chapters in books, or reports of governments, research institutions, or companies. Such information is much less readily accessible; it is sometimes referred to as *grey literature* (white literature is easily accessible, and black literature, such as the internal records of a drug company or government department, is kept confidential). Material that is published in languages other than English, in countries with weaker research bases, or in journals which are not indexed by major indexing systems can all easily be missed. Then of course, some studies may be performed but never published, as discussed above.

## Electronic databases of scientific literature

The two main electronic databases of scientific literature in health are Medline and Embase, which are the electronic versions of *Index Medicus* (published by the US National Library of Medicine) and *Excerpta Medica* (published by Elsevier), respectively. A search of one major database such as Medline, while simple to do, is unlikely to identify all relevant studies. Medline has the great advantage of being freely available on several sites including PubMed (http://www.ncbi.nlm.nih.gov/entrez/query.fcgi). Embase covers European journals more thoroughly, but access requires a subscription (http://www.embase.com). The overlap between these two databases can be quite modest, and they differ in their coverage; one study found that randomized trials reported in Embase had on average smaller effects than trials reported in Medline [24]. Gateway (http://gateway.nlm.nih.gov/gw/Cmd), a database of the US National Library of Medicine, provides searches of PubMed and several other major sources including US clinical trials (http://clinicaltrials.gov/) and presentations at many meetings. PsycInfo (previously PsycLit) is a database of the American Psychological Association which has abstracts from over 2000 journals and other sources on psychological issues (http://www.apa.org/psycinfo/products/psycinfo.html).

The Cochrane Collaboration has given rise to the Cochrane Library, comprising several important databases, accessed through the Cochrane website (www.cochrane.org) and through http://www.mrw.interscience.wiley.com/cochrane/cochrane_search_fs.html.

The Cochrane Library includes several databases. The *Cochrane Database of Systematic Reviews* comprises the detailed reviews of specific clinical questions, mainly on the effectiveness of interventions, which have been produced and published within the collaboration. This database extends to public health policy issues (such as the prevention of tooth decay by fluoridation) and a wide variety of other issues related to clinical care. In December 2005, it included over 2000 full reviews, with over 1400 reviews in progress. Most reviews include a meta-analysis giving the summary effect measure and confidence limits for the combined data from relevant studies.

The *Cochrane Database of Reviews of Effects* includes over 4000 critical assessments and structured abstracts of reviews, dealing with topics that have not yet been covered by a full review and therefore are not in the Database of

Systematic Reviews. The *Cochrane Central Register of Controlled Trials* (CEN-TRAL) is the largest database of randomized controlled trials. Its purpose is to identify randomized studies for further assessment and inclusion in systematic reviews. Considerable effort is being made to produce international registries of active randomized trials, including *Current Controlled Trials* (http://www.controlled-trials.com/mrct/) and *Trials Central* (http://www.trialscentral.org). The *Cochrane Database of Methodology Reviews* provides information on methodological issues.

Another major source of literature is the Centre for Reviews and Dissemination, operated by the British National Health Service and based at the University of York, whose website gives access to DARE (the *Database of Abstracts of Reviews of Effects*) (http://www.york.ac.uk/inst/crd/crddatabases. htm) and to the *Health Technology Assessment Database*, with information on ongoing projects and completed reports from health technology assessment organizations worldwide, and the *NHS Economic Evaluation Database* (NHSEED), which contains structured abstracts of articles describing economic evaluations of health care interventions. These latter two databases are also accessible through the Cochrane site.

Computerized databases record published papers in journals, and increasingly include abstracts from presentations at conferences. Whether abstracts, and also theses, should be included in systematic reviews is a difficult issue. Only about half of abstracts presented at major conferences are later published in full, and probably less than half of doctoral theses eventually result in a publication [20].

## Optimal search strategies

The Cochrane Handbook [9] gives good advice on search strategies. Studies have identified optimal search strategies for use with Medline and other databases to retrieve systematic reviews [25] and scientifically strong studies of treatment [26], and undoubtedly further such papers will follow. These studies were done by applying the logic of screening (described in Chapter 5) to the assessment of the accuracy of specific search strategies. To derive the 'gold standard' for comparison, a substantial team of research staff *hand-searched* each issue of 161 clinical journals for the year 2000. The results of each search strategy were compared with this gold standard in terms of sensitivity, specificity, and overall validity. Using a search strategy with high specificity will yield a relatively small number of articles, most of which will be relevant, which is appropriate for quick searches seeking an immediate answer to a question. Using search strategies with high sensitivity will include almost all relevant material, but also a considerable amount of less relevant material, which will be appropriate for those conducting systematic reviews, for example for the development of clinical guidelines.

Trials in intensively researched mainstream areas of medicine are usually easier to locate. For example, for a meta-analysis of the effects of beta-blockers in treating hypertension, it was sufficient to search the Cochrane library, which of course includes several databases, and PubMed [27]. However, for a meta-analysis of the effect of sedative hypnotics in older subjects with insomnia the authors used Medline/PubMed, Embase, the Cochrane clinical trials database, Psychlit, bibliographies of published reviews, and contacted the manufacturers of the newer drugs; they identified 24 eligible studies [28]. For a meta-analysis of placebo-controlled trials of homeopathy and allopathy, searches were carried out using 19 electronic databases, reference lists of relevant papers, and contacts with experts [29]. In this analysis larger beneficial effects were shown in small trials and in trials judged to be of lower quality.

## Inclusion criteria

The definition of which studies will be included in a systematic review needs to be set. This can be a complex process. The criteria for the inclusion or exclusion of individual studies, applied to the whole systematic review or applied to aspects such as a meta-analysis, should be explicit, well documented, and reproducible. All studies that fulfil the stated inclusion criteria should be accessed and assessed. Typically, a large number of studies are identified and assessed quickly, for example by assessing the title and abstract, and a much smaller group of studies are assessed in more detail. Studies may have major limitations or weaknesses, such as not providing information on the most relevant outcomes, not giving results in sufficient detail for further assessment, presenting results on only a subset of the participants, and so on. The reasons for exclusion of studies from further consideration should be documented, and the process can be described in a flowchart. For example, **Ex. 8.3** refers to the systematic review of SSRI drugs in childhood depression referred to above [22], and shows that 5220 publications were identified and 165 assessed in more detail, to yield only five studies which were included in the meta-analysis. This review follows the principles set out in the QUOROM (Quality of Reporting of Meta-analyses) statement [16], as previously noted.

Each set of data from a study should be counted only once, so multiple publications from the same study can cause difficulties. Only one result from each study should be used in one meta-analysis; if several different outcomes or exposures are to be assessed (for example, an effect of a drug on mortality, and on incidence of a complication), each should be analysed separately. In observational

PROCESS OF A SYSTEMATIC REVIEW

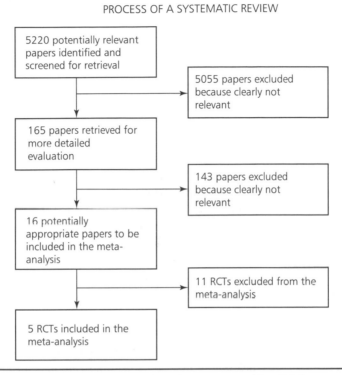

**Ex. 8.3.** Flowchart for a systematic review: the process used by Whittington *et al.* (2004) [22] to identify and select randomized controlled trials (RCTs) of SSRI drugs in the treatment of childhood depression, shown in the flowchart format recommended by QUOROM [16]. Reprinted from *The Lancet* 363 (9418). Whittington CJ, Kendall T, Fonagy P, Cottrell D, Cotgrove A, Boddington E. Selective serotonin reuptake inhibitors in childhood depression: systematic review of published versus unpublished data', 1341–1345, copyright 2004, with permission from Elsevier.

studies, there are often multiple measures of exposure, for example, different methods of assessing a complex exposure such as exercise or sun exposure.

The process should avoid the use of inappropriate exclusion criteria, which sometimes appear in less scientific processes. For example, the association between passive smoking and lung cancer has been of great importance both scientifically and legally. A meta-analysis of all available studies by the US National Research Council gave an overall relative risk of 1.34; a subsequent meta-analysis derived a lower risk of 1.12 based only on the studies which were conducted in the USA, this being justified on the basis that only studies based on the population to which the policy decisions would apply should be used [30]. A similar restriction was suggested in a US Senate report on breast cancer screening, even though most of the randomized trials have been done outside the USA [31,32].

However, the decision to exclude, or place less emphasis on, certain studies because of such methodological criteria may itself introduce more bias, as will be discussed later in this chapter.

## Extraction of data

Once the studies have been identified, the relevant results have to be abstracted from the reports. This requires definition of the comparisons and outcomes to be assessed, and is often a quite complex process. It is also open to subjective influences, and so the extraction of the key data from each study should involve two or more investigators working independently, and disagreements and compromises should be documented. Standardized report forms and computer entry procedures with error checks are desirable. The abstraction of key data could be blinded, with information on, for example, the title of the paper, the journal, the authors, and other aspects removed before the data are abstracted, but the value of this extra investment is not generally accepted.

Care needs to be taken in defining the exposure or intervention and the outcome for each specific comparison. Different studies of the same topic may use different outcome measures or may report a number of outcomes, and for a meta-analysis the outcome must be relevant and consistent.

## Detecting publication bias: funnel plots

From the principle of random variation discussed in Chapter 7, it follows that if there are a number of good (i.e. unbiased) studies of an association, each will give an estimate of the association, subject to chance variation. The results should cluster around the true value of the effect, with the variation being greater in the smaller studies because they have lower precision. Therefore if we plot the estimate given by each study against a measure of the precision of that study, we expect a pattern centred on the true value of the association, with the low-precision studies having greater variability, and therefore more spread on the graph, than the high-precision studies. A funnel plot is a graph with one point for each study; the horizontal axis shows the estimate of the association in the study (with ratios on a log scale), and the vertical axis shows the variability of the estimate (e.g. the standard error). If all the studies are unbiased, and we have information on all the studies, there should be a symmetrical pattern with an overall funnel shape (either an upright or inverted triangle), centred on the true value. Publication bias

FUNNEL PLOT OF 15 TRIALS

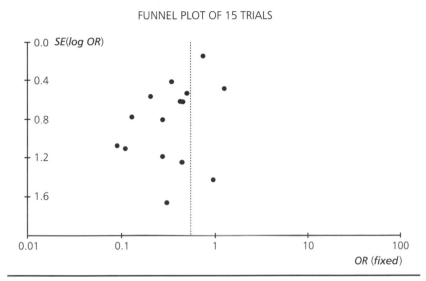

**Ex. 8.4.** Funnel plot: a funnel plot of 15 randomized trials of magnesium in reducing mortality after myocardial infarction. The horizontal axis shows the logarithm of the odds ratio, and the vertical axis shows its standard error; the least precise studies are at the bottom. The asymmetry of the plot suggests publication bias. Data from Sterne and Egger [33]

(usually) means that small low-precision studies that give positive associations tend to be published, but small low-precision studies that show null results or a negative association tend to be ignored. If so, the plot will be asymmetric.

**Exhibit 8.4** shows a funnel plot for 15 randomized trials, published between 1984 and 1995, of magnesium as a treatment to prevent mortality in patients who had or were suspected of having an acute myocardial infarction. The data are from a publication [33] which presents various alternative ways of showing the plot. The odds ratio is shown on the horizontal axis using a logarithmic scale, and compared with its standard error, with the larger studies with greater precision at the top of the graph. The vertical line shows the 'average' odds ratio from the 15 studies shown (calculated by methods that will be described later in this chapter). These are trials of treatment, assessing mortality, and so a beneficial effect (fewer deaths in the treatment arm) is shown by an odds ratio less than 1. If there were no publication bias, and no other variation in the studies other than sample size, the smaller studies with higher standard errors would show a greater spread of results, but this would be symmetric around the average value. Here there are many more data points to the left, representing small studies which show beneficial effects, and very few data points to the right, corresponding to small studies which show negative effects. The implication is that there are other small studies with null or detrimental effects (odds ratios close to or greater than 1), but these have not been published or identified for the review. This example will be described in more detail later in the chapter.

However, asymmetry in a funnel plot could also be due to some studies being biased because of poor design or analysis, or to a true variation in the association between different studies. Visual examination of a funnel plot is obviously a very approximate way to assess publication bias. Various mathematical methods have been suggested, such as estimating the number of extra studies that would be needed to make the plot symmetrical ('trim and fill' methods) or using statistical regression methods, but all these methods have limitations [34].

## Applying quality criteria

The abstracted studies can be assessed using various *quality criteria*. Such criteria have been most fully developed for randomized trials, although various sets of criteria for other types of studies have been proposed. Strong views for [35] and against [36] the use of quality measures have been expressed.

Juni *et al.* [37] note 39 different scales used to assess quality in randomized controlled trials. Some scales are extensive, covering many aspects of study design, and others are relatively limited. One widely used scale for randomized trials is that of Jadad *et al.* [38], which concentrates on the randomization process, double-blind design, indistinguishable placebos, and documentation of patient attrition after randomization. It was developed by a multidisciplinary panel assessing clinical trials in pain research. The scope of these scales varies, their validity is largely untested, and meta-analyses using different scales can produce discordant results. An assessment of the impact of scales in assessing trials relevant to clinical practice guidelines for cancer concluded that the classification of the quality of trials depended largely on the scale used, and concluded that quality assessment was unlikely to change the clinical recommendations produced [39].

The analysis of studies in meta-analyses by particular aspects of quality may be more valuable than using overall scales, as different aspects will have different impacts depending on the topic. Thus, in a meta-analysis of 17 trials comparing types of heparin for the prevention of deep venous thrombosis, the overall relative risk was significantly greater in trials which were not blinded in terms of outcome assessment, but trials with clearly documented concealment of allocation and conduct of an intention to treat analysis did not show different results to trials without these features [37].

The results of quality assessment can be applied in different ways. First, studies that do not fulfil preset quality criteria can be excluded from the analysis completely, but, as noted, it is usually unwise to exclude studies completely because quality criteria are of questionable validity. It may be difficult to ascertain whether a study actually is deficient in a certain area (such as in the checking of validity of information) or whether the relevant information is simply not reported in the papers available. However, the assessment of quality may make a formal meta-analysis inappropriate, or urge caution in its interpretation. Thus a systematic review of cholinesterase inhibitors for patients with Alzheimer's disease assessed cognitive outcome, and most of the trials assessed showed small but positive benefits. However, the authors noted many methodological limitations including multiple testing without appropriate statistical corrections and exclusions of patients after randomization, and therefore did not do a meta-analysis. They concluded that the information was insufficient to support the benefits of these drugs [40].

Secondly, analyses may be carried out comparing studies which differ in terms of an overall quality score or specific components of quality. This is the most generally applicable method as it explores explicitly the aspects of quality that are relevant in a particular context. Where studies can be classified into two or only a few groups in terms of a component (e.g. trials with adequate evidence of double-blind design compared with trials without such evidence), a meta-analysis stratifying on that factor will illustrate its effect. The sensitivity of the overall measure of effect to the exclusion of studies based on the quality criteria can be assessed. Thus Schulz et al. [41] further reviewed 33 meta-analyses, which had themselves involved 250 controlled trials, and analysed the associations between assessments of methodological quality of the trials and the estimated treatment effects. Amongst several results, they found significant differences in outcome in trials which were not double-blind compared with those that were, and in those where the randomization allocation was inadequately concealed, with the weaker studies reporting larger odds ratios. Moher et al. [42] assessed 11 meta-analyses including 127 trials, also finding larger effects in studies with inadequate allocation concealment, but finding no difference in those which were not double-blind.

In a systematic review of glucosamine and condroitin preparations, which are widely promoted for the relief of osteoarthritis, 37 studies were identified, of which 15 were included in a meta-analysis [43]. An assessment of quality was applied, with quality scores ranging from 12 to 55 per cent of the maximum. The meta-analysis demonstrated substantial beneficial effects, but these were reduced when only high-quality or large trials were considered. Furthermore, funnel plots showed significant asymmetry, suggesting publication bias, and so the authors of the review concluded that the estimated effect size in their analysis was probably exaggerated because of the impact of low-quality studies and publication bias.

Some studies show how the measure of effect changes as studies with decreasing quality scores are cumulatively included in the analysis. If the result changes rapidly, this would suggest that the quality scoring is relevant and justifies putting more emphasis on it. Thus, in a meta-analysis of seven randomized trials assessing mammographic screening in women under the age of 50, Glasziou *et al.* [44] presented the results by cumulatively including studies in the rank order of a quality score. This showed that a beneficial result, although non-significant, was seen in the study they regarded as having the best design characteristics, but inclusion of any further studies changed this risk ratio to a null result.

If the component has many ordered categories or is quantitative, for example year of publication or an overall quality score, an analysis can be done assessing the relationship between the results and the quality variable, using *meta-regression* methods. These are discussed later in this chapter.

A third approach is to incorporate information on study quality as weighting factors in the meta-analysis. As will be shown, in meta-analysis the results of different studies are weighted in accordance to their statistical precision. Modification of this weighting by incorporating quality control variables is possible, but the results will depend strongly on the validity of such quality measures, and will often be difficult to interpret.

## Limitations of meta-analysis

If all the studies have a similar limitation, a meta-analysis will not overcome that limitation. An example is the meta-analysis of observational studies assessing the relationship between the practice of breast self-examination and the extent of breast cancer at the time of diagnosis [45]. All the observational studies used suffer from the same problem, that women who choose to practice self-examination differ from those who do not, not only with regard to measurable factors such as age, but with regard to a complex matrix of factors which relates to their own health care practices and use of medical resources. The meta-analysis found that those who practiced self-examination tended to have smaller cancers than those who did not, with the conclusion that self-examination is beneficial. However, none of the studies individually can deal with the confounding problem, that the effect may be due not to the practice of self-examination but to other characteristics which relate to the choice of that method; the meta-analysis does not help with this.

Similarly, a meta-analysis of randomized trials of different surgical methods of hysterectomy identified 27 trials, and reported on the time to return to normal activities after operation and on complications. However, the authors noted that insufficient data were available for many long-term patient outcome measurements, which limited the conclusions that can be reached [46].

## Exploring differences between studies: heterogeneity, effect modification, and meta-regression

One of the main values of meta-analysis is that it can demonstrate differences between study results and lead to explanations of such differences. The interpretation of such results is similar to the situation in a single study where the results differ between subgroups. If the split was anticipated, i.e. if it had been predicted for some logical reason or from other results that there should be this type of variation, the results are reasonably robust. If they are unexpected, their interpretation has to be cautious, and should be looked on as generating a new hypothesis.

Such analyses are assessing effect modification, i.e. the effects of factors which influence the main association that is being studied. The analysis may be by stratification, assessing whether the main effect differs between the strata. Thus, in a meta-analysis of hormone replacement therapy and the incidence of stroke, an excess risk of borderline significance was shown in studies published before 1986, but a significant reduction in stroke in studies published after 1986 [47]. A meta-analysis of nine randomized trials and four case–control studies assessing screening mammography in reducing breast cancer mortality showed that the overall benefit, a 26 per cent mortality reduction, did not vary with the number of mammographic views per screen, the time interval between screenings, or the duration of follow-up, but it did vary with the age of the woman, with no benefit being seen in women entering the studies under age 50 [48]. Statistical methods to assess heterogeneity are discussed in the second part of this chapter.

Whether the factor being considered as an effect modifier has ordered categories or is quantitative, stratification can be augmented by regression analyses relating this factor to the main effect. In the context of meta-analysis, this approach to the study of effect modifying factors is referred to as *meta-regression*. For example, in a meta-analysis of studies reporting operative mortality rates for surgical repair of ruptured abdominal aortic aneurisms, examination by time showed a steady reduction in the operative mortality rate over a 40-year period [49]. In a meta-analysis of 10 cohort studies, the percentage reduction in risk of heart disease for the same reduction in serum cholesterol decreased with increasing age of the subjects, from 54 per cent at ages 35–44 to 19 per cent at ages over 75 [50].

Variables commonly assessed by stratification or meta-regression methods in therapeutic trials include age, sex, previous therapy, aspects of the current therapy such as dose, method of administration, and the time at which the therapy was given. The baseline risk of the patients treated, assessed by the severity or extent of the underlying disease, or by comorbidity and general factors such as clinical performance status, is often of particular interest. The outcome measure used will be relevant. If the therapy has a constant relative risk for different risk categories of patients, i.e. a similar proportional reduction in the underlying hazard, the absolute measure of benefit expressed as a risk difference will be larger in those with a higher baseline risk, and the number needed to treat will be smaller. Also, in subjects with a lower baseline risk of the disease being targeted, other diseases (competing mortality and morbidity) will be more important, and so the effects of the therapy on total mortality or general quality of life may be reduced.

These issues may be explored in a meta-analysis using the results of individual studies, but of course will be limited by the extent of variation in the factors to be assessed in the studies available. Much more powerful and informative analyses can be done in pooled analyses of individual subject data from the various studies.

## Meta-analyses of observational studies

Meta-analysis was first developed for application to randomized trials, on the logic that the chief issue to be overcome was that of the small study size of most trials, using the advantage that randomized trials represent a fundamentally consistent study design, so that the results of different trials could be reasonably combined.

Meta-analytical methods are also appropriate and increasingly widely used for observational studies, both cohort and case–control studies, as well as being applied to studies of screening and diagnostic testing, economic valuations, and other classes of study. The principles and methods are the same, but the objective may be different. Observational studies are often weak not primarily because of small study size, but because of a limited ability to account for confounding and susceptibility to observational bias. Meta-analyses can be very valuable in dealing with confounding and observation bias, but considerable care is needed. If all the studies included in a meta-analysis have the same limitation, for example use the same methods of the assessment or are all inadequate in dealing with confounding factors, a meta-analysis will not necessarily help. As with randomized trials, meta-analyses using individual subject data are particularly powerful in exploring these issues of observation bias and confounder control.

Several important meta-analyses of observational studies have already been mentioned, such as the analyses of aetiological factors in breast cancer. The main advantages of these meta-analyses compared with the individual studies that contribute to them are the reasonably precise measures of association produced and the greatly increased ability to assess confounding and effect modification. For example, the meta-analysis of studies relating previous induced abortions to breast cancer showed that there was no increased risk in studies in which abortions were documented prior to the onset of the breast cancer, and the positive associations came from retrospective case–control studies open to recall bias, as discussed in Chapter 5 [7].

A meta-analysis of observational studies using individual subject data is a complex process. Unless the studies have been designed in common, the methods of assessment of exposures such as diet are often very complex, and it may be difficult or impossible to assess the equivalence of measures used in different studies. For example, there are many studies from different places in the world assessing sun exposure in relationship to skin cancers, but as well as needing to ensure that the questionnaires used in different studies are compatible, there is the issue that a sun exposure of 1 hour in Sydney is not the same as an exposure of 1 hour in London. Often the data need to be considerably simplified to make them consistent between studies. Thus in a meta-analysis of case–control studies of childhood leukaemia related to measured electromagnetic fields, the meta-analysis had to use a simplified assessment which could be obtained from all the studies available, and ignore the more sophisticated, and perhaps more valid, assessment methods used in the most extensive studies [8,51]. However, the advantage of the meta-analysis is that by having greater numbers of subjects the association between increased risk and different levels of exposure can be assessed quite precisely.

An ideal process is to have international collaboration from the study design phase, so that observational studies carried out in different places are designed to be combined in an individual subject data pooled analysis, and use the same questionnaires and methods. This is being done in the Interphone studies relating to use of mobile phones and brain cancers, where an international effort has led to case–control studies being conducted in many different countries using a commonly agreed protocol and data collection methods. The objective is to produce a statistically powerful pooled analysis of all the data, although individual studies are usually funded from each country and also published as separate studies. Even more ambitious are international prospective studies such as the European Prospective Investigation into Cancer and Nutrition (EPIC) [52], which has produced many reports.

# Part 2. Statistical methods in meta-analysis
## Obtaining a measure of overall effect: fixed effects methods

The most widely used statistical methods for meta-analysis are based on a 'fixed effects' model, i.e. they derive a summary estimate of effect only from the data given by the studies included in the analysis.

### Averages weighted by the inverse of variance

The underlying principle of these methods is straightforward. Each study included in the meta-analysis contributes an outcome measurement: relative risk, odds ratio, risk difference, or another measure. The precision of each outcome measurement is indicated by its variance; the more precise the measure, the smaller is the variance. A reasonable overall measure of effect based on all studies is the weighted average of the outcome measurements from each study. The weight is the inverse of the variance of the study. In this way, the studies which have the greatest weight, and therefore contribute the most to the overall measure of effect, are those with the lowest variance and the greatest precision. They will usually be the largest studies.

In mathematical terms, to obtain the weighted average we multiply the measure of effect for each study by its weight, add these terms for all studies, and divide the result by the sum of all the weights. Therefore the summary measure of effect $OR_s$ is given by

$$OR_s = \frac{\sum_i (w_i \times OR_i)}{\sum_i w_i}$$

where $OR_i$ is the odds ratio from each study $i$ and $w_i$ is the weight for that study. The most widely used methods of meta-analysis use this approach; the details vary with the measure of effect and the formula for the variance.

In **Ex. 8.5,** the results of three randomized trials of the treatment of acute conjunctivitis (eye infection) are shown, comparing the antibiotic chloramphenicol with placebo [53]. The outcome assessed here is microbiological remission, assessed by eye swabs taken for culture. The trials were all fairly small, and the result of each trial is shown on one line as the number of successes, i.e. remission, and the number of failures for patients randomized to chloramphenicol (the treated group) and to the placebo control group. The odds ratios range from 2.52 to 11.25. We will show the two most commonly used methods applied to these data. The two methods both use the observed number of successes in the exposed group, the expected number, and the same formula for variance; they use the same statistical test, but different measures of the odds ratios and summary odds ratio.

## Mantel–Haenszel method

The Mantel–Haenszel process is the same as that used in the analysis of stratified data; here the stratification variable is the individual study. Thus, for each study, the quantities $ad/T$ and $bc/T$ are calculated, then these are summed, and the summary odds ratio is calculated as shown. This is the formula given in Chapter 7 and in Appendix Tables 1–3. The summary $\chi$ (or $\chi^2$) statistic is also calculated using the same method as was shown previously. The Mantel–Haenszel calculation gives an odds ratio of 4.77, and a $\chi$ statistic of 6.62, which has a $P$-value of much less than 0.0001.

## Peto method

In the Peto method, the number of observed events in the intervention group $(O_i)$ is known for each trial, and the number of events expected $(E_i)$ is found as shown; the value $O_i - E_i$ is then calculated. The variance of the expected number $(V_i)$ is calculated by the same method as in the Mantel–Haenszel test. As a measure of effect, the differences between the observed and expected numbers in each study are summed. The natural logarithm of the summary odds ratio is given by this term divided by the sum of the variances [54]:

$$OR_s = \exp\left[\frac{\sum_i (O_i - E_i)}{\sum_i V_i}\right]$$

To assess significance, the summary normal deviate statistic is calculated over $i$ trials as

$$\chi = \frac{\sum_i (O_i - E_i)}{\sqrt{\sum_i V_i}}$$

META–ANALYSIS: MANTEL–HAENSZEL AND PETO METHODS

*Results of each study*

| Study | Treated group: Success | Fail | Control group: Success | Fail | Total | Odds ratio |
|---|---|---|---|---|---|---|
| | *a* | *b* | *c* | *d* | *T* | |
| 1 | 24 | 10 | 6 | 26 | 66 | 10.40 |
| 2 | 132 | 8 | 22 | 15 | 177 | 11.25 |
| 3 | 53 | 23 | 32 | 35 | 143 | 2.52 |

*Mantel–Haenszel method*

| | *a* = obs | *E* | *V* | *ad/T* | *bc/T* | Odds ratio | Chi |
|---|---|---|---|---|---|---|---|
| 1 | 24 | 15.45 | 4.15 | 9.45 | 0.91 | 10.40 | 4.19 |
| 2 | 132 | 121.81 | 3.33 | 11.19 | 0.99 | 11.25 | 5.59 |
| 3 | 53 | 45.17 | 8.65 | 12.97 | 5.15 | 2.52 | 2.66 |
| Sum | 209 | 182.44 | 16.12 | 33.61 | 7.05 | | |

| | | |
|---|---|---|
| OR = sum (*ad/T*) / sum (*bc/T*) = | 4.77 | |
| 95% confidence limits for OR | 2.26, 10.07 | |
| Chi = (sum *a* − sum *E*)/sum $V^.5$ = | 6.62 | <0.0001 |
| Heterogeneity chi sq (2 df) | 8.09 | 0.017 |

*Peto method*

| | *a* = obs | *E* | *V* | *O − E* | Odds ratio | *Z* deviate |
|---|---|---|---|---|---|---|
| 1 | 24 | 15.45 | 4.15 | 8.55 | 7.84 | 4.19 |
| 2 | 132 | 121.81 | 3.33 | 10.19 | 21.39 | 5.59 |
| 3 | 53 | 45.17 | 8.65 | 7.83 | 2.47 | 2.66 |
| Sum | 209 | 182.44 | 16.12 | 26.56 | | |

| | | |
|---|---|---|
| Summary results: ln *OR* = sum (*O–E*)/sum *V* = | 1.65 | |
| *OR* = exp (ln *OR*) = | 5.19 | |
| 95% limits for *OR* | 3.19, 8.46 | |
| Normal deviate = sum (*O–E*)/sum $V^.5$ = | 6.62 | <0.0001 |
| Heterogeneity chi sq | 12.13 | 0.002 |

**Ex. 8.5.** Application of the Mantel–Haenszel and Peto methods to a meta-analysis of three randomized trials of chloramphenicol (antibiotic), compared with placebo, for acute conjunctivitis, assessing the outcome of microbiological remission after 2-3 days. Data from Sheik *et al.* [53]

This is the same as the Mantel–Haenszel summary statistic shown earlier (Ex. 7.3).

In this example, the Peto method shows an overall odds ratio of 5.19, and a normal deviate of 6.62 ($P < 0.0001$), showing a highly significant effect. The statistical test is the same in these two analyses. They use different calculations for odds ratio, and in this example the differences in odds ratio are substantial.

## Comparison of Mantel–Haenszel and Peto methods

These two methods are both justifiable on statistical grounds. The Peto method has been very widely applied to large meta-analyses of randomized trials. The measure of effect, dependent on the difference between the observed and expected numbers, is mathematically and intuitively simple to understand and report, which has been advantageous. Where there are considerable differences between the individual studies in the ratios of exposed to unexposed subjects, or of cases to controls, the Mantel–Haenszel method is statistically superior, as the Peto method can produce a biased measure of effect [55]. For this reason, the Mantel–Haenszel method is preferable in the analysis of cohort and case–control studies, where such variation is more likely than in clinical trials. Thus the Peto method was used in the large meta-analysis of the treatment of breast cancer, based on randomized trials using survival data [3], while the Mantel–Haenszel method was used in the meta-analysis of observational studies relating oral contraceptive use to breast cancer incidence [6].

However, both methods have two major disadvantages. The results of each individual study need to be available as a 2 × 2 table. As only these data are used, confounding effects of other variables cannot usually be taken into account (although a simple confounder may be dealt with by using stratified data from each study, for example data by sex, if available). Therefore these methods are of less value where the estimate of effect given by the simple 2 × 2 table is not a good measure of the final result of a study because of confounding or matching. This applies in the diabetes trial referred to in Chapter 6, where a better result is obtained after further analysis incorporating other variables. In randomized trials, this situation is unusual, and so the methods can usually be applied. However, in observational studies, it is less likely that a simple 2 × 2 table gives an adequate summary of the overall result, as adjustment for other confounding factors is often essential. Indeed, for this reason the results may not be published in a form that allows a 2 × 2 table to be constructed. These limitations are overcome by methods based on confidence limits.

## Choice of outcome measures

Most meta-analyses of treatment effects follow the logic that treatment is designed to reduce the frequency of unwanted events, such as deaths, recurrences, or complications, and therefore a beneficial effect is shown by an odds ratio or risk ratio less than 1 and a risk difference less than zero. However, other clinical outcomes may be positive outcomes, such as the achievement of function, discharge from hospital, and so on. Binary outcomes such as survival can be reported as either the proportion of patients surviving or the proportion of patients dying. If analyses are expressed in terms of deaths as distinct from survival, the odds ratios in the two situations are reciprocals of each other, and risk difference measurements will be the same with a reversed sign. However, with risk ratios, i.e. the ratio of incidence rates, the ratio itself will be different, and its statistical significance and heterogeneity between studies may be different.

An example of this is shown by the data presented in Ex. 8.5. We have presented odds ratios to show the application of the Mantel–Haenszel and Peto methods using odds ratios. These methods can also be applied using relative risks. The relative risks for the three studies shown in Ex. 8.5, in the order given, are 3.76, 1.59, and 1.46. They are substantially different from the odds ratios because the outcome is common and the success rates in the control groups vary in the studies, being 19 per cent in study 1, but 60 per cent in study 2 and 48 per cent in study 3. As a result the relative risks for studies 2 and 3 are similar, and lower than the relative risk for study 1. In contrast, as shown in Ex. 8.5, the odds ratios are similar for studies 1 and 2, and higher than the odds ratio in study 3.

## Methods based on the confidence interval for each study

These methods, rather than using a simple $2 \times 2$ table of results from each study, use the published estimate of effect obtained from each study, and its 95 per cent (usually) confidence limits. In observational studies, for example, the overall measure of effect and its confidence limits may be given from the results of a multivariate analysis, a matched analysis, or a Mantel–Haenszel type analysis after controlling for confounding. This method, developed by Prentice and Thomas [56] and by Greenland [57], estimates the variance of each risk estimate from its confidence limits, and then produces a weighted average, using the inverse of the variance. In using this method, care needs to be taken in abstracting the information to ensure that the confidence limits used are correct, and, where possible, these should be checked. In some studies, confidence limits may not be presented, but can be calculated from the raw data or estimated by the test-based method given previously (Ex. 7.7).

**Exhibit 8.6** shows the application of the confidence limits method to a meta-analysis of seven case–control studies that assessed the association between sunburn in childhood and the occurrence of malignant melanoma in later life [58]. In this situation, the studies cannot be reduced to simple $2 \times 2$ tables, as the result of each study is adjusted for various confounders such as ethnic origin and skin type. The best estimate of odds ratio $OR_i$, after appropriate confounder control, and its 95 per cent upper and lower confidence limits, $OR_U$ and $OR_L$ were abstracted from each published study. The variance is calculated as

$$\text{variance } OR_i = \left[ \frac{\ln(OR_U / OR_i)}{1.96} \right]^2$$

or

$$\text{variance } OR_i = \left[ \frac{\ln(OR_i / OR_L)}{1.96} \right]^2.$$

These two expressions should give the same result; it is a useful check to calculate the variance using each of the lower and the upper confidence limits, as variation beyond rounding errors would indicate an error in the abstracted data. The weight $w_i$ for each study is the inverse of the variance, and then the summary odds ratio $OR_s$ is given by

$$OR_s = \frac{\sum_i (w_i \times OR_i)}{\sum_i w_i}.$$

The analysis of the seven studies shows an overall odds ratio of 1.88. The confidence limits are

$$95\% \text{ limits of } OR_s = \exp(\ln OR_s \pm 1.96 \sqrt{Vs})$$

where

$$V_s = \text{variance of } \ln OR_s = 1/\sum_i w_i$$

and here the summary odds ratio of 1.88 has 95 per cent limits of 1.56 to 2.28.

## Display of results: the forest plot

The results of a meta-analysis are often displayed as a *forest plot*. This method has been adopted by the Cochrane Collaboration and built into the RevMan

## META-ANALYSIS: CONFIDENCE LIMITS METHOD

A: *meta-analysis of 7 case-control studies*

| Study $i$ | Odds ratio $OR_i$ | 95% CL lower | 95% CL upper | Variance | weight $w_i$ | $w_i \ln OR_i$ | heterog. $Q_i$ |
|---|---|---|---|---|---|---|---|
| 1 | 1.30 | 0.90 | 1.80 | 0.03 | 31.86 | 8.36 | 4.39 |
| 2 | 1.20 | 0.60 | 2.30 | 0.12 | 8.50 | 1.55 | 1.73 |
| 3 | 3.70 | 2.30 | 6.10 | 0.06 | 16.14 | 21.12 | 7.35 |
| 4 | 2.40 | 0.80 | 7.30 | 0.32 | 3.14 | 2.75 | 0.18 |
| 5 | 6.50 | 3.40 | 12.30 | 0.11 | 9.29 | 17.40 | 14.25 |
| 6 | 1.49 | 0.97 | 2.32 | 0.05 | 20.20 | 8.06 | 1.11 |
| 7 | 1.60 | 1.00 | 2.60 | 0.06 | 16.83 | 7.91 | 0.45 |
| | | | Summation | | 105.97 | 67.14 | 29.47 |

$$\text{summary } \ln OR_s = \frac{\sum_i (w_i \times \ln OR_i)}{\sum_i w_i} = \qquad 0.63$$

Summary $OR_s = \exp(\ln OR) = \qquad 1.88$

95% CI for summary $OR_s$ $\qquad$ lower $\qquad$ 1.56

$$= \exp\left[\ln OR_s \pm 1.96 \Big/ \sqrt{\sum_i w_i}\right] = \qquad \text{upper} \qquad 2.28$$

B: *Excluding studies 3, 5*

| Study $i$ | Odds ratio $OR_i$ | 95% CL lower | 95% CL upper | Variance | weight $w_i$ | $w_i \ln OR_i$ | heterog. $Q_i$ |
|---|---|---|---|---|---|---|---|
| 1 | 1.30 | 0.90 | 1.80 | 0.03 | 31.86 | 8.36 | 0.28 |
| 2 | 1.20 | 0.60 | 2.30 | 0.12 | 8.50 | 1.55 | 0.25 |
| 4 | 2.40 | 0.80 | 7.30 | 0.32 | 3.14 | 2.75 | 0.85 |
| 6 | 1.49 | 0.97 | 2.32 | 0.05 | 20.20 | 8.06 | 0.04 |
| 7 | 1.60 | 1.00 | 2.60 | 0.06 | 16.83 | 7.91 | 0.22 |
| | | | Summation | | 80.54 | 28.63 | 1.64 |

summary $\ln OR_s = \qquad$ 0.36
summary $OR_s = \exp(\ln OR) = \qquad$ 1.43
95% CI for summary $OR = \qquad$ lower $\qquad$ 1.15
$\qquad$ upper $\qquad$ 1.78

**Ex. 8.6.** Meta-analysis using the confidence limits method: results of seven case-control studies relating a history of sunburn in childhood to the incidence of melanoma. Data from Elwood and Jopson [58]

software [14,59]. The results of the meta-analysis just discussed are shown as a forest plot in **Ex. 8.7**. The individual studies are each summarized on one line. The graph for each study shows a square indicating the weight assigned to that study, and a horizontal line showing (in this example) the 95 per cent confidence interval for the odds ratio, on a logarithmic scale. The text shows the odds ratio and its confidence limits, and the weight expressed as a percentage of total weight of all studies. The combined estimate of effect based on the meta-analysis is shown by a diamond, with its width showing the 95 per cent confidence interval. Other data presented are the statistical test for the significance of the overall effect and the statistical test for heterogeneity, which will be discussed later. This output can be produced for odds ratios, relative risks, or risk differences (which are shown with an arithmetic scale), and using Peto, Mantel–Haenszel, or confidence limits calculations, or with the random effects model discussed below.

## Tests of heterogeneity

An important part of any meta-analysis is testing whether the overall summary estimate is an adequate representation of the set of data. To do this a heterogeneity test is used, comparing each of the individual study results with the summary estimate. The demonstration of heterogeneity may be very important, as it will focus attention on why there are differences between studies. If one or two studies stand out from the rest, there may be reasons for this, such as differences in the intervention, the exposure, the study design, or the population studied.

If there is significant heterogeneity between studies, the overall measure of effect cannot be simply interpreted. The studies need to be assessed to see if there is a logical reason for the heterogeneity; if such a reason is found, subdivision of the studies into meaningful groups will be helpful. The heterogeneity statistics produce a value for each individual study, based on the comparison of that study's result to the summary result. Therefore where there is heterogeneity, it is logical to exclude the studies with the highest individual summary values and then repeat the analysis, recalculating the summary measure of effect and the heterogeneity statistics compared with this new summary measure. Often the results have to be presented as showing a summary statistic based on a certain number of studies, and pointing out one or more studies with results which are inconsistent with this overall estimate. This is the technique used, for example, in a meta-analysis of eight studies assessing family history and melanoma [60], where there was considerable heterogeneity with no clear explanation. The heterogeneity may reflect real differences, but may

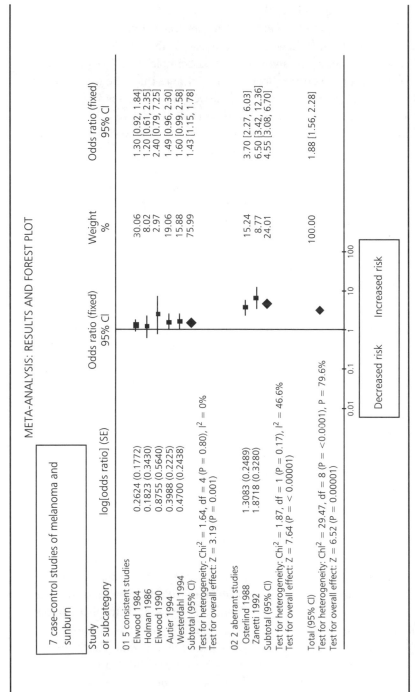

**Ex. 8.7.** Display of meta-analysis of data: data shown in Ex. 8.6, produced by the Cochrane Colloboration RevMan software (version 4.2.8, 2005); the graphical display is a forest plot

also be due to different methods of ascertaining the exposure or of assessing confounders, differences in the definitions of the controls used, and so on.

A widely used test of heterogeneity is analogous to the test used in stratified analysis, shown in Chapter 7. For each study a term $Q_i$ is calculated:

$$Q_i = w_i(\ln OR_i - \ln OR_s)^2$$

so that $Q_i$ depends on the weight $w_i$, and the difference between the odds ratio $OR_i$ for that study and the summary odds ratio $OR_s$.

Then the sum $\Sigma_i Q_i$ is a $\chi^2$ statistic on $(n-1)$ degrees of freedom, where $n$ is the number of studies. For the analysis of the seven studies of sunburn and melanoma (Exs 8.6 and 8.7), the overall heterogeneity statistic is 29.5 on six degrees of freedom, which is highly significant ($P < 0.001$). Examination of the heterogeneity statistics for each study shows that the major contributors to this are studies 5 and 3, which have the highest odds ratios. Exclusion of these studies allows the calculation of a summary odds ratio based on the remaining five studies, which is 1.43, and the heterogeneity statistic (recalculated using this revised summary odds ratio) is no longer significant. The next step in the analysis is to consider why two of the studies give considerably higher odds ratios than the remaining five studies. This may relate to a real difference in the populations studied or to a difference in method, for example in the methods used to ascertain sunburn. It would be unwise to assume that the discrepancy necessarily means that the studies which are in the minority are in error; they may be as or more valid than the rest. Heterogeneity statistics for the Mantel–Haenszel and Peto methods are shown in Appendix Table 12, and for confidence limits methods in Appendix Table 13 (pp. 542 and 548).

The quantity $I^2$ is calculated as $100 \times [Q - (k-1)]/Q$, where $Q$ is the sum of all $Q_i$ given above and $k$ is the number of studies in the analysis. It is approximately the proportion of total variation attributable to between-study heterogeneity, the remainder being sampling error.

## Random effects models

The methods described above are all *fixed effects* models, i.e. they estimate the overall measure of effect given the studies which have been included in the analysis. A different approach assumes that the studies which have been included are a representative sample of a hypothetical larger population of studies, and therefore uses a different method of estimation—a *random effects* model. Where there is no heterogeneity between studies, these two approaches give the same results. Where there is heterogeneity, the random effects model may give substantially different results [61,62]. It gives a greater importance (weight) to the smaller studies in the set, and this can be criticized as the smaller studies may be more likely to suffer from methodological limitations or from publication bias (in the presence of publication bias, it is the smaller studies that are a biased sample). Given the different views about the relevance of these methods, and the fact that the random effects models give different results only if there is heterogeneity of effect, they are less widely used.

The calculations for the most widely used random effects model, the DerSimonian–Laird method [63], are shown in Appendix Table 14. The fixed effect models (the Mantel–Haenszel and Peto methods) and the random effects model (the DerSimonian–Laird method) both produce weighted averages of the results from the individual studies. The fixed effect models use as weights the inverse $1/v_i$ of the within-study variance for each study. The DerSimonian–Laird method weights the studies by the inverse of a combination of within-study and between study-variation $1/(v_i + D)$; as this variance will be larger, the confidence interval of the summary measure of effect will be wider. The term $D$ depends on the heterogeneity between studies (it includes the sum $Q_i$ mentioned above) and is zero if this is small, in which case the results given are the same as for fixed effect models; $D$ cannot be negative. When there is substantial between-study variance, i.e. heterogeneity, the DerSimonian–Laird method gives relatively more importance to the smaller studies within the set. With this difference, the random effects model can be applied to count data and to confidence limits data.

For the data shown in Exs 8.6 and 8.7, using all seven studies, the random effects model gives a summary odds ratio of 2.1 with 95 per cent confidence limits of 1.36 to 3.23; the calculations are shown in Appendix Table 14. The odds ratio is higher than the fixed effects estimate, as some small studies have high odds ratios and are given more weight in the random effects model, and the confidence interval is wider as between-study variation is incorporated.

## An example of heterogeneity and publication bias

A study shown earlier in this chapter shows what is now recognized as a classic example of publication bias. The funnel plot shown in Ex. 8.4 is for 15 randomized controlled trials of magnesium treatment to reduce deaths following myocardial infarction, published between 1964 and 1975 [33]. The forest plot for these trials is shown in **Ex. 8.8,** with the studies in order of their weight in the analysis (the forest plot has the larger studies at the bottom; the funnel plot has them at the top). Most of these trials were small, with nine of them having less than 100 patients and less than 10 deaths in the treated group. One trial published in 1992 was much larger than the rest, with over 1000 patients

META-ANALYSIS: RESULTS AND FOREST PLOT (2)

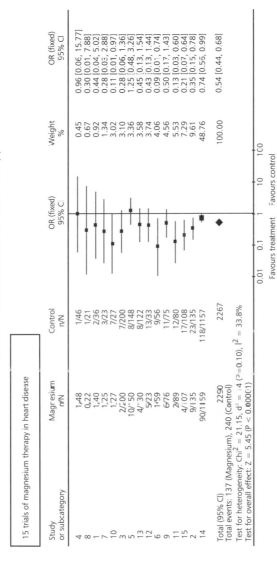

15 trials of magnesium therapy in heart disease

| Study or subcategory | Magnesium n/N | Control n/N | OR (fixed) 95% CI | Weight % | OR (fixed) 95% CI |
|---|---|---|---|---|---|
| 4 | 1/48 | 1/46 | | 0.45 | 0.96 [0.06, 15.77] |
| 8 | 0/22 | 1/21 | | 0.67 | 0.30 [0.01, 7.88] |
| 1 | 1/40 | 2/36 | | 0.92 | 0.44 [0.04, 5.02] |
| 7 | 1/25 | 3/23 | | 1.34 | 0.28 [0.0, 2.88] |
| 10 | 1/27 | 7/27 | | 3.02 | 0.11 [0.01, 0.97] |
| 3 | 2/200 | 7/200 | | 3.10 | 0.28 [0.06, 1.36] |
| 5 | 10/150 | 8/148 | | 3.36 | 1.25 [0.48, 3.26] |
| 13 | 4/150 | 8/122 | | 3.58 | 0.45 [0.13, 1.54] |
| 12 | 5/23 | 13/33 | | 3.74 | 0.43 [0.13, 1.44] |
| 6 | 1/59 | 9/56 | | 4.06 | 0.09 [0.0, 0.74] |
| 9 | 6/76 | 11/75 | | 4.56 | 0.50 [0.17, 1.43] |
| 11 | 2/89 | 12/80 | | 5.53 | 0.13 [0.03, 0.60] |
| 15 | 4/107 | 17/108 | | 7.29 | 0.21 [0.07, 0.64] |
| 2 | 9/135 | 23/135 | | 9.61 | 0.35 [0.15, 0.78] |
| 14 | 90/1159 | 118/1157 | | 48.76 | 0.74 [0.56, 0.99] |
| Total (95% CI) | 2250 | 2267 | | 100.00 | 0.54 [0.44, 0.68] |

Total events: 137 (Magnesium), 240 (Control)
Test for heterogeneity: Chi² = 21.15, d² = 14 (P=0.10), I² = 33.8%
Test for overall effect: Z = 5.45 (P < 0.00001)

0.01  0.1  1  10  100
Favours treatment    Favours control

**Ex. 8.8.** Display of meta-analysis of data: forest plot for 15 trials of magnesium therapy in heart disease, also shown in Ex. 8.4, produced by the Cochrane Colloboration RevMan software (version 4.2.8, 2005). Addition of one much larger trial changed the summary odds ratio from 0.54 to 1.01 (see text)

in each arm and about 100 deaths, and appears at the bottom of the forest plot. The meta-analysis for these 15 studies shows a statistically significant benefit of magnesium therapy, with an approximately 50 per cent reduction in deaths, shown by the odds ratio of 0.54, with 95 per cent confidence limits of 0.44 to 0.68, using the Mantel–Haenszel method shown earlier. However, there is substantial heterogeneity (shown by the $I^2$ value of 33.8 per cent). The larger studies have results closer to the null value, and the smaller studies show a pattern of results extending mainly to the left, representing results showing benefits of magnesium therapy. There is a noticeable absence of results on the right-hand side, suggesting publication bias.

Subsequently (published in 1995) a very large randomized trial was performed [64], which involved almost 30 000 patients treated with magnesium and 30 000 controls, with over 2000 deaths in each group. Its statistical weight is sufficient to outweigh all the other trials combined by a large margin. This large study showed no benefit from magnesium therapy; indeed there was a slight excess of mortality in the magnesium-treated subjects (Mantel–Haenszel odds ratio 1.06, 95 per cent limits 1.00 to 1.13). Adding this large trial to the previous meta-analysis changes the combined odds ratio to 1.01 (limits 0.95 to 1.07), showing no effect of magnesium. The overwhelming results from the large trial shows that the meta-analysis based on the previous 15 studies had given an erroneous conclusion because of publication bias.

The publication bias could be suspected from the funnel plot shown in Ex. 8.4. If there is no publication bias, as mentioned earlier, the spread of points from the studies with poor precision should be symmetrical around the overall odds ratio estimate. A statistical method of assessing publication bias is to fit a regression model on the points given in the funnel plot, showing the estimated linear relationship between the log odds ratio and its standard error. In the absence of publication bias there should be no relationship between these, and the line fitted to the plot would be vertical. Fitting a line and measuring its slope allows a statistical test of whether the slope varies from the null hypothesis that the odds ratio does not change as the standard error changes. Several such methods have been described [65]; for example one was used in a large meta-analysis comparing trials of homeopathic interventions and trials of conventional medical approaches for similar conditions, which demonstrated substantial publication bias in both sets of trials [29].

## Meta-regression

The tests of heterogeneity so far discussed apply to stratified analyses. As well as the situation where each study forms one stratum, strata may be formed by, for example, studies carried out over different time periods, with male or female subjects, and indeed any variable for which sufficient data are available. As mentioned earlier in this chapter, where the effect-modifying factor has ordered categories (such as extent of disease) or is quantitative (such as age), meta-regression methods may be used. These are particularly powerful in pooled analyses using individual study data contributed by the studies making up the meta-analysis. Thus, as mentioned earlier, a meta-regression of the age of the subjects against the relative risk of ischaemic heart disease with lowered cholesterol levels showed that the extent of the risk reduction decreased with increasing age. This was shown by a regression of the relative risk against age, and also by stratification by age [50].

The statistical methods for meta-regression will not be discussed in any detail. They are basically a regression analysis, where the measure of effect such as odds ratio or relative risk (on a log scale) or risk difference is the dependent variable, the other factors which are being assessed, such as age, are the independent variables, and the analysis assesses the relationships between the measure of effect and the other factors. Single-factor analyses are analogous to regression with one variable, and methods analogous to multivariate regression can be used. However, the appropriate estimation of variances, appropriate weighting, and other statistical issues may be complex. Specialized software packages are available.

## Self-test questions (answers on p. 503)

**Q8.1** What is publication bias, and what effect is it likely to have on a review of published data?

**Q8.2** What are the main arguments for and against including all possible studies in a meta-analysis?

**Q8.3** In a review of personal versus group counselling for alcohol-related problems, two randomized trials were found. In one, there were 40 'successes' out of 70 clients given individual therapy compared with 20 successes in 60 clients treated in groups; in the other trial the success rates were 60/75 for individual intervention compared with 20/35 for group intervention. Use the Peto and Mantel–Haenszel methods to estimate the overall odds ratio and the associated statistical test.

**Q8.4** In reviewing studies of environmental smoke and asthma, you find four cohort or case–control studies, with the following results, given as odds ratios and 95% confidence limits: 3.0 (2.2, 4.1); 6.0 (2.6, 13.8); 3.22 (2.78, 3.73); 1.40 (0.34, 5.76). What is the summary odds ratio and its confidence limits? Is there significant heterogeneity?

# References

1. Daniels M, Hill AB. Chemotherapy of pulmonary tuberculosis in young adults. An analysis of the combined results of three Medical Research Council trials. *BMJ* 1952; **1**: 1162–1168.

2. Winkelstein W. The first use of meta-analysis? *Am J Epidemiol* 1998; **147**: 717.

3. Early Breast Cancer Trialists' Collaborative Group. Systemic treatment of early breast cancer by hormonal, cytotoxic, or immune therapy. Part 1. *Lancet* 1992; **339**: 1–15.

4. Early Breast Cancer Trialists' Collaborative Group. Effects of chemotherapy and hormonal therapy for early breast cancer on recurrence and 15-year survival: an overview of the randomised trials. *Lancet* 2005; **365**: 1687–1717.

5. Clarke M, Collins R, Darby S, *et al*. Effects of radiotherapy and of differences in the extent of surgery for early breast cancer on local recurrence and 15-year survival: an overview of the randomised trials. *Lancet* 2005; **366**: 2087–2106.

6. Collaborative Group on Hormonal Factors in Breast Cancer. Breast cancer and hormonal contraceptives: collaborative reanalysis of individual data on 53 297 women with breast cancer and 100 239 women without breast cancer from 54 epidemiological studies. *Lancet* 1996; **347**: 1713–1727.

7. Collaborative Group on Hormonal Factors in Breast Cancer. Breast cancer and abortion: collaborative reanalysis of data from 53 epidemiological studies, including 83 000 women with breast cancer from 16 countries. *Lancet* 2004; **363**: 1007–1016.

8. Greenland S, Sheppard AR, Kaune WT, Poole C, Kelsh MA. A pooled analysis of magnetic fields, wire codes, and childhood leukemia. *Epidemiology* 2000; **11**: 624–634.

9. Higgins JPT, Green S (Eds). *Cochrane Handbook for Systematic Reviews of Interventions* 4.2.5 (updated May 2005), 2005. Available online at: http://www.cochrane.org/resources/handbook/

10. Cochrane AL. *Effectiveness and Efficiency: Random Reflections on Health Services*. Oxford: Nuffield Provincial Hospitals Trust, 1972.

11. *Non-Random Reflections on Health Services Research: On The 25th Anniversary of Archie Cochrane's 'Effectiveness and Efficiency'*. London: BMJ Publishing Group, 1997.

12. Antes G, Oxman AD. The Cochrane Collaboration in the 20th century. In: Egger M, Davey Smith G, Altman DG (eds). *Systematic Reviews in Health Care. Meta-analysis in Context* (2nd edn). London: BMJ Publishing Group, 2001, pp. 447–458.

13. Volmink J, Siegfried N, Robertson K, Gulmezoglu AM. Research synthesis and dissemination as a bridge to knowledge management: the Cochrane Collaboration. *Bull World Health Organiz* 2004; **82**: 778–783.

14. The Cochrane Collaboration. RevMan 4.2 User Guide (updated April 2004), 2004. Available online at: www.cochrane.org/resouces/

15. The Cochrane Collaboration. Glossary of Terms in The Cochrane Collaboration (updated May 2005), 2005. Available online at: http://www.cochrane.org/resources/glossary.htm

16. Moher D, Cook DJ, Eastwood S, Olkin I, Rennie D, Stroup DF. Improving the quality of reports of meta-analyses of randomised controlled trials: the QUOROM statement. Quality of Reporting of Meta-analyses. *Lancet* 1999; **354**: 1896–1900.

17. Turnbull F, Blood Pressure Lowering Treatment Trialists' Collaboration. Effects of different blood-pressure-lowering regimens on major cardiovascular events: results of prospectively-designed overviews of randomised trials. *Lancet* 2003; **362**: 1527–1535.

18. Rosenthal R. The file drawer problem and tolerance for null results. *Psychol Bull* 1979; **86**: 638–641.

19. Peto R, Pike MC, Armitage P, *et al.* Design and analysis of randomized clinical trials requiring prolonged observation of each patient. II. analysis and examples. *Br J Cancer* 1977; **35**: 1–39.

20. Egger M, Dickersin K, Davey Smith G. Problems and limitations in conducting systematic reviews. In Egger M, Davey Smith G, Altman DG (eds), *Systematic Reviews in Health Care. Meta-analysis in Context* (2nd edn). London: BMJ Publishing Group, 2001, pp. 43–68.

21. Melander H, Ahlqvist-Rastad J, Meijer G, Beermann B. Evidence b(i)ased medicine: selective reporting from studies sponsored by pharmaceutical industry: review of studies in new drug applications. *BMJ* 2003; **326**: 1171–1173.

22. Whittington CJ, Kendall T, Fonagy P, Cottrell D, Cotgrove A, Boddington E. Selective serotonin reuptake inhibitors in childhood depression: systematic review of published versus unpublished data. *Lancet* 2004; **363**: 1341–1345.

23. Anonymous. Depressing research. *Lancet* 2004; **363**: 1335.

24. Sampson M, Barrowman NJ, Moher D, *et al.* Should meta-analysts search Embase in addition to Medline? *J Clin Epidemiol* 2003; **56**: 943–955.

25. Montori VM, Wilczynski NL, Morgan D, Haynes RB. Optimal search strategies for retrieving systematic reviews from Medline: analytical survey. *BMJ* 2005; **330**: 68.

26. Haynes RB, McKibbon KA, Wilczynski NL, Walter SD, Werre SR. Optimal search strategies for retrieving scientifically strong studies of treatment from Medline: analytical survey. *BMJ* 2005; **330**: 1179.

27. Lindholm LH, Carlberg B, Samuelsson O. Should beta blockers remain first choice in the treatment of primary hypertension? A meta-analysis. *Lancet* 2005; **366**: 1545–1553.

28. Glass J, Lanctot KL, Herrmann N, Sproule BA, Busto UE. Sedative hypnotics in older people with insomnia: meta-analysis of risks and benefits. *BMJ* 2005; **331**: 1169.

29. Shang A, Huwiler-Muntener K, Nartey L, *et al.* Are the clinical effects of homoeopathy placebo effects? Comparative study of placebo-controlled trials of homoeopathy and allopathy. *Lancet* 2005; **366**: 726–732.

30. Fleiss JL, Gross AJ. Meta-analysis in epidemiology, with special reference to studies of the association between exposure to environmental tobacco smoke and lung cancer: a critique. *J Clin Epidemiol* 1991; **44**: 127–139.

31. Committee on Government Operations. *Misused Science: The National Cancer Institute's Elimination of Mammography Guidelines for Women in their Forties.* Washington: US Government Printing Office, 1994.

32. Elwood JM. Breast cancer screening in younger women; the need for evidence based medicine. *NZ Med J* 1995; **108**: 239–241.

33. Sterne JAC, Egger M. Funnel plots for detecting bias in meta-analysis: guidelines on choice of axis. *J Clin Epidemiol* 2001; **54**: 1046–1055.

34. Sterne JAC, Egger M, Davey Smith G. Investigating and dealing with publication and other biases. In Egger M, Davey Smith G, Altman DG (ed), *Systematic Reviews in Health Care. Meta-analysis in Context* (2nd edn). London: BMJ Publishing Group, 2001, pp. 189–208.

35. Chalmers TC. Problems induced by meta-analyses. *Stat Med* 1991; **10**: 971–980.

36. Greenland S. Quality scores are useless and potentially misleading. Reply to 'Re: A critical look at some popular analytic methods'. *Am J Epidemiol* 1994; **140**: 300–302.

37. Juni P, Altman DG, Egger M. Assessing the quality of randomised controlled trials. In Egger M, Davey Smith G, Altman DG (ed), *Systematic Reviews in Health Care. Meta-analysis in Context* (2nd edn). London: BMJ Publishing Group, 2001, pp. 87–108.

38. Jadad AR, Moore RA, Carroll D, *et al.* Assessing the quality of reports of randomized clinical trials: is blinding necessary? *Control Clin Trials* 1996; **17**: 1–12.

39. Brouwers MC, Johnston ME, Charette ML, Hanna SE, Jadad AR, Browman GP. Evaluating the role of quality assessment of primary studies in systematic reviews of cancer practice guidelines. *BMC Med Res Methodol* 2005; **5**: 8.

40. Kaduszkiewicz H, Zimmermann T, Beck-Bornholdt HP, van den BH. Cholinesterase inhibitors for patients with Alzheimer's disease: systematic review of randomised clinical trials. *BMJ* 2005; **331**: 321–327.

41. Schulz KF, Chalmers I, Hayes RJ, Altman DG. Empirical evidence of bias. Dimensions of methodological quality associated with estimates of treatment effects in controlled trials. *JAMA* 1995; **273**: 408–412.

42. Moher D, Pham B, Jones A, *et al.* Does quality of reports of randomised trials affect estimates of intervention efficacy reported in meta-analyses? *Lancet* 1998; **352**: 609–613.

43. McAlindon TE, LaValley MP, Gulin JP, Felson DT. Glucosamine and chondroitin for treatment of osteoarthritis: a systematic quality assessment and meta-analysis. *JAMA* 2000; **283**: 1469–1475.

44. Glasziou PP, Woodward AJ, Mahon CM. Mammographic screening trials for women aged under 50. A quality assessment and meta-analysis. *Med J Aust* 1995; **162**: 625–629.

45. Hill D, White V, Jolley D, Mapperson K. Self examination of the breast: is it beneficial? Meta-analysis of studies investigating breast self-examination and extent of disease in patients with breast cancer. *BMJ* 1988; **297**: 271–275.

46. Johnson N, Barlow D, Lethaby A, Tavender E, Curr L, Garry R. Methods of hysterectomy: systematic review and meta-analysis of randomised controlled trials. *BMJ* 2005; **330**: 1478.

47. Grady D, Rubin S, Petitti DB, *et al.* Hormone therapy to prevent disease and prolong life in postmenopausal women. *Ann Intern Med* 1992; **117**: 1016–1037.

48. Kerlikowske K, Grady D, Rubin SM, Sandrock C, Ernster VL. Efficacy of screening mammography. A meta-analysis. *JAMA* 1995; **273**: 149–154.

49. Bown MJ, Sutton AJ, Bell PR, Sayers RD. A meta-analysis of 50 years of ruptured abdominal aortic aneurysm repair. *Br J Surg* 2002; **89**: 714–730.

50. Law MR, Wald NJ, Thompson SG. By how much and how quickly does reduction in serum cholesterol concentration lower risk of ischaemic heart disease? *BMJ* 1994; **308**: 367–372.

51. **Elwood JM.** Childhood leukemia and residential magnetic fields. Are pooled analyses more valid than the original studies? *Bioelectromagnetics* 2006; **27**: 112–118.

52. **Riboli E, Kaaks R.** The EPIC Project: rationale and study design. European Prospective Investigation into Cancer and Nutrition. *Int J Epidemiol* 1997; **26** (Suppl 1): S6–S14.

53. **Sheikh A, Hurwitz B, Cave J.** Antibiotics for acute bacterial conjunctivitis. *Cochrane Database Syst Rev* 2000; (2): CD001211.

54. **Yusuf S, Peto R, Lewis J, Collins R, Sleight P.** Beta blockade during and after myocardial infarction: an overview of the randomized trials. *Prog Cardiovasc Dis* 1985; **27**: 335–371.

55. **Greenland S, Salvan A.** Bias in the one-step method for pooling study results. *Stat Med* 1990; **9**: 247–252.

56. **Prentice RL, Thomas DB.** On the epidemiology of oral contraceptives and disease. *Adv Cancer Res* 1987; **49**: 285–401.

57. **Greenland S.** Quantitative methods in the review of epidemiologic literature. *Epidemiol Rev* 1987; **9**: 1–30.

58. **Elwood JM, Jopson J.** Melanoma and sun exposure: an overview of published studies. *Int J Cancer* 1997; **73**: 198–203.

59. **The Cochrane Collaboration.** RevMan 4.2.8 software (released July 2005), 2005. Available online at: http://www.cc-ims.net/RevMan

60. **Ford D, Bliss JM, Swerdlow AJ, et al.** Risk of cutaneous melanoma associated with a family history of the disease. *Int J Cancer* 1995; **62**: 377–381.

61. **Petitti DB.** *Meta-analysis, decision analysis, and cost-effectiveness analysis. Methods for Quantitative Synthesis in Medicine* (2nd edn). New York: Oxford University Press, 2000.

62. **Berlin JA, Laird NM, Sacks HS, Chalmers TC.** A comparison of statistical methods for combining event rates from clinical trials. *Stat Med* 1989; **8**: 141–151.

63. **DerSimonian R, Laird N.** Meta-analysis in clinical trials. *Control Clin Trials* 1986; 7: 177–188.

64. **ISIS-4 (Fourth International Study of Infarct Survival Collaborative Group)** ISIS-4: A randomised factorial trial assessing early oral captopril, oral mononitrate, and intravenous magnesium sulphate in 58 050 patients with suspected acute myocardial infarction. *Lancet* 1995; **345**: 669–685.

65. **Sterne JAC, Egger M, Smith GD.** Systematic reviews in health care: investigating and dealing with publication and other biases in meta-analysis. *BMJ* 2001; **323**: 101–105.

Chapter 9

# The diagnosis of causation

*What is more unwise than to mistake uncertainty for certainty, falsehood for truth?*

—Cicero (106–43 BC); De senectute, XIX

## Part 1: The assessment of causation in one study or in a set of studies

We have now come to the point where we can summarize how to assess whether a particular study or set of studies allows us to decide whether a relationship is causal. As was pointed out in Chapter 1, the question of absolute proof is irrelevant. It can be argued that no amount of data on past experience can ever allow us to predict with absolute certainty the outcome of situations in individuals we have not studied, such as future patients. In health care there are few situations where there is not another factor that could be considered, another study that could be done, or a variation of the hypothesis which could be suggested. To balance this, we have to be able to make judgements in order to make decisions, whether these are decisions about the diagnosis and treatment of an individual patient, or whether they are policy decisions which may affect many people. These decisions must be made by a process of judgement, and that judgement must be based on an objective consideration of the evidence.

In this chapter we present a scheme for assessing causal relationships in human health. The approach is that the diagnosis of causation depends on the consideration of both causal and non-causal explanations for the association seen. A reasoned judgement must be reached as to the likelihood of the association seen being produced by causality rather than by any other mechanism. The conclusion as to whether a particular association reflects causation is not a simple yes or no, but requires reasoned and probabilistic judgements.

An overall scheme to assess causality is shown in full in **Ex. 9.1**, and in a shorter form in **Ex. 9.2**. The questions shown will be dealt within turn.

---

A SCHEME FOR THE ASSESSMENT OF CAUSATION

A. *Description of the evidence*
 1 What was the exposure or intervention?
 2 What was the outcome?
 3 What was the study design?
 4 What was the study population?
 5 What was the main result?

B. *Internal validity: consideration of non-causal explanations*
 6 Are the results likely to be affected by observation bias?
 7 Are the results likely to be affected by confounding?
 8 Are the results likely to be affected by chance variation?

C. *Internal validity: consideration of positive features of causation*
 9 Is there a correct time relationship?
10 Is the relationship strong?
11 Is there a dose–response relationship?
12 Are the results consistent within the study?
13 Is there any specificity within the study?

D. *External validity: generalization of the results*
14 Can the study results be applied to the eligible population?
15 Can the study results be applied to the source population?
16 Can the study results be applied to other relevant populations?

E. *Comparison of the results with other evidence*
17 Are the results consistent with other evidence, particularly evidence from studies of similar or more powerful study design?
18 Does the total evidence suggest any specificity?
19 Are the results plausible in terms of a biological mechanism?
20 If a major effect is shown, is it coherent with the distribution of the exposure and the outcome?

---

**Ex. 9.1.** Twenty questions relevant to the assessment of evidence relating to a causal relationship

# What evidence do we have?

Consider the practical situation with initially one set of evidence, such as a published study or raw data from our own or others' work. We must critically evaluate the methods used and the results given, and decide whether a causal relationship seems a likely explanation for the results. The questions to be asked are as follows.

## Questions 1–5. Description of the evidence

Question 1.   What was the exposure or intervention?

Question 2.   What was the outcome?

Question 3.   What was the study design?

---

THE ASSESSMENT OF CAUSATION

A. *Description of the evidence*
1  Exposure or intervention
2  Outcome
3  Study design
4  Study population
5  Main result

B. *Non-causal explanations*
6  Observation bias
7  Confounding
8  Chance

C. *Positive features*
9  Time relationship
10  Strength
11  Dose–response
12  Consistency
13  Specificity

D. *Generalizability*
14  Eligible population
15  Source population
16  Other populations

E. *Comparison with other evidence*
17  Consistency
18  Specificity
19  Plausibility
20  Coherence

---

**Ex. 9.2.** A scheme for the assessment of causation in note form

Question 4.   What was the study population?

Question 5.   What was the main result?

The first and often overlooked step is to understand for the particular study exactly what relationship is being evaluated, or, to put it another way, what hypothesis is being tested. We should be able to reduce every study to a consideration of a relationship between an *exposure* or intervention and an *outcome*. It is also necessary to categorize the study in terms of the *design* used; comparative studies of individuals will be intervention studies, randomized or non-randomized, or observational studies of the survey, case–control or cohort design. As was shown in Chapter 3, understanding the design shows what type of analysis is appropriate and indicates which methodological issues will be most important. Then we need to consider the *subjects* studied, in terms of the source populations, the eligibility criteria, and the participation rates of the different groups compared, as was discussed in Chapter 4.

More than occasionally, describing a published study in this way requires a critical perusal of the methods section rather than simply a glance at the title, because the question which has actually been answered may be somewhat different from the one the investigators would like to have answered.

Two advantages arise from this systematic consideration. First, before getting caught up in the particular details of the study, which may be quite complex, reviewing these questions will give us a clear idea of the overall purpose and relevance of the study. Secondly, it will help us decide whether indeed the study is sufficiently relevant and important for us to review it in more detail. This early consideration of the study design and study population may make it clear that this particular study is not relevant to the question we wish to assess; for example, we may be interested in the use of chemotherapy as part of the primary management of a newly diagnosed cancer patient, but we may find that the study describes the use of the drug in palliation. Thirdly, if there is a great deal of literature available on the topic, this may help us decide which studies are worthy of most attention. Later in this chapter, a system of classifying different types of study in order of their likely relevance will be given; for example, if the question has been addressed in several randomized trials, there is little value in reviewing an uncontrolled descriptive study in any detail.

Having defined the topic of the study, it is very useful to summarize the *main result*: what is the result in terms of the association between exposure and outcome? This step forces us to distinguish the main result from subsidiary issues, which should be considered only after the main result has been dealt with. It should be possible to express the main result in a simple table, and obtain from the paper or calculate ourselves the appropriate measure of association (usually relative risk, odds ratio, or a difference in proportions).

In much current literature, the main result will come from a complex analysis, such as a multivariate analysis. Even so, the raw data are usually available, from which a simple $2 \times 2$ table of the primary crude result can be generated. Although of course this crude result should not be used in preference to the published more complex analysis, assuming that the analysis is appropriate, it is often a great help in understanding the study and giving us some feeling for the essential content. Moreover, if the simply derived crude result differs dramatically from the published result based on a more complex analysis, it is useful to look at that more complex analysis very carefully.

## Internal validity: consideration of non-causal explanations

Having described the study, we assess its *internal validity*, i.e. for the subjects who were studied, does the evidence support a causal relationship between the exposure and the outcome? This assessment is in two parts; first, we consider the three possible non-causal mechanisms which could produce the result seen. The questions are as follows.

## Questions 6 to 8: non-causal explanations

Question 6.   Are the results likely to be affected by observation bias?

Question 7.   Are the results likely to be affected by confounding?

Question 8.   Are the results likely to be affected by chance variation?
These have been dealt with in detail in Chapters 5, 6, and 7. For each, we need to consider how the main result of the study may be influenced. It is useful to consider each separately, making our assessment of the likelihood of the study result being produced by that mechanism compared with a causal effect. Thus, for a study which shows an association between exposure and outcome, the questions can be summarized as follows.

◆ Could the results seen have arisen by observation bias, if there were no true difference between the groups being compared?

◆ Do the results show a true difference, but is it due to a confounding factor rather than to the putative causal factor?

◆ Do the results show a true difference, but one which has occurred through chance, there being no general association between exposure and outcome?
As mentioned previously, while our final assessment will take all these factors into account, and the problems in a particular study may involve all three, considering each in the extreme case of it alone explaining the results seen will often clarify our judgement. The order of these non-causal explanations is relevant. If there is severe observation bias, no manipulation of the data will overcome the problem. If there is confounding, an appropriate data analysis may be able to demonstrate it and control for it; we need to assess if such analysis has been done. The assessment of chance variation should be made on the main result of the study, after considerations of bias and confounding have been dealt with.

## Internal validity: consideration of positive features of causation

So far we have considered the recognition of a causal relationship only by the exclusion of non-causal explanations. The new material in this chapter is a consideration of features which when present can be regarded as positive indicators of causality. At this point we will discuss the assessment of these features within a particular study, and later we will discuss them with regard to all available information relevant to the hypothesis under assessment.

The relevant questions are as follows.

9. Is there a correct time relationship?

10. Is the relationship strong?

11. Is there a dose–response relationship?

12. Are the results consistent within the study?

13. Is there any specificity within the study?

## Question 9. Time relationship

For a relationship to be causal, the putative exposure must act before the outcome occurs. In a prospective design where exposed and non-exposed subjects are compared, this is established by ensuring that the subjects do not already have the outcome when the study is commenced. The ability to clarify time relationships is obviously weaker in retrospective studies, and care must be taken to avoid considering as possible causal factors events which took place after the outcome had developed. For this reason, in retrospective studies of disease it is best to enrol incident subjects (those who have just been found to have the outcome), to interview subjects fairly rapidly, and to record only information related to events preceding the outcome.

A difficulty in all study designs, but particularly in retrospective studies, is that the occurrence in biological terms of the outcome of interest may precede the recognition and documentation of that outcome by a long and variable time; often some arbitrary assumption about this time is used. For example, in the retrospective study described in Chapter 14, drug histories of case and control subjects were taken from medical records, but excluding the time period of 1 year prior to clinical diagnosis in the cases, and an equivalent time in the controls. In the cohort study described in Chapter 12, it is suggested that differences between studies may be due to the key association changing with the time since exposure.

A similar issue may arise in the definition of exposure. For example, in assessing an association between an occupational exposure and disease, it may be reasonable to define exposure as a minimum of, say, 5 years in a particular occupation. In that event, the follow-up period begins immediately the 5-year period is completed.

A study may show no association because the time scale is inadequate; a treatment comparison may give irrelevant results if based on a short follow-up, and long-term effects of an exposure factor such as radiation or oral contraceptive use will be missed by studies with a short time scale.

## Question 10. Strength of the association

A stronger association, i.e. a larger relative risk, is more likely to reflect a causal relationship. One reason is that as the measured factor approaches the biological event in the causal pathway more closely, the relative risks will become larger. The deterministic ideal is that the factor is the necessary and sufficient cause, which gives a risk of zero in the unexposed and 100 per cent in the exposed, and a relative risk of infinity. However, this is a very rare situation in health issues. Suppose that a rare disease is in fact caused totally by exposure to a specific chemical used in the manufacture of photographic film. In sequential studies, we might detect a weak association with employment in a photographic plant, a stronger one with working in the film manufacture process, and a very strong association with heavy exposure to the particular chemical.

However, a true causal factor may be related to a small increase of risk, as the factor may be one of a number of such factors operating. Consider the role of air pollution in the causation of chronic bronchitis. Where there are few other factors operating to cause the disease, for example in non-smoking subjects who are not exposed to occupational hazards, the role of air pollution may be major, producing a high relative risk which is relatively easy to demonstrate. However, in a heavy smoker, the smoking factor is of such overwhelming importance that the extra risk contributed by atmospheric air pollution will be relatively small; if the attributable risk of air pollution is similar to that in a non-smoker, the relative risk will be small because of the very high baseline risk produced by smoking. This does not alter the causal nature of the relationship, but it does make the strength of the relationship less and makes it more difficult to demonstrate.

The fact that a relationship is strong does not protect against certain noncausal relationships. Severe observational bias may produce very strong relationships. Suppose we identify mothers who have recently been delivered of babies with abnormalities, ask them about exposure to drugs in early pregnancy, and compare their responses with those of mothers of healthy babies. We should anticipate that bias in selective recall might be very considerable. If it operated at all, there is little reason to assume that the bias it could produce would be small; it could quite easily be very large. Similarly, strength does not protect against confounding caused by closely associated factors. An example of this is where a disease risk may be related to a previous drug exposure, or to the reason for that exposure. There may be a close relationship between the indication and the drug, and therefore if one of them is a true causal factor the association of disease with the other factor will be strong despite the fact that it is due only to confounding.

However, if a strong relationship is due to bias, the bias must be large and so should be relatively easy to identify. If a strong relationship is due to confounding, either the association of the exposure with the confounder must be very close, or the association of the confounder with the outcome must be very strong. For example, the relative risk of lung cancer in heavy smokers compared with non-smokers is of the order of 30. It has been suggested that this relationship is due to confounding by a genetic predisposition to lung cancer, linked to a genetically determined personality trait leading to smoking. If so, that genetic predisposition factor must have a relative risk of about 30 for lung cancer. Even given the difficulties of assessing personality, it should be possible to demonstrate the existence of such a relationship.

## Question 11. Dose–response relationship

The consideration of a dose–response relationship is similar to that of strength. The major issue which it does not protect against is the relationship being due to a confounding factor closely related to the exposure, such as in the drug versus indication for drug situation. In some circumstances the demonstration of a smooth dose–response relationship may be a strong argument against the relationship being due to bias. For example, it could be argued that women who use oral contraceptives might be more likely to have certain symptoms recorded, simply because they visit their general practitioners more frequently than women who do not use oral contraceptives. However, it is less likely that there is a close relationship between the oestrogen dose of the oral contraceptive and the frequency of visits. Therefore, if the outcome under study shows a regular dose–response relationship with the oestrogen dosage, this bias is unlikely to be the explanation.

We usually expect unidirectional dose–effect relationships. Obviously other types of associations, showing a threshold or all-or-none effect, or a complex relationship may be in fact the true situation. However, the general assumption that if a causal relationship holds, the frequency of the outcome should show a unidirectional increase with increasing exposure, even though the relationship may not be linear, seems very reasonable—so reasonable, that evidence that that is not the case should be considered carefully. For example, the age distribution of Hodgkin's disease does not show the common unidirectional increase of incidence with age as is seen in many other cancers, but instead shows a complex pattern with a peak at younger ages followed by a decrease followed by a further increase. On the general assumption that complex relationships are unlikely, this pattern suggested that there are two distinct diseases, of which one shows the steady increase of incidence with age characteristic of many other cancers, and the other shows a peak incidence at young ages.

This suggestion, made in the 1950s simply from descriptive data [1] was later confirmed by the demonstration of differences in clinical and pathological features between the previously unseparated types of disease [2]. The demonstration of a dose–response relationship is an important component of the study presented in Chapter 14, and is one of the prime objectives of the study described in Chapter 15.

## Question 12. Consistency of the association

A causal relationship will be expected to apply across a wide range of subjects. If a new painkiller is effective, it is likely to be effective in patients of both sexes and different ages, for a wide variety of causes of pain. In other circumstances, specificity (see below) rather than consistency might be predicted; for example, a hormonal treatment for breast cancer might be expected to work best for cancers which are positive for hormone receptors. If an association within one study is seen to be consistent in different groups of subjects, that may well be regarded as support for causality, particularly if the likely sources of bias and confounding are different in those subgroups. Similarly in reverse: when a new study showing a positive association between the consumption of artificial sweeteners (mainly saccharine) and bladder cancer was published, the association was seen only in males, and in the absence of a biological explanation for that lack of consistency, it weakened the case for causality [3]. The international trial described in Chapter 11 demonstrates consistency of the main effect with regard to different geographical areas and the main subtypes of the outcome.

The difficulty with consistency is that large data sets are required to assess the similarity or otherwise of associations in different subgroups of subjects, the effective sample size is the number of observations in each subset. Even with adequate numbers, the subgroups to be compared need to be defined on a priori grounds, and not merely generated from the analysis. In a large analysis where many subgroups are defined, it is to be expected that some will show different results by chance alone. This has been a major problem in clinical trials; even where no overall benefit of a new treatment is shown, a benefit may be apparent in one subgroup of patients. Such post hoc analysis is misleading and best avoided; such findings should be regarded as new hypotheses which require testing.

## Question 13. Specificity of association

It has been argued that a specific association between one causal factor and one outcome is good evidence for causality. This may be misleading; some took the view that the fact that smoking was shown to be associated with the occurrence of a number of cancers and other serious diseases, and therefore demonstrated non-specificity of action, made the hypothesis of a causal link with lung cancer less likely. In the medical area specificity is often contrived by definition. If we define tuberculosis as a clinical disease comprising various signs and symptoms, which is produced by infection by the tubercle bacillus, we end up with a specific association between that disease so defined and the infectious agent. Without that definitional convenience, the associations between infection with tubercle bacillus and chronic meningitis, swollen joints, and lung disease do not appear to be specific.

However, in many situations demonstration of specificity may be valuable, as it may show that bias or confounding is unlikely to explain the results. For example, consider a retrospective study in which recently delivered mothers are interviewed, which shows that use of a certain drug is much more frequently reported by mothers of infants with cardiac malformations than by mothers of healthy babies. We would have to question whether recall bias is the explanation of that association. However, if mothers of babies with a range of other defects were questioned, and their reported histories of drug use were similar to the mothers of the healthy babies, this would be a strong argument against recall bias being the explanation of the association seen with cardiac disease. In a study of birth defects in relation to vitamin A intake, an excess risk was found with high intakes only before pregnancy and in early pregnancy, but there was no association with high intake after 6 weeks of pregnancy; this specificity of exposure is consistent with causality and provides some protection against both confounding and observation bias [4]. The trial described in Chapter 11 was set up to distinguish the effects of two different exposures, and showed a result specific to one of the exposures. Previous observational studies could not separate the effects of these two related exposures. The study described in Chapter 15 also illustrates specificity, as an association between breast cancer and alcohol intake was found for only certain types of alcohol intake, but further work on this result has produced conflicting evidence.

A hospital based study showed that women who had developed endometrial cancer had a higher frequency of past use of oestrogenic drugs than did patients who had cervical cancer [5]. Endometrial cancer is more common in high socio-economic groups, while cervical cancer is less common. The use of this drug is likely to be greater in the higher socio-economic groups, and so the association seen may be due to confounding. However, patients with ovarian cancer, which has a similar socio-economic distribution to endometrial cancer, were also assessed, and their usage of oestrogen drugs was also much lower than that of the endometrial cancer patients. This makes confounding by socio-economic status a less likely explanation for the association seen.

Therefore specificity may be useful if we do not make it an absolute criterion, as one causal agent may in truth produce various outcomes, and one outcome may result from various agents. The concept is often useful in study design; as a check on response bias we may deliberately collect information on factors which we expect to be the same in the groups compared, as similar results will indicate a lack of observation bias. We may choose control groups to capitalize on similar effects, as noted above.

## Summary of internal validity

By this point, we should be able to decide whether the internal validity of the study is adequate. A positive decision means that we accept the results to be a valid measure of the true association in the subjects studied, and if an association between exposure and outcome is present, we regard it as likely to be due to a causal relationship.

A negative decision means that we decide that one or more of the non-causal explanations is likely to hold; the association seen is due to observation bias, to confounding, or to chance, and we should be able to specify the likely biases or confounding factors. Often we will be able to eliminate some but not all of the options, and decide for example that the result is likely to be due to either causation or to confounding; such a conclusion is very valuable as it makes clear what further information is necessary.

Observation bias is discussed in all the studies presented in the later chapters, but is of particular interest in the studies described in Chapters 11, 12, and 14; all these studies demonstrate efforts to minimize observation bias. In the studies described in Chapters 12 and 14, the major question of interpretation is whether the association is causal or is due to confounding; for the studies discussed in Chapters 10 and 13, the main issue is whether the result is causal or due to chance variation.

## External validity: generalization of the results

If the internal validity of the study is very poor, there is no point in proceeding further, for if the study result is not valid even for the subjects studied, its application to other groups of subjects is irrelevant. However, if we conclude that it is a reasonably valid result and that a causal relationship is a reasonably likely explanation, we need to go on to consider the external validity of the result. The relevant questions are as follows.

Question 14. Can the study results be applied to the eligible population?

Question 15. Can the study results be applied to the source population?

Question 16. Can the study results be applied to other relevant populations?

The relationship between the study participants and the population of eligible subjects should be well documented. Losses due to non-participation have to be considered carefully as they are likely to be non-random, and the reasons for the losses may be related to the exposure or to the outcome. These issues were discussed in Chapter 4.

Beyond this, it is unlikely that the study participants will be a 'representative sample' of a definable source population, and even if they were, we would want to extrapolate the results further, for example to our own community, future patients, and so on. The issue is not whether the subjects studied are 'typical' or 'representative', but whether the *association* between outcome and exposure given by the study participants is likely to apply to other groups. In assessing the applicability of results, we need to be specific about the factors which are likely to affect the association. Most clinical trials are done on patients in teaching hospitals. If a new therapy for breast cancer is shown to be effective in such a trial, we would readily apply the results to patients in a district hospital who had a similar stage and type of tumour and were of similar age, even though the trial patients cannot be said to be 'representative' of district hospital patients in a general or statistical sense. Similarly, women in the USA and Japan have very different incidence rates of breast cancer, and very different diets; but if a causal relationship exists between saturated fat intake and breast cancer incidence, we should expect to see it in both populations, even though its strength might be modified by the relative importance of other factors. However, other considerations may apply. If we read of a clinical trial of a new drug therapy used for severe depression in a well-known teaching centre, we should not apply the results to patients in general practice uncritically; the general practice patients, even with the same diagnosis, are likely to be different (e.g. in the severity and duration of disease) from those in the teaching centre, and the effects of the therapy may well differ in inpatients and in ambulant patients. In general, the difficulties of applying results from one group of subjects to another will be minimal for issues of basic physiology and genetics, and maximal for effects in which cultural and psychosocial aspects are dominant. The generalizability of the results is important for all the studies discussed in subsequent chapters, but is particularly interesting for the trial discussed in Chapter 11, where generalization from a high-risk population to a general population is a major issue. The applicability of the results of the trial described in Chapter 10, and of the cohort study described in Chapter 12, are important issues in the interpretation.

## Comparison of the results with other evidence

We have now made a critical assessment of the evidence presented by one study. We have assessed the internal validity, and come to a reasoned judgement as to whether the results of the study are consistent with a cause and effect relationship. We have explored the external validity of the study, and come to a decision concerning how far we can generalize the result beyond the subjects who participated in the study.

We can now move to the issue of comparing the result of this particular study with the evidence from other studies and other types of experience. As we did with the evidence from within the study, we shall make these comparisons with specific questions in mind. In comparing the results of a particular study with those of other studies, we will ask the following questions.

Question 17. Are the results consistent with other evidence, particularly evidence from studies of a similar or more powerful study design?

Question 18. Does the total evidence suggest any specificity?

Question 19. Are the results plausible, in terms of a biological mechanism?

Question 20. If a major effect is shown, is it coherent with the distribution of the exposure and the outcome?

## Question 17. Consistency with other studies

This is the most important characteristic used in the judgement that an association is causal. To say that the result is consistent requires that the association has been observed in a number of different studies, each of which individually can be interpreted as showing a causal explanation, and which have enough variation in their methodology and study populations to make it unlikely that the same biases or confounding factors apply in all the studies. For example, when a British case–control study demonstrated a new relationship between hormone replacement therapy and venous thromboembolism [6], the interpretation of this was aided by the simultaneous publication, because of cooperation between investigators, of a case–control study and a cohort-based study from the USA [7,8] with consistent results.

Consistency of results between studies, each of which is individually unsatisfactory, is of little value, as is consistency between studies which all suffer from the same design defect. For example, it is difficult to assess the effect of breast self examination in producing early diagnosis of breast cancer from observational studies, because women who practise self-examination are likely to have many other characteristics which may lead them to an earlier diagnosis of a tumour. A meta-analyses of such studies has been performed [9], but it is still open to the alternative explanation of confounding due to other factors associated with earlier diagnosis. Lack of consistency argues against causality, but care must be taken in its assessment also. The failure to find an association in a study which is limited in its methodology and size so that it has very little power to detect an association, if one were present, is of no value. When a new and controversial result is published, weak, badly designed, and small studies which show no association are often presented to refute it; these studies have to be examined with the same critical approach as is applied to the original.

Consistency is assessed statistically within meta-analyses by the assessment of heterogeneity, testing by methods such as those described in Chapter 8 whether the results for each study are consistent with the overall pooled result. The difficulty arises when there is significant heterogeneity. Often, the studies with outlying results are simply noted and then removed from the overall analysis, and a summarized result based on the rest is published. It is more satisfactory if the reasons for these discrepancies can be explored, as was discussed in Chapter 8. Consideration of the quality of the studies and their specific characteristics, using meta-regression methods if appropriate, may be valuable.

## Question 18. Specificity

Specificity relates closely to consistency. Whether a difference in results between two studies is interpreted as inconsistency or specificity depends on whether the difference is anticipated by a hypothesis set up before the comparison is made. If not, but a plausible mechanism can be found or if the difference is itself found consistently, then the hypothesis may be modified to take into account the specificity which has been shown. This creates a new hypothesis which should be assessed by a further independent study.

For example, the two congenital defects of spina bifida and anencephalus have similar embryological and epidemiological features, and both are prevented by folic acid, as discussed in Chapter 11. However the antiepileptic drug valproic acid shows a strong and apparently specific association with spina bifida, while no excess of anencephalus has been recorded. If this is not due to some observation bias, it suggests a specificity of effect, showing one substantial difference in the aetiology of the two conditions [10]. A highly specific association is easier to recognize; an example quoted by Bradford Hill in a celebrated paper [11] was that of nickel miners in South Wales, where there were 16 deaths from lung cancer and 11 from cancer of the nasal sinuses, compared with expected numbers of about 1 and much less than 1, respectively; deaths from all other causes numbered 67, similar to the expected number of 72, pointing to a risk specific to these two cancer types.

## Question 19. Plausibility

Plausibility refers to the observed association being biologically understandable on the basis of current knowledge concerning its likely mechanisms. The consideration of plausibility is useful, particularly as it may indicate biases or confounding factors which should be considered. The interpretation of the positive association between ice-cream sales and drowning at summer holiday resorts is an example, as a consideration of its plausibility will suggest a confounding factor.

However, any dramatically new observation may be in advance of current biological thinking and its lack of plausibility may reflect deficiencies in biological knowledge rather than an error in the observation. John Snow effectively prevented cholera in a district of London 25 years before the isolation of the cholera bacillus and acceptance of the idea that the disease could be spread by water. Percival Pott demonstrated the causal relationship between exposure to soot and scrotal cancer some 150 years before the relevant carcinogen was isolated and the mechanism further understood. The greatest value of the concept of plausibility is to emphasize that where an association does not match a known biological mechanism, further studies are indicated to clarify this, but these need not necessarily delay appropriate action if the evidence for causality is strong enough.

There has been considerable debate on the possible relationship between exposure to electromagnetic fields at low frequencies from electric power sources and the occurrence of childhood leukaemia. One of the major reservations about accepting such an association is the lack of plausibility. Even after extensive research, there is little evidence from cellular or animal studies that indicates a mechanism for a carcinogenic effect. On the other hand, meta-analyses of several epidemiological studies shows an empirical association with the highest level of exposure found in the home environment [12,13]. At present, it is unclear whether these epidemiological investigations are the first indication of an important effect, with the elucidation of a biological mechanism to follow, or whether these observations are explicable by non causal relationships such as confounding and selection biases.

The dramatic reduction in the frequency of a major developmental defect by a relatively low dose of a common vitamin is described in the study in Chapter 11. Although plausible in general terms, this empirical demonstration of effect preceded specific knowledge of a mechanism, but has stimulated extensive work to identify the key biochemical process and its genetic aspects [14].

Lists of the expected features in causality often include the concept of *analogy*, meaning that a relationship is regarded as more acceptable if it is analogous to some other well-established relationship, but clearly this concept comes within the overall concept of plausibility.

## Question 20. Coherence

An association is regarded as coherent if it fits the general features of the distribution of both the exposure and the outcome under assessment; thus if lung cancer is due to smoking, the frequency of lung cancer in different populations and in different time periods should relate to the frequency of smoking in those populations at relevant earlier time periods. The concept of coherence has several limitations: it is assumed that the exposure and the outcome are the same in different populations, and it holds only if a high proportion of the outcome is caused by the exposure, and if the frequency of the outcome is fairly high in those exposed. If the factor causes only a small proportion of the total disease, the overwhelming influence of other factors may make the overall pattern inconsistent. A comparison of an exposure such as smoking in different countries, or a general category of disease such as lung cancer, may not take sufficient note of differences in types of smoking and in types of lung cancer.

As an example of an argument based on coherence, it was suggested some years ago that neural tube defects were caused by a teratogen in damaged potatoes. In support, the high frequency of the defects in Ireland and the strong association with low social class were quoted, on the argument that these populations had a high consumption of potatoes. However, it was also noted that the condition is fairly common in Taiwan, and is also more common in the poor, although potato consumption is probably higher in the upper social classes [15]. The case–control study described in Chapter 14 shows an association between a drug and a disease outcome, and in this instance the question of coherence is of great importance in separating a causal relationship from the alternative explanation of confounding. However, in the other studies described in subsequent chapters, coherence is not particularly helpful, either because the association suggested is not strong enough, or the information on the distribution of the relevant exposure and outcome is inadequate.

## Assessing causal relationships and making decisions

A general method has now been set out which should assist the reader to assess written evidence, his or her own experience, and the experience of colleagues. The system is obviously only a framework, and issues specific to each subject will influence the relative importance of different aspects of the process; a minor issue in one subject may be a major issue in others. The entire process is summed up in **Ex. 9.3.** Presented with new results from a study of a putative causal relationship, the question we must ask is: 'Does the evidence given in this study support a causal relationship?' This involves the assessment of the internal and external validity of the study, and its relationship to other evidence, as expressed in the scheme given in this chapter.

If our judgement is that the evidence does support a causal relationship, we should be able to reinforce this by answering the question: 'What is this

THE DECISION PROCESS

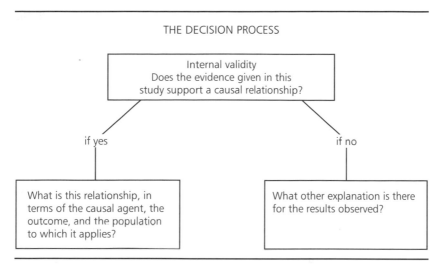

**Ex. 9.3.** Assessment of causal relationships: the decision process

relationship, in terms of the causal agent, the outcome, and the population to which it applies?'

If the answer to our question is in the negative, we need to be able to answer the question: 'What other explanation is there for the results observed?' The results we have been presented with do not go away; they are the facts from which we are arguing. If we reject a causal explanation, we must be able to propose an alternative hypothesis. The specification of the alternative hypothesis, or hypotheses, will help us to see the weaknesses in the evidence we have and guide us in how to search for better information.

## Some further applications of the assessment of causality

In this book, we have concentrated on the assessment of cause and effect relationships, and almost exclusively on evidence provided by studies of groups of individuals. There are many important relationships which are not necessarily of a cause and effect type, and there are other types of data which can be considered. While there is no intention to go into these fully, a few comments on the relevance of the concepts expressed in this approach to these other questions may be helpful.

### Associations can be useful even if not causal

If we can establish that an association exists, even if it is not causal, this information may be very valuable. In particular, *diagnosis* is dependent on the reliable demonstration of associations which are not causal associations. Diagnosis, the separation of subjects with a pathological condition from subjects who do not have that condition, is based on the features associated with that condition; whether they are part of the causation of the condition is irrelevant. Diagnostic symptoms, signs, and laboratory-measured abnormalities are usually features which are produced by the same causal mechanism as produces the disease which we are trying to diagnose, or are produced by the disease process. Despite that, many of the principles outlined in this volume are applicable to the study of diagnostic concepts, particularly the issues of observation bias and external validity.

Similarly, in the social sciences the emphasis has generally been on exploring associations between factors, for example whether attitudes to health care are different in different social groups, without of necessity considering cause and effect relationships. Often, however, assumptions and judgements about cause and effect relationships lie not far below the surface, and again the principles set forth in this volume should be of assistance in assessing such questions.

## Application to studies of populations, and of physiological or biochemical parameters

This book is primarily about studies of individuals, where each contributes one exposure and one outcome event. Causal relationships may often be suggested, and sometimes be assessed, by data comparing different population groups; e.g. routine statistics of disease incidence, morbidity, or case fatality. Such studies yield comparisons between rates of exposure and rates of outcome in populations, without having data showing which individuals within those populations are involved. While such studies are inherently weaker than studies of individuals, they can be analysed in the same way. Most can be considered as cross-sectional surveys or cohort studies. For example, in a correlation study it was shown that populations (Canadian provinces) with more intense programmes of cervical cytology (the exposure) showed a larger decrease in mortality from uterine cancer (the outcome) [16]. The comparisons of firearm-related outcomes in Seattle and Vancouver [17], noted in Ex. 3.11, page 70, is similar. The analysis of these associations is conceptually the same as for a study of individuals: Is the association likely to be due to bias, confounding, or chance? Does it show the positive features of causation? The same logical approach can be applied.

Similarly, we have not dealt directly with the other main group of human studies, those where the results are based on series of physiological or biochemical measurements within an individual. Thus, to show the causal relationship between external temperature and peripheral blood flow, measurements could be made in different subjects at different temperatures, but it is much more efficient to compare the same individuals, making a series of measurements of peripheral blood flow while varying the external temperature. The logic of causal inference presented here is totally applicable: bias, confounding, and chance must be considered, and the positive indicators of causality sought. Such studies can be considered as matched cohort studies, with each group of subjects under one set of conditions being one study cohort.

While the logic can be applied to both descriptive epidemiological and physiological studies, often the outcome and/or exposure factors will be continuous rather than discrete variables, such as temperature, peripheral blood flow, and morbidity rate. The statistical methods applicable are those for continuous variables, including Student's $t$-test, correlation and regression methods, analysis of variance, multiple linear regression, and non-parametric methods such as rank correlation techniques. Such methods are well described in most statistical textbooks.

## Applications in designing a study

This scheme can also be used in the design of studies. A useful general approach to the design of a study is that the investigator should attempt a *forward projection* to the point where the study has been completed and the results have been compiled. It is useful for the investigator to consider all possible results, i.e. a positive association or one in the direction expected, no association or a negative one, or an association in the opposite direction from that expected. The investigator can then ask the question, given that those results arise, 'How will I assess this study in terms of its internal and external validity?' or in simpler terms, 'Will I believe the results that I have obtained?' A good test of a well-designed study is that the investigator will be willing to accept and act on the results, even if they are different from the anticipated result. This is also a useful question to ask colleagues who wish you to be involved in their research. By projecting yourself to the point of assessing the possible results of the study, you as investigator can consider the major issues of bias, confounding, and chance variation, and consider methods by which these issues can be recognized and dealt with. You can also consider the desirability of being able to demonstrate strong associations, dose–response effects, specific relationships, and so on. By doing this, you give yourself the opportunity to incorporate into the design of the study the potential for demonstrating such features. The discussion of the study design with colleagues who are prepared to adopt a similar critical approach and who bring to bear specialist knowledge of the issues involved will be a major safeguard against embarking on a study which is inadequately designed.

# Part 2. The application of causal reasoning to clinical care and health policy

## Hierarchies of evidence

In appraising the science relevant to an issue, each piece of evidence has three relevant dimensions: What type of study is it? Is it a high-quality study? Is it relevant to the question? So far in this text we have concentrated on assessing the quality of studies within the major study types, and in assessing their external validity, which will determine whether they are relevant to a particular question.

For most clinical and policy questions, a large amount of evidence from different types of study is available, and so it is useful to consider a hierarchy of evidence. Given that the studies are adequately performed within the limitations of the design used, the reliability of the information from them can be ranked in the manner shown in **Ex. 9.4.** Most generally accepted classifications follow this format.

At the top are randomized intervention trials, if properly performed on adequate numbers of subjects and, of course, in the human situation. Evidence from such studies should be given the greatest weight because of the unique advantages of these studies in overcoming the problems of bias and confounding.

Second come observational studies of appropriately selected groups of subjects, i.e. the cohort and case–control designs. There is logic in placing cohort studies somewhat ahead of case–control studies because, if well performed, cohort studies should have less observation bias, give clearer evidence of the time relationships of the association, and have a comparison group whose results are more easily interpreted. However, both these observational designs can have severe problems, and a well-performed case–control study may be of more value than a poorly performed cohort study.

---

### A SIMPLE HIERARCHY OF EVIDENCE

| Level 1 | Randomized trials | 1m: Results from a meta-analysis of trials<br>1s: One or more individual trials |
|---|---|---|
| Level 2: | Cohort and case-control studies | 2m: Results from a meta-analysis of such studies<br>2s: One or more individual studies |
| Level 3: | Other comparative studies | |
| Level 4: | Case series, descriptive studies, professional experience, etc. | |

**Ex. 9.4.** A simple hierarchy of types of evidence relevant to human health studies: as well as the level of evidence, the consistency or otherwise of the results, the quality and detail of the studies, and the relevance of the studies to the situation and question of interest have to be assessed

As we have seen in Chapter 8, the data from many randomized trials can be summarized in a meta-analysis, and meta-analyses can also be done for cohort and case–control studies, although they are generally more difficult as there are usually greater methodological differences between the studies. Thus in categories 1 and 2 in Ex. 9.4 we can give higher ranking to an appropriately performed meta-analysis which combines the results of several relevant trials. The best possible evidence relating to an intervention would come from a clear result from a well-performed meta-analysis of all available randomized trials.

The third level of evidence comes from studies comparing groups of subjects not chosen specifically for the purpose of the study but representing different population or subject groups. This includes correlation studies of populations in which data on each individual are not assessed separately, and also informal comparisons between patients in different hospitals, patients treated at different time periods, and so on.

In the fourth category there is evidence which is largely anecdotal, based on the unsystematic recollection of personal or group experience (sometimes referred to as 'clinical judgement' or 'experience'), conclusions based on traditional practice, and information derived from other species, *in vitro* testing, physiological principles, and other indirect assessments. Meta-analyses may also be applied to evidence in the third and fourth categories; this is less frequently done, but undoubtedly more efforts will be made in the future.

This hierarchy is useful in assessing the very large amounts of information that may be available on a particular topic. It is sensible to concentrate on the best possible evidence. If there are randomized trials available on the question, they should be evaluated first, and if they provide strong evidence for or against causality, the results of the other less rigorous types of study may add little. For many topics, randomized trial evidence will not be available, and therefore we must look particularly at the results of well-performed cohort and case–control studies.

This general hierarchy of evidence is followed in the now numerous specific versions of hierarchies, some of which are becoming quite complicated. It has become quite customary for people to refer to 'level 1 evidence', generally meaning randomized trials, 'level 2 evidence', generally meaning comparative observational studies, and so on. This quite useful shorthand may disappear as more complex systems develop. For example, because the best source of evidence for studies of the effects of hazardous exposures comes from cohort and case–control studies, some feel that such studies should be referred to as level 1 evidence in this context; but this would lose the attractive simplicity of the overall framework described here. Of course, many systematic reviews use an even simpler ranking system, concentrating solely on randomized trials and ignoring other evidence.

The value of such ranking systems is now widely accepted. One of the first uses of such a system was in the reports, starting in 1979, of a Canadian multidisciplinary group on the effectiveness of procedures for inclusion in regular medical examinations [18,19]. The group concerned itself only with clinical efficacy, not with economic value or social acceptability. They assessed 88 suggested procedures including testing newborn babies for phenylketonuria, routine tests for urinary tract infection in pregnancy, and screening of preschool children for hearing impairments and adolescents for spinal deformity. Of the 88 situations, evidence from randomized trials was available in only 20 (of these 12 were questions of immunization), for 17 conditions evidence from cohort or case–control studies was available, for 22 only descriptive or uncontrolled observations were available, and for 29 there was nothing other than subjective opinion and 'experience'. The relationship between the type of evidence available and the final decision of the multidisciplinary committee (**Ex. 9.5**) shows, as we would expect, that where the quality of evidence was high, a firm recommendation on whether to include or to exclude the procedure could be made. The situation where a firm recommendation was based on only category 3 evidence was one with a long clinical tradition—the use of silver nitrate drops in a neonate's eyes to prevent ophthalmia neonatorum.

This report was unusual at that time because it documented both the committee's recommendations and the type of evidence available for each procedure. This was done in terms of both the hierarchical system of classification of evidence, which is a gross measure of internal validity, and its applicability

| | | EVIDENCE AND DECISION | | | | | |
|---|---|---|---|---|---|---|---|
| Best evidence | | Recommendation | | | | Total | With firm recommendation |
| | include | | | exclude | | | |
| | firm | weak | none | weak | firm | | |
| 1. Randomized trials | 11 | 0 | 1 | 2 | 6 | 20 | 17 |
| 2. Cohort, case-control | 3 | 5 | 1 | 8 | 0 | 17 | 3 |
| 3. Other comparative | 1 | 11 | 2 | 8 | 0 | 22 | 1 |
| 4. Other types | 0 | 0 | 29 | 0 | 0 | 29 | 0 |
| | | | | | | 88 | |

**Ex. 9.5.** Evidence and decision: relationship between decisions of a multidisciplinary group regarding regular health examinations and the best type of evidence available for 88 procedures for the general population. Derived from Canadian Task Force on the Periodic Health Examination [18]

to the relevant population, patients in primary care in Canada, giving a measure of external validity. Since then many groups have used such ranking systems, including the US Preventive Services Task Force [20].

## From evidence to recommendations

The classification of the type of evidence needs to be taken together with an assessment of the quality and relevance of the study in coming to an overall decision as to whether the evidence supports, rejects, or is neutral concerning a specific intervention or recommendation. Clinical and health policy groups have come up with various schemes to summarize this process. For example, the US Preventive Services Taskforce presents its recommendations in five categories [21] (**Ex. 9.6**). Many other groups have schemes which are similar in their objectives, while differing in the details.

The recommendations result from a detailed assessment of individual studies and the use of a hierarchy of evidence as has been described, to assess the overall quality of evidence on a five category scale, with an approximate estimate of the relative size of the expected net benefits (**Ex. 9.7**). Thus to give an 'A' recommendation, the US Preventive Services Taskforce scheme requires

---

### GRADES OF CLINICAL RECOMMENDATIONS

A.  The USPSTF strongly recommends that clinicians provide [the service] to eligible patients. *The USPSTF found good evidence that [the service] improves important health outcomes and concludes that benefits substantially outweigh harms.*

B.  The USPSTF recommends that clinicians provide [the service] to eligible patients. *The USPSTF found at least fair evidence that [the service] improves important health outcomes and concludes that benefits outweigh harms.*

C.  The USPSTF makes no recommendation for or against routine provision of [the service]. *The USPSTF found at least fair evidence that [the service] can improve health outcomes but concludes that the balance of benefits and harms is too close to justify a general recommendation.*

D.  The USPSTF recommends against routinely providing [the service] to asymptomatic patients. *The USPSTF found at least fair evidence that [the service] is ineffective or that harms outweigh benefits.*

I.  The USPSTF concludes that the evidence is insufficient to recommend for or against routinely providing [the service]. *Evidence that [the service] is effective is lacking, of poor quality, or conflicting, and the balance of benefits and harms cannot be determined.*

---

**Ex. 9.6.** The U.S. Preventive Services Task Force (USPSTF) grades of recommendations: these are based on the strength of evidence and magnitude of net benefit (benefits minus harms). From US Preventive Services Task Force [21] (www.ahrg.gov/clinic/pocketgd.pdf)

## DERIVATION OF CLINICAL RECOMMENDATIONS

1. *Rating of quality of the overall evidence in three categories:*

   Good: Evidence includes consistent results from well-designed well-conducted studies in representative populations that directly assess effects on health outcomes.

   Fair: Evidence is sufficient to determine effects on health outcomes, but the strength of the evidence is limited by the number, quality, or consistency of the individual studies, generalizability to routine practice, or indirect nature of the evidence on health outcomes.

   Poor: Evidence is insufficient to assess the effects on health outcomes because of limited number or power of studies, important flaws in their design or conduct, gaps in the chain of evidence, or lack of information on important health outcomes.

2. *Assessment of size of net benefit (benefit–harm) in four categories: comparison with rating of quality of evidence determines the final recommendation as A, B, C, D or I.*

| Rating | Estimate of Net Benefit (Benefit Minus Harms) | | | |
|---|---|---|---|---|
| | Substantial | Moderate | Small | Zero/Negative |
| Good | A | B | C | D |
| Fair | B | B | C | D |
| Poor | I – Insufficient Evidence | | | |

**Ex. 9.7.** Derivation of the overall grades of recommendations shown in Ex. 9.6. From: US Preventive Services Task Force [21] (www.ahrg.gov/clinic/pocketgd.pdf)

high-quality evidence which shows a substantial net benefit for the intervention in relevant populations [20]. Such recommendations include chemoprevention by aspirin for adults at increased risk of coronary heart disease, and routine screening for blood lipids in adults. A 'B' recommendation may have good evidence of a moderate benefit, or fair evidence of a moderate or substantial benefit; an example is counselling and behavioural interventions for weight reduction in obese adults, where the main caution is around the evidence for effectiveness of the interventions, which is mixed. In many situations the evidence is judged insufficient to yield clear recommendations, for example in screening for prostate cancer, and in others, the evidence is firm enough to recommend that such interventions have a zero or negative net benefit and should not be used, for example routine screening of adolescents for scoliosis.

For clinical interventions, many specialist and professional groups produce clinical guidelines, which vary considerably in their content and presentation, but inherently they all assess the available evidence according to a process involving critical appraisal and using a hierarchy of evidence similar to that in Ex. 9.4.

The type of advice can range from specific advice on particular issues representing the consensus of the group producing the guidelines, to the more sophisticated approach of encouraging practitioners to assess and use the evidence efficiently themselves. The latter approach is shown by the manuals for evidence-based clinical practice produced by the Evidence-based Medicine Working Group of the American Medical Association and the Centre for Health Evidence, which has a valuable website (www.userguides.org) [22].

## Conflicting recommendations

In many controversial issues, different conclusions are reached not because of fundamental disagreements about the evidence available, but because of different methods of ranking different types of evidence. For example, there has been much controversy about breast cancer screening at younger ages, with some expert groups recommending it as a beneficial procedure, while others have concluded that the evidence for benefit is unclear and do not recommend it. In general, those less willing to support such screening argue primarily from the results of randomized trials, which have not shown clear benefits. Some of the groups reaching a different conclusion, such as the American Cancer Society, make it clear that they put considerable emphasis on the results of other types of study, such as a large uncontrolled demonstration project carried out in the USA [23]. The inherently different rankings given to different types of evidence influence the conclusion reached, and cultural differences in different societies are important [24,25]; for example, some argue that if the evidence is unclear, an established intervention like screening should be continued unless there is clear evidence of lack of benefit, and some argue that it should not proceed until there is clear evidence of benefit. This issue came to a head in 1993, when the National Cancer Institute in the USA assessed the available randomized trial evidence on breast cancer screening in women under age 50, concluded that the benefits were uncertain, and changed its previous recommendation which supported screening in this age group. This decision resulted in a report from a US Senate subcommittee, which criticized the dependence on randomized trial results, pointing to the uncontrolled demonstration projects in the USA, and argued that screening should continue unless the absence of benefit could be proven. A similar scene was repeated when a consensus conference was held by the National Institutes of Health in 1997; again, this group, putting most emphasis on randomized trial results, concluded that there was no clear evidence of a mortality reduction and did not recommend screening [26]. This decision was rejected by the director of the National Cancer Institute and again by the US Senate, which voted unanimously in favour of the value of mammograms for younger women, using what one journalist described as 'some mysteriously acquired medical insight' [27]. The result seemed to be that in this context a scientific conclusion that mammography in younger women was not effective was not politically acceptable, whereas in some other countries it was more accepted that it was necessary to prove the benefits of screening, rather than to prove the lack of benefit [24].

## The application of critical appraisal to clinical medicine and health care policy

In this book we have reviewed a system for the critical appraisal of evidence relating to cause and effect relationships in health. The application of critical appraisal methods to health care issues is often described as *evidence-based medicine*, with a primarily clinical orientation, or as *knowledge-based health care* or *evidence-based policy* with a wider community perspective. Of course, these are both huge topics about which only a few words can be said here. What follows is a brief comment on the development of evidence-based medicine and health policy, rather than any attempt at a comprehensive approach to the area.

### The development of evidence-based medicine

Clinical decision-making has had three main influences: authority and tradition, laboratory-based science, and empirical assessment. The predominant influence through most of the twentieth century was authority and tradition: the viewpoint of accumulated experience and consensus. Many such 'consensus' views are not supported by empirical evidence. In 1991, a *British Medical Journal* editorial concluded that 'only about 15 per cent of medical interventions are supported by solid scientific evidence' [28], noting several previous similar estimates. More eloquently, David Naylor, head of the medical school and subsequently President of the University of Toronto, said 'clinical medicine seems to consist of a few things we know, a few things we think we know (but probably don't), and lots of things we don't know at all' [29].

Many health interventions arise from a consideration of mechanisms studied in the laboratory, but this can be dangerous if empirical testing in a whole person and community situation is not done. One of the worst examples of this was the use of drugs to suppress cardiac arrhythmias that were observed in patients who had had a myocardial infarction. The logic was that patients with such arrhythmias had a higher risk of death, the drugs could effectively suppress the arrhythmias, and therefore the drugs should reduce mortality. The drugs were developed, marketed, approved, and widely used on this basis, before large randomized trials demonstrated that although reducing the ectopic heartbeats, the drugs produced an increase in mortality [30]. Similarly, the evidence from basic science and observational epidemiological studies that beta-carotene should protect against cancer was strong, and led to its widespread use as a preventive factor outside mainstream medicine. However, randomized trials of beta-carotene have shown no benefit or even higher risks of cancer, so that supplementation in these trials has had to be stopped, as was discussed in Chapter 6 [31].

The tensions between different sources of wisdom are not new. In the nineteenth century pioneers such as the French physician Louis promoted empirical methods of assessing therapies using the 'numerical' method, i.e. observing and counting the results in patients, which demonstrated amongst other things that the popular use of leeches in therapy was unsupported by evidence of efficacy [32]. The contrast between assessments based on clinical experience and on numerical observations was shown in the debates about thyroid immunization in the early part of the twentieth century. Supporting immunization was Sir Almroth Wright, a prominent pathologist (and later mentor of Alexander Fleming, of penicillin fame), who put his faith in what he called the 'experiential' method. He described this as 'unconscious automatic induction by an expert', or more fully: 'we let the two streams of experience which correspond to the two series of substantive and controlled experiments filter through our minds and then compare the impressions which have been imprinted' [33,34]. Opposing him was Karl Pearson, one of the pioneers of statistical methods, arguing from empirical data that the efficacy of vaccination was unproven; Pearson used correlation techniques, having written that 'this new conception of correlation brought psychology, anthropology, medicine and sociology in large parts into the field of mathematical treatment' [35]. In this debate, described eloquently by Susser [36], Wright was correct, because his clinical experience showed him that some of the data used by Pearson was poorly collected and unreliable. In our terminology, he was aware of the problems of observation bias and error, whereas Pearson's statistical technique gave equal weight to all the observations he had available, irrespective of their quality. However, subsequently, Wright's methodological weakness showed in his development of, and fervent support for, an autoimmunization process for treating infections, which gained immense popularity but was not subjected to empirical trial and led to a great deal of inappropriate and probably dangerous therapy [37]. His process, and the issues it raised in terms of the use of resources and access to care, were described by George Bernard Shaw, a close friend, in his play *The Doctor's Dilemma*, first performed in 1906.

In 1937, introducing a series of articles on statistics by Bradford Hill, which later emerged as an important textbook [38], the editor of *The Lancet* wrote: 'in clinical medicine today there is a growing demand for adequate proof of the efficacy of this or that form of treatment'. Bradford Hill's papers, which embodied most of the principles of assessment of causality covered in this book, went beyond arithmetical methods to the assessment of observation bias, confounding, and the evidence for causality [39].

Evidence-based medicine was developed prominently at the McMaster Medical School, in Canada, led by David Sackett, and was expressed in *Clinical Epidemiology*, first published in 1985 [40]. It was firmly rooted in individual patient care, with four steps described in 1995 [41]: to formulate a clear clinical question of a patient-based problem, search the literature for relevant clinical articles, critically appraise the evidence for its validity and usefulness, and implement useful findings in clinical practice. The focus of this development was on the efficacy of clinical interventions. Sackett and his colleagues reported that, in contrast with the estimates given earlier, the great majority of interventions in a specialist medical unit at Oxford under Sackett's direction were demonstrated to be based on empirical evidence [42]. However, this experience in a pioneering academically based unit cannot be generalized to clinical medicine as a whole.

Critical appraisal threatens the traditional approach. The *Lancet* editorial in 1937 commented on the threat which doctors saw from statisticians: 'It is exasperating, when we have studied a problem by methods which we have spent laborious years in mastering, to find our conclusions questioned, and perhaps refuted by, someone who could not have made the observations himself' [39]. The development of meta-analyses, the insistence on systematic standards even for review articles, and the extension of evidence-based medicine to policy and management may be viewed by many as further threats. Some may feel vulnerable if individual professional experience counts for little in comparison with a well-planned study, and if an individual cannot even be trusted to collate experience, that also requiring an objective and systematic process. Even in 2005, a Canadian contributor to *The Lancet* wrote: 'Yet if everything has to be double-blinded, randomized, and evidence-based, where does that leave new ideas?' [43], and more scholarly papers have asked if evidence-based practice does more good than harm [44]. The authoritarian tradition is still dominant in many cultures, such as that of Japan [45]. However, there is no doubt that the greater attention paid to the justification of policies from empirical evidence has been beneficial, and the requirements for such objectivity will continue to increase.

## From clinical efficacy to health policy

The individual patient-based approach has been criticized as paying insufficient attention to issues of efficiency, cost, and other social considerations;

it has been labelled 'narrow scienticism'. The prominent British health econo-
mist Alan Maynard wrote: 'If evidence- based medicine and the individual
ethic are allowed to determine treatment choices, resources will be used ineffi-
ciently and unethically' [46], and a leading social science commentator bor-
rowed the traditional clinical criticism of empirical scientific evidence,
arguing that the heterogeneity of individual patient problems requires the
mysterious process of 'clinical judgement' [47].

However, a wider concept of evidence-based medicine allows for the consideration of cost and utility in addition to clinical efficacy [48]. The emphasis in
this book is on the assessment of a causal relationship between an exposure
and an outcome. Where we are dealing with an intervention, this is the question of *efficacy*: does the intervention produce the outcome desired? In clinical
and policy decision-making, efficacy is the most important but not the only
component. *Efficiency*, i.e. efficacy in comparison with the resources necessary,
is also relevant, and so is *acceptability*, which brings in many other considerations from cultural approaches to ethical questions. Efficacy is central, and
arguments about efficiency or acceptability are rather pointless where efficacy
is dubious. Efficiency and acceptability will be of overriding importance
where a choice has to be made between different efficacious approaches.

The evidence-based approach can now be applied to the appraisal of all
health interventions, and terms such as *knowledge-based health care* have been
used. While John Swales, a national director of research and development for
the British National Health Service, noted [49] 'in the 1980's, it was inconceiv-
able that purchasers of health services would enquire in any but the most
rudimentary way about scientific evidence before funding new developments',
such assessments have since become an essential part of NHS development,
and other countries have followed to various extents.

Methods have been developed which combine the critical appraisal of scientific evidence with cost–benefit or cost–utility analysis, and can incorporate
considerations of equity, acceptability, and feasibility. For example, one such
method is programme budgeting marginal analysis, which has been used to
compare options in health care development in several countries [50–52].
These methods take into account more of the various influences which impact
on decision-making in our societies. However, the relationships between
objective appraisal of evidence and the realities of policy-making are far from
simple. Just as proponents of evidence-based clinical medicine may assume
that decisions will be driven only by the quality of scientific evidence, most
economic models assume that decision-makers are pure and rational; they are
'benevolent and unbiased, seeking to maximise efficiency and equity subject
to budgetary constraints'. In a more cynical (or realistic) view, it has been said
that 'just as companies seek to maximise profits and consumers seek to

maximise utility, clinicians seek to maximise their autonomy, bureaucrats seek to maximise control, and politicians seek to maximise support' [53].

Decision-makers operate in a different environment from clinicians, researchers, or indeed economists. Politicians and bureaucrats need to make decisions under time pressure and with incomplete information, must take account of the perceived urgency and importance of the issue, and must operate with short time horizons. Indeed, these characteristics are often used to criticize research evidence or researchers and to dismiss them as irrelevant [54]. Some regard the gaps between decision-makers and researchers as insurmountable. Comments include 'Researchers are from Mars; policymakers are from Venus' and 'research is actually a dirty word to many policymakers' [55]. On the other hand, health care professionals may feel that policy-makers set the policy first and use scientific evidence, if at all, only to support already agreed policies; they use policy-based evidence rather than evidence-based policy.

Such gaps may be attributed to the poor communication skills of researchers, or to the lack of consultation by policy-makers, but such blame attribution is unhelpful. Researchers need to be aware of the constraints policy-makers work under, and anticipate the counter-arguments that will arise. Approaches that will be more likely to bridge the gaps include an emphasis on presenting solutions rather than problems, and paying attention to wide consultation and to gaining broad professional and consumer support. Policy-makers generally have neither the time nor the expertise to assess the value of a proposal, and so they often assess who is promoting an idea and who would be opposed to it. In this context, the consumers' voice has become very important in health planning in most countries. Decision-makers will accept decisions that appear good enough, ('satisficing' decision-making), rather than seeking the optimum, and they like incremental decisions, in which options are kept open and irrevocable commitments are not made, to keep an escape route open. Risk assessment is an integral part of any policy development, including the assessment of financial and political hazards. Doing something new has more risks than continuing current policy: starting friction is greater than sliding friction. The greatest political risks are in taking something away; witness the almost inevitable outcry over the closure of a facility, even if a good argument has been made on grounds of clinical efficacy or efficiency. It has been found that systematic attempts based on good scientific and economic logic to reduce ineffective care in several countries have not been successful [53].

An elegant synthesis is given by Dobrow et al. [56], who consider decision-making in terms of the importance of scientific evidence and the importance of context, which includes economic, social, and political considerations (**Ex. 9.8**). The evidence-based clinical model rates high on the evidence axis but low on the context axis, while the traditional political process rates high on the context axis but low on the evidence axis. They argue for an ideal situation where these are balanced. The challenge is how to achieve this. Even recently, in a major review of several massive social interventions in the UK, the King's Fund group concluded that these multi-million pound programmes were developed 'on the basis of informed guesswork and expert hunches, enriched by some evidence and driven by political and other imperatives' [57,58].

This was in part because the necessary research had not been done. The choice of what research is done is haphazard, and if we base programmes only on the existing research our scope is very limited. The further development of evidence-based policy requires identifying key questions that require new research. A good example of this is screening for neuroblastoma, a cancer affecting young children. It can be detected by a urine test in infancy, and screening has been advocated, especially in Japan. Before routine screening was accepted in Canada or the USA, a trial was done in Canada. This was not a randomized trial, but a comparison of a screening programme applied to births in Quebec, with control groups unscreened in Ontario. The results showed that screening produced a great increase in the incidence rate of

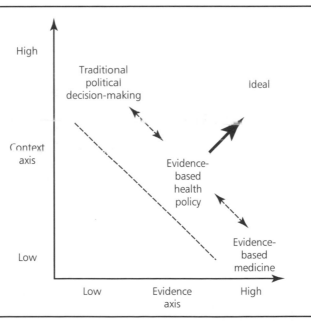

**Ex. 9.8.** The context and evidence axes of evidence-based decision-making as given by Dobrow et al. [56] Reprinted from Social Science in Medicine, **58,** Dobrow et al. Evidence based health policy: context and utilization, pp. 207–17, 2004, with permission from Elsevier.

diagnosed neuroblastoma, but the mortality rate was not reduced. The interpretation was that screening produced a substantial number of false-positive diagnoses, and also 'silent tumours', which are tumours which were diagnosed as neuroblastoma and treated, but which if left alone would not have produced any clinical problems. The trial cost $US 8.8 million. If a screening programme had been set up, the costs for the USAand Canada would have been $570 million over a 12-year period [59]. Thus as well as avoiding substantial morbidity, the trial investment showed a rate of return of 6400 per cent, which even the most cynical policy-maker would regard as impressive.

## Finale

The appraisal of evidence is an essential component of any wider decision-making process. Like any other process, it can sometimes be misused. It is important that the central issue in evidence-based health care, the critical appraisal of the available evidence, receives adequate attention. This indeed is the purpose of this book.

The remaining six chapters of this book present the application of this method of critical appraisal to six studies, illustrating a range of study designs and topics. The reader is encouraged to work through these and apply the system which has been presented.

## References

1. **MacMahon B.** Epidemiological evidence on the nature of Hodgkin's disease. *Cancer* 1957; **10**: 1045–1054.

2. **Glaser SL, Jarrett RF.** The epidemiology of Hodgkin's disease. *Baillieres Clin Haematol* 1996; **9**: 401–416.

3. **Howe GR, Burch JD, Miller AB,** *et al.* Artificial sweeteners and human bladder cancer. *Lancet* 1977; **ii**: 578–581.

4. **Rothman KJ, Moore LL, Singer MR, Nguyen US, Mannino S, Milunsky A.** Teratogenicity of high vitamin A intake. *N Engl J Med* 1995; **333**: 1369–1373.

5. **Smith DC, Prentice R, Thompson DJ, Herrmann WL.** Association of exogenous estrogen and endometrial carcinoma. *N Engl J Med* 1975; **293**: 1164–1167.

6. **Daly E, Vessey MP, Hawkins MM, Carson JL, Gough P, Marsh S.** Risk of venous thromboembolism in users of hormone replacement therapy. *Lancet* 1996; **348**: 977–980.

7. **Jick H, Derby LE, Myers MW, Vasilakis C, Newton KM.** Risk of hospital admission for idiopathic venous thromboembolism among users of postmenopausal oestrogens. *Lancet* 1996; **348**: 981–983.

8. **Grodstein F, Stampfer MJ, Goldhaber SZ,** *et al.* Prospective study of exogenous hormones and risk of pulmonary embolism in women. *Lancet* 1996; **348**: 983–987.

9. **Hill D, White V, Jolley D, Mapperson K.** Self examination of the breast: is it beneficial? Meta-analysis of studies investigating breast self-examination and extent of disease in patients with breast cancer. *BMJ* 1988; **297**: 271–275.

10. **Elwood JM, Little J, Elwood JH.** *Epidemiology and Control of Neural Tube Defects.* Oxford: Oxford University Press, 1992.

11. **Hill AB.** The environment and disease: association or causation? *Proc R Soc Med* 1965; **58**: 295–300.

12. **Crumpton MJ.** The Bernal Lecture 2004. Are low-frequency electromagnetic fields a health hazard? *Philos Trans R Soc Lond B Biol Sci* 2005; **360**: 1223–1230.

13. **Ahlbom IC, Cardis E, Green A, Linet M, Savitz D, Swerdlow A.** Review of the epidemiologic literature on EMF and Health. *Environ Health Perspect* 2001; **109** (Suppl 6): 911–933.

14. **Mitchell LE, Adzick NS, Melchionne J, Pasquariello PS, Sutton LN, Whitehead AS.** Spina bifida. *Lancet* 2004; **364**: 1885–1895.

15. **Emanuel I, Sever LE.** Questions concerning the possible association of potatoes and neural-tube defects, and an alternative hypothesis relating to maternal growth and development. *Teratology* 1973; **8**: 325–332.

16. **Miller AB, Lindsay J, Hill GB.** Mortality from cancer of the uterus in Canada and its relationship to screening for cancer of the cervix. *Int J Cancer* 1976; **17**: 602–612.

17. **Sloan JH, Kellermann AL, Reay DT,** *et al.* Handgun regulations, crime, assaults, and homicide. *N Engl J Med* 1988; **319**: 1256–1262.

18. **Canadian Task Force on the Periodic Health Examination.** The periodic health examination. *Can Med Assoc J* 1979; **121**: 1193–1203.

19. **Woolf SH, Battista RN, Anderson GM, Logan AG, Wang E.** Assessing the clinical effectiveness of preventive maneuvers: analytic principles and systematic methods in reviewing evidence and developing clinical practice recommendations. A report by the Canadian Task Force on the Periodic Health Examination. *J Clin Epidemiol* 1990; **43**: 891–905.

20. **Sibbald B, Addington-Hall J, Brenneman D, Freeling P.** Telephone versus postal surveys of general practitioners: methodological considerations. *Br J Gen Pract* 1994; **44**: 297–300.

21. **U.S Preventive Services Task Force.** *The Guide to Clinical Preventive Services 2005.* Washington, DC: Agency for Healthcare Research and Quality, 2005.

22. **Guyatt GH, Rennie D** (eds). *Users' Guide to the Medical Literature: A Manual for Evidence-Based Clinical Practice.* Chicago, IL: JAMA & Archives Journals, American Medical Association, 2002.

23. **Mettlin C, Smart CR.** Breast cancer detection guidelines for women aged 40 to 49 years: rationale for the American Cancer Society reaffirmation of recommendations. *CA Cancer J Clin* 1994; **44**: 248–255.

24. **Elwood JM.** Breast cancer screening in younger women: evidence and decision making. *J Eval Clin Pract* 1997; **3**: 179–186.

25. **Jatoi I, Baum M.** American and European recommendations for screening mammography in younger women: a cultural divide? *BMJ* 1993; **307**: 1481–1483.

26. **National Institutes of Health Consensus Development Conference.** *National Institutes of Health Consensus Development Statement: Breast Cancer Screening for Women ages 40–49: January 21–23, 1997.* Washington: National Institutes of Health, 1997.

27. Begley S. The mammogram war. *Newsweek* [Feb 24], 55–59. 1997.

28. Smith R. Where is the wisdom...? *BMJ* 1991; **303**: 798–799.

29. Naylor CD. Grey zones of clinical practice: some limits to evidence-based medicine. *Lancet* 1995; **345**: 840–842.

30. The Cardiac Arrhythmia Suppression Trial II Investigators. Effect of the antiarrhythmic agent moricizine on survival after myocardial infarction. *N Engl J Med* 1992; **327**: 227–233.

31. Omenn GS, Goodman GE, Thornquist MD, *et al.* Effects of a combination of beta carotene and vitamin A on lung cancer and cardiovascular disease. *N Engl J Med* 1996; **334**: 1150–1155.

32. Armitage P. Trials and errors: the emergence of clinical statistics. *J R Statist Soc Ser A* 1983; **146**: 321–334.

33. Wright AE, Morgan WP, Colebrook L, Dodgson RW. Observations on the pharmacotherapy of pneumococcus infections. *Lancet* 1912; **ii**: 1701–1705.

34. Wright AE. *The Unexpurgated Case Against Women's Suffrage*. London: Constable, 1913.

35. Pearson ES. *Karl Pearson: An Appreciation of Some Aspects of His Life and Work*. Cambridge: Cambridge University Press, 1938.

36. Susser M. Judgment and causal inference: criteria in epidemiologic studies. *Am J Epidemiol* 1977; **105**: 1–15.

37. Nachbar J, (Ed.). *Vaccine Therapy: Its Administration, Value and Limitations. A Discussion Opened by Sir Almroth E. Wright, MD, FRS*. London: Longmans, Green, 1910.

38. Hill AB. *Principles of Medical Statistics*. London: The Lancet Ltd, 1937.

39. Anonymous. Mathematics and medicine. *Lancet* 1937; **i**: 31.

40. Sackett DL, Haynes RB, Tugwell P. *Clinical Epidemiology: A Basic Science for Clinical medicine*. Boston, MA: Little, Brown, 1985.

41. Rosenberg W, Donald A. Evidence-based medicine: an approach to clinical problem-solving. *BMJ* 1995; **310**: 1122–1126.

42. Ellis J, Mulligan I, Rowe J, Sackett DL. Inpatient general medicine is evidence based. *Lancet* 1995; **346**: 407–410.

43. Wu J. Could evidence-based medicine be a danger to progress? *Lancet* 2005; **366**: 122.

44. Hammersley.M. Is the evidence-based practice movement doing more good than harm? Reflections on Iain Chalmers' case for research-based policy making and practice. *Evid Policy* 2005; **1**: 85–100.

45. Yokota T, Kojima S, Yamauchi H, Hatori M. Evidence-based medicine in Japan. *Lancet* 2005; **366**: 122.

46. Maynard A. Evidence-based medicine: an incomplete method for informing treatment choices. *Lancet* 1997; **349**: 126–128.

47. Klein R. The NHS and the new scientism: solution or delusion? *Q J Med* 1996; **89**: 85–87.

48. Sackett DL, Rosenberg WMC. The need for evidence-based medicine. *J R Soc Med* 1995; **88**: 620–624.

49. Swales J. Scientific basis of health services. Science and medical practice: the turning tide. *J Health Serv Res Policy* 1996; **1**: 61–62.

50. Mitton C, Donaldson C. *Priority Setting Toolkit: A Guide to the Use of Economics in Healthcare Decision Making*. London: BMJ Publishing, 2004.

51. **Peacock S, Ruta D, Mitton C, Donaldson C, Bate A, Murtagh M.** Using economics to set pragmatic and ethical priorities. *BMJ* 2006; **332**: 482–485.

52. **Mitton C, Donaldson C.** Twenty-five years of programme budgeting and marginal analysis in the health sector, 1974–1999. *J Health Serv Res Policy* 2001; **6**: 239–248.

53. **Hauck K, Smith PC, Goddard M.** *The Economics of Priority Setting for Health Care: A Literature Review*. Washington, DC: Health, Nutrition, and Population Family (HNP) of the World Bank's Human Development Network, 2003.

54. **Innvaer S, Vist G, Trommald M, Oxman A.** Health policy-makers' perceptions of their use of evidence: a systematic review. *J Health Serv Res Policy* 2002; **7**: 239–244.

55. **Greenlick MR, Goldberg B, Lopes P, Tallon J.** Health policy roundtable—view from the state legislature: translating research into policy. *Health Serv Res* 2005; **40**: 337–346.

56. **Dobrow MJ, Goel V, Upshur RE.** Evidence-based health policy: context and utilisation. *Soc Sci Med* 2004; **58**: 207–217.

57. **Coote A, Allen J, Woodhead D.** *Finding Out What Works: Building Knowledge About Understanding Complex, Community-Based Initiatives*. London: King's Fund, 2004.

58. **Bowen S, Zwi AB.** Pathways to 'evidence-informed' policy and practice: a framework for action. *PLoS Med* 2005; **2**: e166.

59. **Soderstrom L, Woods WG, Bernstein M, Robison LL, Tuchman M, Lemieux B.** Health and economic benefits of well-designed evaluations: some lessons from evaluating neuroblastoma screening. *J Natl Cancer Inst* 2005; **97**: 1118–1124.

# Critical appraisal in action: introduction to Chapters 10–15

The following chapters present examples of the application of the scheme for critical appraisal to six studies of different types: randomized trials of interventions, observational cohort studies, and case–control studies.

These studies have been chosen because they were published in prominent medical journals (*The Lancet*, the *New England Journal of Medicine*, and the *Journal of the National Cancer Institute*), and the summaries and usually the full text can be obtained through the internet. An extract from each study has been reproduced, with the permission of the journal and the first author. The main elements of the study and the key results are described in these appraisals, and so it is possible to follow the study from the material presented here.

However, to gain most value from these appraisals, you are urged to find the original paper and work through it, applying the scheme for critical appraisal presented in this book, and summarized in Ex. 9.1 (p. 324). You should prepare a summary of your own appraisal, with brief answers to each of the questions in Ex. 9.1. This includes summarizing the key result of the study in as simple a table as possible. You are encouraged to calculate for yourself the key measure of effect and an appropriate statistical test, even if a more sophisticated analysis is given in the original paper. You should be able to summarize the main conclusions in terms of the internal and external validity of the study: What does it show? Is it true? Is it relevant? You can then compare your appraisal with the one given here; undoubtably, you will note several points that may not be covered here.

The assessment of any study involves specific subject matter knowledge as well as a methodological framework. The subject matter issues of these various studies are not dealt with here in any detail, although some comments on their substantive importance are made. At the end of each of these chapters there is a brief summary of the situation since the study was published up to the time of writing (early 2006). The general system of critical appraisal is a framework which helps to identify the major strengths and weaknesses of any study, so that you can then concentrate on the particular issues of critical importance.

These studies have been chosen for their accessibility, because they address important issues, and because they are good examples of the research methods. All represent important research contributions. In some of these chapters, the end conclusion will be that the association seen is due to either causation or confounding; for others, observation bias or chance variation are the main alternative explanations. All have questions of generalizability.

In each of the following six chapters, we will go through the 20 questions set out in Ex. 9.1 in sufficient detail to illustrate the key points. The approach is not exhaustive; the reader may be able to add more to each particular issue. The major aspects of each study are summarized in exhibits, referred to as Ex. 10.1 and so on, whereas the tables and figures in the original paper are referred to by their original numbers.

# Chapter 10

# Critical appraisal of a randomized clinical trial

The first of our critical assessments deals with a randomized clinical trial, published in *The Lancet*, 2 July 2005, **366**, 37–43 [1]. The summary is reproduced here, with permission from Elsevier and the first author, and the full paper can be accessed at http://www.thelancet.com.

## Chloramphenicol treatment for acute infective conjunctivitis in children in primary care: a randomised double-blind placebo-controlled trial

Peter W Rose, Anthony Harnden, Angela B Brueggemann, Rafael Perera, Aziz Sheikh, Derrick Crook, David Mant

Summary

**Background.** One in eight schoolchildren have an episode of acute infective conjunctivitis every year. Standard clinical practice is to prescribe a topical antibiotic, although the evidence to support this practice is scarce. We undertook a randomised double-blind trial to compare the effectiveness of chloramphenicol eye drops with placebo in children with infective conjunctivitis in primary care.

**Methods.** Our study included 326 children aged 6 months to 12 years with a clinical diagnosis of conjunctivitis who were recruited from 12 general medical practices in the UK. We assigned 163 children to receive chloramphenicol eye drops and 163 to receive placebo eye drops. Eye swabs were taken for bacterial and viral analysis. The primary outcome was clinical cure at day 7, which was assessed from diaries completed by parents. All children were followed up for 6 weeks to identify relapse. Survival statistics were used for comparison, and analysis was by intention to treat.

**Findings.** Nine children were lost to follow-up (one in chloramphenicol group; eight in placebo group). Clinical cure by day 7 occurred in 128 (83%) of 155 children with placebo compared with 140 (86%) of 162 with chloramphenicol (risk difference 3·8%, 95% CI −4·1% to 11·8%). Seven (4%) children with chloramphenicol and five (3%) with placebo had further conjunctivitis episodes within 6 weeks (1·2%, −2·9% to 5·3%). Adverse events were rare and evenly distributed between each group.

**Interpretation.** Most children presenting with acute infective conjunctivitis in primary care will get better by themselves and do not need treatment with an antibiotic.

## A. **Description of the evidence**

1. What was the exposure or intervention?
2. What was the outcome?
3. What was the study design?
4. What was the study population?
5. What was the main result?

As stated in the summary, this trial was undertaken to assess whether using antibiotic eye drops (chloramphenicol) in children with conjunctivitis is any more effective than a placebo. The background explained in the paper is that conjunctivitis in children is a common complaint presenting to general practitioners, and it is usually treated with antibiotic eye drops although there is no strong evidence that such treatment is beneficial. This results in extensive prescribing of antibiotics at considerable costs, and some schools require children to be treated before they return to school. It is noted that there has been a Cochrane systematic review of the treatment of conjunctivitis in adults and children [2], which showed superiority of antibiotic treatment to placebo, but it is noted that all the trials included in that review were based on hospital populations, with patients who are likely to have more severe infections. It is not stated if the review was of all ages, and if results specific to children are available.

The intervention tested was regular use of 0.5 per cent chloramphenicol eye drops, compared with placebo eye drops containing water, boric acid, and borax, which could have a soothing effect.

The definition of the outcome is important. The primary outcome measure, decided in advance, was the clinical cure rate at 7 days, as stated by the parents who were asked to keep a diary. The time of cure was defined as the first recorded time in the diary after which none of the three symptoms of pain, redness, or discharge was recorded. There was also an assessment by a research nurse at study entry and at 7 days, and the nurse took two conjunctival swabs from the more affected eye at these times; microbiological cure or improvement was defined on these results, but the clinical cure was defined as the primary endpoint.

The study design was a randomized control trial, comparing the active agent with a placebo, and the study was double-blind, with neither the treating doctors nor the children or their parents being aware of whether the active drug or placebo was used. Although the family doctors identified the eligible patients, they were then seen by a research nurse either at the doctor's premises or at home. The study was explained to parents and children old enough to understand, with standard information sheets designed for children being used, and written consent was obtained. The full paper has quite a long section describing the procedures. A research nurse assessed the clinical severity of the conjunctivitis, assessing the degree of redness by comparison with validated photographs, and then the active drug or placebo was provided. These had been prepared to be in identical bottles, labelled A or B, with the persons knowing the code not participating in the trial. Parents were given instruction for administration of the drugs, and also given a symptom sheet to fill in every time drops were given. The research nurse saw the children again at 7 days follow-up, and further swabs were taken for laboratory examination. Finally, parents were telephoned 6 weeks after the trial had started to identify any further problems or recurrences. Further details of the laboratory techniques and data were given, which need not concern us here.

The study population, as is usual in clinical trials, is specified in detail and has some restrictions. The target population comprises children in the UK or a similar country presenting to a primary care practitioner with conjunctivitis. The source population was 12 general practices in Oxfordshire, UK. Eligible subjects were children aged between 6 months and 12 years, who presented during office hours and had a diagnosis of acute infective conjunctivitis. There were some exclusions for clinical reasons—children allergic to chloramphenicol, those with evidence of severe infection that would necessitate active treatment, those who were immunocompromised, and those who were taking an antibiotic currently or within the previous 48 hours—to avoid modification of the intervention. The restriction to children who presented during office hours was for logistical reasons. The study was done over the winter period of October to April in three consecutive years from 2001 to 2004. Participants are those eligible children who were identified, and whose parents gave written consent to their participation.

The main result of the study is the proportion of children clinically cured, i.e. symptom free, at 7 days, as assessed by the parents' diaries. The key result is shown in **Ex. 10.1,** in the format previously shown for a prospective study. This shows that 140 of the 163 children randomized to treatment with chloramphenicol were clinically cured (85.9 per cent) compared with 128 out of the 163 children randomized to placebo (78.5 per cent). Thus there is a somewhat higher cure rate in the actively treated group, but this is not statistically significant at the 5 per cent level. The result shown in the paper (in Table 3) is the risk difference, 7.4 per cent, and its 95 per cent confidence limits, which were –0.9 per cent and

RESULTS OF A RANDOMIZED TRIAL

*Result shown in paper, for primary outcome of clinical cure at day 7*

| | clinical cure | not cured | total randomized | proportion cured | percentage cured |
|---|---|---|---|---|---|
| chloramphenicol | **140** | 23 | **163** | 0.859 | 85.9 |
| placebo | **128** | 35 | **163** | 0.785 | 78.5 |
| Total | 268 | 58 | 326 | 0.822 | 82.2 |

*Risk calculations:*

| | | | |
|---|---|---|---|
| relative risk | = 0.859 / 0.785 | | 1.09 |
| odds ratio | = 140*35/(128*23) | | 1.66 |
| risk difference | = ( 0.859 - 0.785 )*100 | | 7.36% |
| Number needed to treat = 1 / (risk difference) | | | 13.6 |

*Statistical test (Mantel–Haenszel):*

| $a = 140$ | $E = 134$ | $V = 11.95692$ |
|---|---|---|
| $\chi^2 = 3.01$ | $\chi = 1.74$ | $P = 0.083$ |

*Confidence limits* are calculated based on the standard deviation of ln *RR*, ln *OR*, or *RD*, following Appendix Table 2.

| | value | ln | std dev | 95% confidence limits | |
|---|---|---|---|---|---|
| relative risk | 1.09 | 0.0896 | 0.0518 | 0.99 | 1.21 |
| odds ratio | 1.66 | 0.5095 | 0.2950 | 0.93 | 2.97 |
| risk difference (%) | 7.362 | | 4.217 | −0.9 | 15.6% |
| Number needed to treat = 1 / (risk difference) | | | | infinity | 6.4 |

**Ex. 10.1. Main outcome of trial** comparing antibiotic treatment with placebo for conjunctivitis in children. Adapted from Table 3 of Rose *et al.* [1]

15.6 per cent. Using the 95 per cent standard, the result is compatible with no difference, but also with a difference as large as 15.6 per cent. The number needed to treat, which is the inverse of the risk difference of 7.4 per cent, is 13.6.

Also shown in Ex. 10.1 are the full calculations for this 2 × 2 table, using the methods described in Chapters 3 and 7. The relative risk and odds ratio are quite different as the frequency of the outcome is high; for a ratio measure, relative risk is easier to interpret here. The risk difference and number needed to treat are as shown above, and the confidence limits for the risk difference, calculated as shown in Ex. 7.3 and Appendix Table 2, are as given in the paper. The approximate limits calculated by the method shown in Ex. 7.7 are virtually identical.

This outcome examines only if children had a clinical cure or not at one point in time, i.e. 7 days. The first time at which the children were symptom-free could be assessed from the parents' diaries, and **Ex. 10.2** shows the cumulative

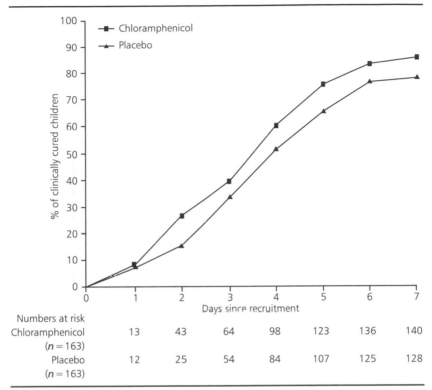

| Numbers at risk | | | | | | | |
|---|---|---|---|---|---|---|---|
| Chloramphenicol (n = 163) | 13 | 43 | 64 | 98 | 123 | 136 | 140 |
| Placebo (n = 163) | 12 | 25 | 54 | 84 | 107 | 125 | 128 |

**Ex. 10.2.** Cumulative incidence curve of percentage cured by day, from trial comparing antibiotic treatment with placebo for conjunctivitis in children. Figure 3 of Rose *et al.* [1]

proportion of children with clinical cure at each day after recruitment. This is presented as a cumulative incidence curve for clinical cure, using the Kaplan–Meier calculation shown in Chapter 7. This adds extra information as it assesses not simply the proportion of children with clinical cure at day 7, but the time at which cure occurred. Exhibit 10.2 shows that the time to cure, i.e. the duration of the conjunctivitis, tended to be shorter in the group receiving chloramphenicol; for example, the median time, at which 50 per cent of the children were cured, was around 3.5 days for the chloramphenicol group and around 4 days for the placebo group.

Further outcome data are given for the subgroup of children with confirmed bacterial pathogens and full follow-up, in whom the risk difference was in fact smaller than in the intention to treat analysis (**Ex. 10.3**). This shows that there was no larger effect in confirmed bacterial cases. Results for 'microbiological cure', i.e. the eye swabs at day 7 being free from pathogens, are also shown. These give a higher cure rate in the chloramphenicol group; the risk

OUTCOMES IN A RANDOMIZED TRIAL

| Outcome | Basis of comparison | chloramphenicol | | | placebo | | | Risk difference % | 95% confidence limits |
|---|---|---|---|---|---|---|---|---|---|
| | | No. events | No. children assessed | Rate % | No. events | No. children assessed | Rate % | | |
| Clinical cure at day 7 | Intention to treat | 140 | 163 | 85.9 | 128 | 163 | 78.5 | 7.4 | -0.9  15.6 |
| | Excluding lost to follow up | 140 | 162 | 86.4 | 128 | 155 | 82.6 | 3.8 | -4.1  11.8 |
| | Children with bacteria isolated, and full information | 101 | 119 | 84.9 | 94 | 117 | 80.3 | 4.5 | -5.1  14.2 |
| Microbiological cure at day 7 | Only subjects with information | 50 | 125 | 40.0 | 29 | 125 | 23.2 | 16.8 | 5.5  28.1 |
| Adverse clinical events, day 1 to 7 | Excluding lost to follow up | 3 | 162 | 1.9 | 3 | 155 | 1.9 | -0.1 | -2.9  2.9 |
| Further episodes of conjunctivitis within 6 weeks | Only subjects with information on 6 weeks' follow up | 7 | 157 | 4.5 | 5 | 150 | 3.3 | 1.1 | -2.9  5.3 |

**Ex. 10.3.** Several outcomes assessed in the randomized trial.

From Tables 1 and 2 of *Rose et al.* [1]

difference is 16.8 per cent, which is statistically significant (Ex. 10.3). Further results are given in the original paper.

## B. Internal validity: consideration of non-causal explanations

### 6. Are the results likely to be affected by observation bias?

Observation bias is obviously a critical issue in this study, as the outcome is defined as 'cure', based on observations by each child's parents, and is open to observer variation. Several steps are taken to ensure that the study results are still valid. First, cure was defined in advance: as an absence of the key symptoms of pain, redness, or discharge, and as recorded by the parents' diaries. The parents were asked to keep a regular record of symptoms, recording them each time the drops were given, rather than being asked to state when symptoms resolved. It might be thought that a more 'scientific' outcome would be, for example, the rate of bacteriological or viral clearance as detected by the eye swabs at day 7, or the clinical observations by the nurse at day 7, and these outcomes were also assessed, but there is wisdom in the definition of clinical cure used in the study. It allows constant observation; the parents are acting as unpaid researchers in recording the study endpoint. More importantly, this definition of clinical cure is what is used in normal practice in primary care, and is what affects activities such as return to school. In the paper there is discussion of this, and it is pointed out that the relationship between clinical state and bacteriological findings is mixed, as bacteria and viruses can be isolated from normal eyes, and are isolated from only a proportion of eyes with clinical conjunctivitis. Thus clinical cure can occur without microbiological clearance. Therefore the outcome chosen is clinically relevant, and can be observed continuously in time. However, it is still weak methodologically; the outcome is assessed by laypersons, and a different person makes the observations of outcome for each child in the study. There will be considerable observer variation, which may be random but could vary with the characteristics of the parents or the child (e.g. some parents will be health professionals, and the observations may be more difficult in younger children). If the parents' assessment of symptoms were compared with a definitive standard, many differences would be seen.

The chief defence against this is the fact that the study is randomized, a placebo is used, and the essential element is that the trial is double-blind. Some of the parents may have suspected or assumed that the treatment their child was receiving was either active or placebo, but as long as the blindness is preserved that protects against any systematic observation bias between the two groups.

This method of recording the clinical outcome would be very inadvisable in a study which was not double-blind and placebo-controlled.

Results are also presented for microbiological cure, which interestingly enough show a statistically significant difference in favour of chloramphenicol, and the results for microbiological improvement, or for the combination of cure or improvement, while not statistically significant, show larger effects than the results based on the clinical cure. This could be because the drug is more effective at producing a biological cure than a clinical cure, or because of the larger degree of random observation error with respect to the clinical data. The children were also assessed clinically by the research nurse at the beginning of the study and to day 7, and those results would be interesting in this respect, but are not given. In later correspondence, the authors state that the clinical cure rate assessed by the nurses was 79 per cent in the chloramphenicol group and 78 per cent in the placebo group [3]. In summary, we must accept that there will be some random error in the clinical cure information, which might impact to reduce the observed difference, but bias in the clinical observations is unlikely to be important.

## 7. Are the results likely to be affected by confounding?

The prime protection against confounding is the randomized design, applied to a reasonably large number of study entrants, and the correct intention to treat analysis. Of course, randomization does not guarantee that the two groups are comparable on all relevant factors, and information is presented on demographic factors, clinical features, and results of microbiological assessment at baseline, as shown in **Ex. 10.4**. These show very similar distributions, demonstrating the value of the randomization process. The group receiving the chloramphenicol includes slightly more children with unilateral disease and a slightly higher social class distribution shown by a greater proportion in the professional or managerial groups, but there are very similar distributions in terms of other factors and bacterial and viral results. The relevant factors are those that are related to the natural history and the outcome of treatment of acute conjunctivitis in children, and a literature review or specialist knowledge would be needed to assess if there are other important relevant factors. If there had been substantial differences in recorded potential confounding factors despite the randomization, stratification or multivariate analysis could be used, as described in Chapters 6 and 7.

Confounder control in a randomized trial depends on the randomization being done appropriately. The randomization process should be clearly described, and should be free from any possible compromise. Both those enrolling the subjects and the subjects themselves should have no means of knowing the treatment assignment until after the eligibility and consent

COMPARISONS AT BASELINE IN A RANDOMIZED TRIAL

|  | Randomized to: | |
|  | chloramphenicol | placebo |
| --- | --- | --- |
| Number | 163 | 163 |
| Age, mean | 3.3 | 3.3 |
| Age, standard deviation | 2.8 | 2.6 |
| % male | 51 | 53 |
| % higher social class (maternal) | 56 | 49 |
| *Clinical features (%)* | | |
| moderate or severe redness | 24 | 26 |
| purulent discharge | 83 | 81 |
| pain or soreness | 50 | 48 |
| unilateral | 36 | 31 |
| *Bacteria isolated* | | |
| Any | 78 | 77 |
| *H.influenzae* | 61 | 60 |
| *S.pneumoniae* | 20 | 20 |
| *M.catarrhalis* | 12 | 10 |
| *Viruses isolated* | | |
| Any | 15 | 12 |
| Adenovirus | 7 | 5 |
| Picornavirus | 8 | 7 |

**Fx. 10.4.** Features of children with conjunctivitis randomized to the two treatments. Adapted from Tables 1 and 2 of Rose *et al.* [1]

processes are complete, and the subject has agreed to participate. The randomization process is not very clear in the paper. It is stated that family doctors recruited eligible children and gave them an information sheet. Then the children and families were seen by a research nurse, and the study explained and consent received. Identical bottles of the active and the placebo agent were prepared and were 'randomized centrally by use of random number tables in blocks of ten'. The recruiting nurse gave a bottle to the family, chosen according to the next available number; the block system ensured that for each 10 children, five received active drug and five received placebo. It is stated that the main analysis of the study was undertaken before the randomization code was broken, which would allow the study to be described as having a triple-blind design.

The protection against confounding is given by the fact that the analysis was done on an intention to treat basis, i.e. the group randomized to active treatment (not just the children who received the treatment) was compared with the group randomized to placebo, as discussed in Chapter 6. As anyone who has given eye drops to a baby or child knows, there is likely to be considerable variation in the actual regime of treatment; some parents may be very rigorous, and others much less attentive. Again, this mirrors normal practice, and the double-blind trial design should ensure that such variations are similar in the two groups. Some children may have had very little treatment; others may have had other treatment in addition to the study treatment. One child was found not to fulfil the eligibility criteria (by being too old) after randomization, and was withdrawn from the study. This is acceptable, but if a large number of children were found to be ineligible after randomization, that would raise questions about the quality of the study process.

Any comparison other than that performed—comparing the groups as originally randomized—loses the value of the randomization. Some children entered the study but did not complete it, being 'lost to follow-up'. In general in a clinical trial, those lost to follow-up are likely to be substantially different in terms of factors recorded as potential confounders, and also other aspects of clinical condition, lifestyle, or social and medical support which could be related to outcome. The use of the intention to treat analysis is the only way in which the advantages of randomization for confounder control are realized. Thus the intention to treat analysis still includes these children. The problem is that to include them in the analysis some assumptions must be made about their outcome.

In this study only nine of the 326 children did not complete the follow-up examinations and have missing outcome data. This is a very small number and testifies to the care taken in the practical aspects of this study. However, presumably simply by chance, one child was in the active treatment group and eight in the placebo group. The predetermined routine was to that assume children lost to follow-up were failures of treatment, and this has been done in the main results that have been discussed. If, instead, they are excluded from the results, the proportion in the placebo group with clinical cure rises from 79 to 83 per cent, becoming closer to the result in the active treatment group which remains at 86 per cent. If it had been assumed that all children lost to follow-up were in fact cured, that would have a similar effect to exclusions. Given that the overall cure rate was high, at 83 per cent, an assumption that those lost to follow-up were cured would probably be more accurate than the assumption that they were treatment failures. Therefore although the numbers of children lost to follow-up are very small, because the numbers are unevenly distributed this does influence the results, and larger numbers lost to follow-up could make the results very difficult to interpret.

There is an error in the way the paper is presented. In the summary, shown at the start of this chapter, although it is stated that analysis was by intention to treat, the results given for clinical cure are the results excluding those children lost to follow-up. The results by intention to treat are given in the results section, and shown in Ex.10.1, but are not used in the summary. The fact that more children were lost to follow-up in the placebo group also raises a question about whether the blinding could have been compromised. Could families which received the placebo have guessed that, and therefore have lost interest in the study more readily than families with active treatment? We have the authors' assurance that the drops and bottles were identical and the same numbers were prescribed extra antibiotics (see next paragraph), and the overall results of the trial would suggest that the clinical course of the disease was similar, so the inequity of distribution of loss to follow-up is probably just chance variation. However, the exclusion of children lost to follow-up does compromise the randomization, and could introduce confounding if those lost to follow-up differ systematically from the rest. The reliance on the intention to treat comparison will avoid these confounding effects.

Some children were prescribed antibiotic eye drops during the trial; presumably their parents or practitioners were concerned or impatient. These children were correctly included in the main analysis, as excluding them would compromise the randomization. This extra treatment could be associated with the outcome, and if unevenly distributed between the two groups, would be a confounding factor. However, this only applied to 12 children, six in each group. If a large number had received extra treatment outside the protocol, and if the numbers had been unequal in each group, this would raise questions of interpretation. The effect of an equal distribution of such extra treatment would tend to decrease any real difference in effectiveness between the chloramphenicol and placebo groups in the trial, but only if the extra treatment were effective; otherwise it would have no effect on the study.

Thus because the study was reasonably large, the groups compared were obtained by randomization, and the data on recorded factors suggest no major differences between the groups in the intention to treat analysis, confounding is unlikely to have any substantial influence on the results.

## 8. Are the results likely to be affected by chance variation?

These results show the problems of concentrating on a conventional significance level of 5 per cent. On the primary outcome of clinical cure, with the intention to treat analysis, the results as shown in Ex. 10.1 show confidence limits which come close to the conventional 5 per cent significance level but overlap the null value, so that they are not statistically significant. More information is given by the analysis taking the time to cure into consideration, and the log-rank statistic (calculated by the method shown in Chapter 7) for the data shown in Ex. 10.2 showed a $P$-value of 0.025, which is statistically significant by the usual criterion. Thus the probability that the difference seen could be due only to chance, with the real situation being that the clinical cure rate is the same with either active or placebo treatment, is reasonably substantial. However, the results do show an increased cure rate with chloramphenicol, and the likelihood that this reflects a real effect cannot be dismissed.

The graph in Ex 10.2 also raises the question of whether the small difference in cure rate at 7 days persists, with the two curves remaining separate, or whether they come together. There was a telephone follow-up with the parents at 6 weeks, which is reported in terms of adverse clinical events and further episodes of conjunctivitis, which were experienced by 4 per cent of children with active treatment and 3 per cent of those on placebo. It is not clear whether the conjunctivitis resolved in all other children, or when it did, which would be useful information.

In assessing chance variation we need to assess both whether appropriate tests have been used, and whether they have been done at the appropriate time. In clinical trials the issues of multiple testing, and perhaps publication of results or termination of studies on the basis of one of a series of tests, are relevant. With regard to this study, there is a clearly stated protocol setting the follow-up at 7 days, and there is no issue with interim or frequent analyses.

Thus we cannot exclude chance variation in this study, nor can we be sure that chance variation explains the results. The difference in outcome at 7 days and the more sensitive analysis of time to cure give results close to the conventional 0.05 significance level.

This raises a question of whether the trial has sufficient statistical power. It is stated that it was designed with reference to an earlier study, which showed a 19 per cent improvement in outcome with antibiotics, and this difference was accepted as clinically important. The study was initially planned to have 80 per cent power to detect a 19 per cent difference, assuming a cure rate in the placebo arm of 72 per cent, and using a two-sided test at the 5 per cent significance level. It was further assumed that 60 per cent of children would have a bacterial aetiology, and only in these would a difference be seen. The precise method by which the sample size was calculated is not given or referenced; there are many such methods. If the relatively simple method described in Chapter 7 is applied, setting the cure rate in the placebo group as 72 per cent and in the active treatment group as 91 per cent, and using the given statistical parameters ($K = 7.9$), gives a sample size estimate of 124 in each group. Increasing this by 100/60 gives 207 in each group, 414 in total. Sample sizes are only approximate, and it is best to increase the size to account for losses to follow-up; therefore the sample size of

500 given in the paper seems reasonable, although we do not know exactly how it was calculated. Then the sample size was recalculated when the ongoing trial showed that the overall cure rate was more than 80 per cent and there was evidence of bacterial infection in almost 80 per cent. The first point is not really different, and on the first calculation the overall cure rate would be 81 per cent, but the higher bacterial component increases the power of the study. It was then calculated that randomization of 326 children gave 80 per cent power to detect a 12–14 per cent difference, and therefore recruitment to the trial was stopped. Using the same method as above, and reducing the inflation factor to 100/80 gives 155 in each group, 310 in total, as giving 80 per cent power. Considering that this trial took 3 years to complete recruitment, and was obviously quite difficult logistically, this may be reasonable, although in fact the results are somewhat unsatisfactory in statistical terms and a larger sample size would have been advantageous. However, as noted in the paper, the power does not increase much with an increase in size.

## C. Internal validity: consideration of positive features of causation

### 9. Is there a correct time relationship?

This is not a problem in an intervention study; the outcomes follow the randomization. Note that, to preserve the value of randomization, we employ criteria that are somewhat illogical in terms of timing. An analysis based on intention to treat must include events from the time of randomization, even if they occur prior to the intervention. If there is a time interval between randomization and the start of treatment, this can occur. In this trial, the precise timing of the randomization and the start of treatment is not quite clear, although the whole process was quite quick. It is stated that children were recruited to the study by the family doctors, and seen by a research nurse usually within 4 hours. At that time information was given and informed consent was obtained. The research nurse assessed clinical severity and took conjunctival swabs from one eye. Then a bottle of either active or placebo drops was given to the parents with instructions to use them initially every 2 hours. It is not clear if the randomization was done on recruitment by the doctor, or when seen by the nurse, and it is not clear if the first eye drops were given when the nurse was present or left to the parents. Although there is no problem in interpretation, greater clarity is desirable. As noted already, the timing of the outcome events is important and forms part of the analysis. There was active follow-up over 7 days. As discussed already, some information on events in subsequent days would be useful. There was a 6-week telephone follow-up, completed by an impressive 307 children, 94 per cent of study entrants, and at this time a further episode of conjunctivitis was recorded for 4 per cent of the children on active treatment and 3 per cent of those on placebo. All trials have time limitations; obviously, no statements can be made about events later than 6 weeks.

## 10. Is the relationship strong?

The value of a strong relationship in an observational study is largely because bias or confounding should be readily detected. In a randomized double-blind trial, such issues can be dealt with firmly, and so the strength of the relationship is less crucial to internal validity, although still helpful. The relationship observed here is weak, with a small difference in clinical cure rate and somewhat larger differences in the time to cure and the microbiological cure rate. All these differences show better outcomes in the active treatment group, but the small size of the difference means that the differences could simply be due to chance. The weak association also means that small differences in confounding factors could be a reason, despite the randomization. Observation bias can be excluded from the double-blind design, but a substantial amount of non-differential misclassification in the clinical outcome assessment may have occurred, which would diminish the observed difference if there were true difference in outcome between the two groups. The fact that the difference in microbiological cure rate was greater might be because of less non-differential error. The more important aspect in this study is the clinical implications of the size of the difference, as will be discussed.

## 11. Is there a dose–response relationship?

This is not a relevant question, as a fixed dose of the chloramphenicol eye drops was used. In other randomized trials more than one dose or time course of treatment is often used, and consideration of dose–response may be relevant. We might be tempted to ask whether the patients who received the drug according to the protocol, rather than in smaller amounts or perhaps not at all, had better outcomes, and if the drug is active it is logical that they should. However, such a comparison may be misleading, as patients who accept full doses of treatment are likely to be very different to patients who do not. An example of this has been given in a study in adults in Chapter 6. In this study the compliance issue may relate more to the parents than to the children, but the issue is still relevant. No information on compliance in the trial is presented in this study, which is surprising as the design would allow some assessment of compliance. The implication is that compliance was good, and perhaps the requirement of the parents both to give the treatment and to record symptoms in the diary every time treatment was given has ensured that.

12. **Are the results consistent within the study?**
and

13. **Is there any specificity within the study?**

As consistency and specificity are often related, they can be discussed together. Consistency is often a relevant issue in clinical trials, as we wish to know whether the intervention has different effects in some groups of patients. However, this requires the trial to be specifically designed to answer questions about subgroups of patients. The use of post hoc analysis looking at subgroups of patients defined after the trial has been done is open both to the problems of multiple comparisons and comparisons between non-randomized groups. Such analyses are appropriately avoided in this paper.

The one pre-planned subgroup analysis was in terms of microbiological cause, although this is limited because few children did not have a bacterial pathogen. The results for those who did are given in Ex. 10.3, and are similar to the overall result; this result excludes children lost to follow-up and they did not have the further swab taken. If the results for those without bacteria isolated are calculated by subtraction, the result is similar, with wider confidence limits as the numbers are small. This is consistent with no overall effect. It might be expected that if chloramphenicol were effective, this effect would be restricted to, or increased in, children in whom bacterial pathogens were isolated. The demonstration of such specificity would strengthen the evidence for a real effect. It would also depend on the validity of the isolation of pathogens as showing the aetiology of the child's condition; it cannot be assumed that children from whom bacteria were not isolated were in fact free from bacteria. The results compared are consistent within the trial in that there is reasonable consistency between microbiological and clinical cure, although the effect on microbiological cure is larger, and the pattern of time to cure shows a smooth trend.

The results give the overall effect of the treatment in all the patients randomized. It does not follow that the same effect holds within subgroups, for instance within particular age or gender categories. Other relevant assessments of consistency could be, for example, in terms of the age of the children, differences between boys and girls, and differences between children with different bacterial or viral results or different clinical features. However, such assessments have the major problem of being subgroup analyses in a relatively small study, and if any differences were seen they could well be due to chance.

## Conclusions with regard to internal validity

This is a well-designed and carefully performed randomized trial, and so we can be reasonably confident about its internal validity. We can dismiss with considerable certainty observation bias and confounding as explanations of the differences seen. As is often the case with randomized trials, statistical variation is an issue, and we cannot firmly conclude whether the differences in outcome between the active treatment and placebo groups are simply due to chance variation or are reflecting real differences.

## D. **External validity: generalization of the results**

The next few questions relate to the generalizability of the results from the study participants to the populations from which they are derived, following the approach set out in Chapter 4. A profile of the trial, following the CONSORT principles [4], was given in the paper and is shown as **Ex. 10.5**.

In the first question, we must first assess if there are any differences between the study participants—those who complete the study and provide data for the analysis—and the study entrants. Then we assess issues comparing the study entrants with the eligible population.

### 14. **Can the study results be applied to the eligible population?**

Almost all children entering the study completed it. There were 327 study entrants, i.e. children who were randomized, and of these one was found after randomization to be too old to be eligible. Finding subjects to be ineligible after they have been randomized is obviously a problem of study procedures, but is not uncommon. In principle, any exclusions after randomization compromise the validity of the randomization, but keeping an ineligible subject in the trial analysis also breaches the protocol. With only one subject affected, the choice to withdraw that subject is reasonable. The remaining 326 children were divided equally by the randomization process, and all appear in the main analyses. However, nine were lost to follow-up and so the outcomes for these children were unknown. The remaining 317 completed the main trial, with outcomes assessed at 7 days. There was a telephone follow-up 6 weeks later, completed for 307 children, with 10 not assessed. Subjects who enter but do not complete a trial present issues in interpretation, and so the fact that very few study entrants did not complete this study is a major strength. If the study losses are equal in each group, that is helpful as any biases are likely to affect each treatment group similarly. Here, there were five children in each group for whom the 6-week follow-up information was not available. However, of the nine children lost to follow-up earlier, one had been allocated to chloramphenicol and eight to placebo, and so the handling of these can affect the results.

A strong aspect of this study is that the generalizability is explicitly considered and addressed in the study design. During one week of each month during

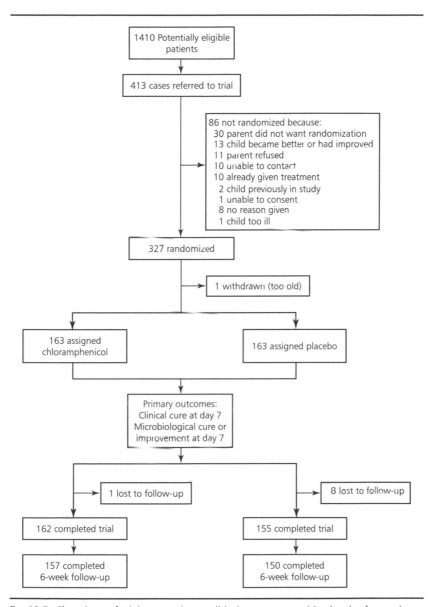

**Ex. 10.5.** Flowchart of trial comparing antibiotic treatment with placebo for conjunctivitis in children. Figure 1 from Rose *et al.* [1]

active recruitment for the trial, the records of the practitioners involved in the study were audited to find all children in the eligible age group who presented with acute infective conjunctivitis, including those presenting out of working hours. Thus it was established that during the recruitment period, 29 per cent of all eligible children entered the study. It would also be helpful to know the reasons for non-participation: How many were out of hours? How many of the rest were not approached? How many were invited to participate but declined? The authors point out that children presenting out of working hours may have had more severe symptoms, and also that family doctors may have tended to exclude children with more severe symptoms, feeling that they required antibiotics; therefore the participants may have had less severe conjunctivitis than a representative sample. However, the fact that for 78 per cent of the children recruited, bacteria were cultured from the eye swabs shows that the participants had significant pathology. It is reasonable to assume that the results can be applied to the eligible population.

## 15. Can the study results be applied to the source population?

The source population is children coming to these 12 general practices in Oxfordshire, with a quite limited list of contraindications which seem clinically justified. One issue that could be raised is that the recruitment period was the winter months, and it is possible that children with conjunctivitis presenting in the summer months have a different spectrum of aetiological agents and so the results could conceivably be different. It is stated in the methods that the study was done in the winter because conjunctivitis is more likely to be infectious than allergic in origin in the winter months. However, in general, the study results should be applicable to the source population.

## 16. Can the study results be applied to other relevant populations?

The diagnostic criteria used in this study are clinical, and are consistent with those used in normal clinical practice. The results are similar for the children with positive bacterial cultures, and so this study also applies to clinical practice where topical chloramphenicol is used only after laboratory tests. If the results of this study reflect a causal relationship with the intervention, it seems likely that such a relationship will hold in similar patients seen in other areas of the UK, and even in similar patients elsewhere in the world, at the current time and into the future.

We should be cautious in applying the results to any groups in which the natural history of conjunctivitis might be substantially different; this might include older patients, patients with concomitant clinical conditions, even if these are not listed in the eligibility criteria, and patients in different environments. Whether the results apply to patients outside the age range chosen for this study will depend on how the aetiology and natural history of conjunctivitis varies by age. A major factor governing the natural history is the bacterial or viral agent present. Information is given in the paper on the details of bacteria and viruses cultured (Ex. 10.4), and a comparison is given with the results of two other studies, presented as the risk ratio for the presence of specific bacteria in swabs from children with conjunctivitis compared with asymptomatic controls in the same population. This shows some consistency, for example in the occurrence of *Haemophilus influenzae*, but also some substantial differences between the studies in, for example, the frequency of different types of Staphylococcus; the authors suggest that as there are many staphylococci species, the isolation rates of particular species will vary in different laboratories. In assessing whether the results were generalizable to a quite different population, for example children in Africa, an assessment of the bacteriological and viral characteristics of acute conjunctivitis in that country would be useful.

The authors point out that the study area had a more privileged social class distribution than the UK in general, but state that this is more likely to effect the transmission of the disease than change its causation or prognosis. They conclude that the results are probably generalizable to most primary care settings in developed countries.

Whether the ethnic background of the patient would influence the result is not mentioned. The results may not apply to patients with other major conditions, especially any that would affect their susceptibility to infection. However, unless there is other evidence to suspect that the results would be substantially different in some groups, it is most reasonable to assume consistency of the results. One of the main results of the study is the high rate of clinical cure in the placebo group, which is generalizable to other populations with similar underlying aetiology.

The trial was restricted to the use of one agent and one dose, 0.5 per cent chloramphenicol eye drops. This agent is commonly used in clinical practice on the basis of its broad-spectrum activity against several bacterial pathogens. The authors point out in the discussions that the other agent commonly used in the UK is fusidic acid, and clinical trials show similar effectiveness for this drug as for chloramphenicol. The results are likely to apply to other agents with similar efficacy, but clearly may not apply to substantially different or new agents with different effectiveness.

## E. Comparison of these results with other evidence

### 17. Are the results consistent with other evidence, particularly evidence from studies of similar or more powerful study design?

The consistency of information with other studies is not discussed in the paper, implying that there are no other relevant clinical trials. In the background to the study a Cochrane systematic review of antibiotic treatment of conjunctivitis is noted, dated 1999, but it is not stated if that incorporated many studies of children. If there are other relevant studies, it would be useful to compare these results, and it may be appropriate to add these results to the others in a meta-analysis and estimate the combined result. Given that this is a well-designed randomized trial, with great strength in the double-blind design, studies such as non-randomized comparisons or case reports on similar topics are much less reliable, and their results are probably not helpful.

## 18. Does the total evidence suggest any specificity?

Because there is no comparison made with other trials, no conclusions can be reached on this point. Meta-analysis of several studies could provide the large numbers of observations needed to make more reliable assessments of specificity.

## 19. Are the results plausible in terms of the biological mechanism?

In clinical trials the issue of a biological mechanism has usually been answered before the trial is initiated, and that certainly applies to this trial. The results are plausible in terms of biological mechanism, in that the main result is that most of these infections are self-limiting, with clinical cure of around 80 per cent within 7 days without active antibiotic intervention. The results show a small increase in this cure rate with an active antibiotic, which is a plausible result. There is still debate about the key pathogens in conjunctivitis.

## 20. If a major effect is shown, is it coherent with the distribution of exposure and the outcome?

In the context of a randomized trial, this is better applied as the question of whether the results will influence the outcome in a substantial way. If the results show a true effect, is the effect substantial enough to be clinically important?

The key issue in this study is whether the small difference in cure rate observed is a real difference or a chance finding, and, if real, whether this is clinically important and justifies treatment. On the intention to treat analysis based on clinical cure, predefined as the key analysis, the difference in cure rates at 7 days was 7.4 per cent, which translates to a number needed to treat of 14. If the children lost to follow-up were excluded, the difference in cure rate is only 3 per cent, resulting in a number needed to treat of 25. On an individual basis this means that for a patient being treated the probability that their cure is related to the treatment is small, and on a population basis it means that considerable numbers of children need to be treated for an extra cure by day 7. Whether this is valuable or not depends on the importance of an extra cure by day 7.

This is where the further information beyond day 7 would be very valuable. For example, the graph shown in Ex. 10.3 could imply the curves are parallel beyond day 7, meaning that children not cured by day 7 may have a long continuation of conjunctivitis; if so, an extra individual cured at day 7 may be quite important. On the other hand, if the curves both continue to increase with the sort of time difference which was seen earlier, those not cured at day 7 may well be cured at day 8, and therefore the extra advantage of a cure at day 7 would be small. The finding on the 6-week follow-up that the proportion of children with further episodes of conjunctivitis within the 6 weeks was small and similar in the two groups is reassuring in this regard. In terms of microbiological cure, the difference seen in the study is larger (16.8 per cent), and the number needed to treat is correspondingly smaller at around six.

The result stressed by the authors is that most children presenting with acute infective conjunctivitis in primary care will recover by themselves and do not need treatment with an antibiotic. The authors' interpretation is that treatment should not be used routinely. Whether parents, or the older children, presented with the same data would come to that conclusion is uncertain. The coherence issue could be envisaged as stating that if that became clinical policy, and treatment with antibiotics was greatly reduced, would that occur without any increase in the incidence of conjunctivitis (which might represent cross-infection), without any increase in the complications of conjunctivitis, and without any increase in concern about the disease and its treatment. The last point may be the more difficult issue, as a major effect of giving antibiotics may be to decrease parental or the child's own concern about the disease, and reassure them that cure will come quickly. In practice, this may be a major barrier to reducing antibiotic prescribing. In contrast, other parents may be aware of the dangers of using unnecessary antibiotics (e.g. the development of resistance) and may be pleased not to use them.

## Summary of external validity

This study was carried out in a primary care setting in England, and the results should be applicable in general to children presenting to primary care facilities in that country and under that time. The results are likely to be applicable much more widely, the main issue being whether the causal agents and clinical presentation of acute conjunctivitis in children differs substantially in different places and at different times. There is the possibility that children with more severe conjunctivitis may have been excluded from the study, and children with severe infection such as periorbital cellulitis were excluded according to the protocol. However, that is not a severe constraint, as the study does not set out to address the issue of treatment of conjunctivitis in unusually severe cases. What it does assess is the treatment of the more typical case. Although the results show a slightly increased cure rate for active treatment compared with placebo, which is statistically significant in terms of microbiological remission, and significant when assessed by cumulative analysis, the prime conclusions is that cure rates assessed clinically are very high with either placebo or antibiotic, and that the small increase in cure rate with antibiotic treatment, even if it does apply, does not justify the costs and potential complications of prescribing antibiotics. As a result the paper challenges widely held normative practice.

## Conclusions

In summary, this study illustrates both the strengths and weaknesses of randomized trials. A summary of the appraisal is shown in **Ex. 10.6**. The strengths are that, with reasonable confidence, we can exclude confounding and observation bias as explanations for the results seen. The main weakness is that, despite the enormous effort involved, the study is still limited in terms of size, and the main results are close to the conventional 5 per cent cut-off for statistical significance. As is typical of randomized trials, there were strict eligibility

---

ASSESSMENT OF A RANDOMIZED TRIAL

Chloramphenicol eye drops for conjunctivitis in children: Rose *et al.* [1]

*A. Description of evidence*

| | | |
|---|---|---|
| 1 | Intervention | Chloramphenicol 0.5% eye drops, compared with placebo drops |
| 2 | Outcome | Clinical cure at 7 days |
| 3 | Design | Double-blind randomized trial |
| 4 | Study population | Children aged 6 months to 12 years attending 12 general practices in England, with diagnosis of acute infective conjunctivitis |
| 5 | Main result | Clinical cure in 86% of those randomized to antibiotic and 79% of placebo group; relative risk 1.09, 95% confidence limits 0.99 to 1.21. |

*B. Non-causal explanations*

| | | |
|---|---|---|
| 6 | Observation bias | Outcome based on parents' diaries — relevant outcome, probably some error, but double-blind design protects against bias; error would make the results conservative. Differences based on microbiological clearance greater; less error potential, but less relevant outcome. |
| 7 | Confounding | Randomized design protects against confounding |
| 8 | Chance | Main result close to the 0.05 probability level; could be due to chance |

**Ex. 10.6. cont'd**

*C. Positive features of causation*

| | | |
|---|---|---|
| 9 | Time relationship | The small difference in outcome is seen by day 2 and persists with little change. Further follow-up to 6 weeks shows no differences |
| 10 | Strength | Main result weak; not large enough to be clinically important, even if not due to chance |
| 11 | Dose–response | Not assessed as only one dose was used |
| 12 | Consistency | One subgroup defined in protocol, those with a bacterial pathogen isolated; showed similar result to whole group |
| 13 | Specificity | Not assessed as only one intervention–outcome combination is assessed |

Summary of internal validity: high, result shows a small effect, which may be due to chance or causation. Effect may be weakened by error in observations of outcome. No likely confounders

*D. External validity*

| | | |
|---|---|---|
| 14 | To the eligible population | Very high completion rate by randomized subjects. Some 29% of eligible subjects entered study; more severe cases possibly excluded, but main result should apply to eligible population |
| 15 | To the source population | Few contraindications to eligibility; result should apply to source population |
| 16 | To other populations | Source population is children presenting in primary care in winter months. Likely to be applicable to similar contexts in other places. Extension of results to other age groups unknown |

*E. Other evidence*

| | | |
|---|---|---|
| 17 | Consistency | Few other studies; but result is consistent with most other less rigorous evidence |
| 18 | Specificity | Result may be generalizable to other antibiotic treatments, or may be specific to the treatment assessed — little evidence that other antibiotics would give different result |
| 19 | Plausibility | Shows that antibiotic clearance of bacteria is not necessary for clinical cure; plausible and suggests role of bacterial agents is minor |
| 20 | Coherence | Little information on coherence; size of effect suggests that clinical cure will vary with level of antibiotic treatment |

Summary of external validity: study has been done in a relevant setting (primary care and home treatment), and result is widely generalizable; it suggests topical antibiotic treatment has only a small, or no, effect, and is unnecessary for cases similar to those included in this trial

**Ex. 10.6. cont'd** Assessment of causality in a randomized trial: trial of chloramphenicol eye drops, compared with placebo, in the treatment of acute infectious conjunctivitis in children, by Rose *et al.* [1]

criteria for the subjects, and therefore we have to be careful about the generalizability of the results, although here the eligibility criteria were not very restrictive, and are clearly set out and could be reproduced in clinical practice. We are told what proportion of the source population was eventually entered into the trial, information that is all too often not recorded.

Any study can be interpreted in different ways, some of which are more reasonable than others. As an exercise, consider these different statements: are they accurate, and are they a fair interpretation?

- In children with acute conjunctivitis, treatment with antibiotic resulted in a 74 per cent increase in cure rates within 7 days, confirmed by laboratory testing.

- If your child has a painful red eye, treatment with simple and safe antibiotic eye drops may decrease the risk of treatment failure by 40 per cent.

- In children with conjunctivitis, treatment with antibiotic eye drops may increase the cure rate by 10 per cent.

- The use of antibiotic eye drops may increase clinical cure at day seven from 79 per cent to 86 per cent.

- In children with conjunctivitis, treatment with antibiotic eye drops has no statistically significant effect on the cure rate.

- Most children presenting with an acute infective conjunctivitis in primary care will get better by themselves and do not need treatment with an antibiotic.

All these statements are factually accurate, with the quantitative statements derived from the information in Ex. 10.3. The last statement is the authors' conclusion expressed in the summary of the paper, and approved by the peer review process. A paper published in a clinical journal needs to report both the factual results and the implications in practical terms. Not all the statements above are reasonable summaries of the study. You may wish to reflect on the different impacts of these statements, and how they could be used to support different points of view.

## Subsequent development

At the time of writing (April 2006) this study is still recent, and it will be interesting to observe its impact on clinical practice. Almost simultaneously with the publication of this paper, in June 2005, chloramphenicol eye drops were approved for over-the-counter sales, being the first antibiotic available without a doctor's prescription in the UK [5]. The regulatory authority knew about the results of this trial before they made this decision (P. Rose, personal communication). This implies that policy had been influenced by general practitioners' workloads and costs, but not by the danger of emerging antibiotic resistance; the authors of this paper mention both these issues as justification for doing the trial. This wider availability was followed by an aggressive television marketing campaign from pharmaceutical companies promoting the use of chloramphenicol eye drops for conjunctivitis [6].

In correspondence in *The Lancet* following publication of this paper, several of the points discussed in this chapter were raised, and some more information was given, such as the data on the nurses' evaluation given under question 6. There is great pressure to keep published papers as short as possible, and there are often issues that can be resolved by reporting further data from the study. For example, we queried the lack of information on compliance under question 11; in correspondence, the senior author said that the bottles were weighed to find how much of the eye drops had been used, but this was not helpful as they were often spilt or lost. Discussions of the results of this trial have raised the question of whether other antibiotics would be more effective, but there is no good evidence that they would. In contrast, a possible beneficial lubricant or washing-out effect of eye drops has been suggested, implying that both the antibiotic and placebo eye drops could be beneficial; to assess this, a trial which also compared the effect of chloramphenicol eye ointment could be helpful (P. Rose, personal communication).

The authors of this study carried out interviews with general practitioners and a questionnaire survey of parents of children with conjunctivitis, and of nurseries and primary schools, addressing knowledge about conjunctivitis and beliefs about its management [7]. This survey showed that parents were certain about the benefits of antibiotic treatment, and sought early consultations with their general practitioner to ensure good treatment results and the ability to get the child back to school quickly. The survey also found that general practitioners would sometimes prescribe the antibiotic to enable school attendance.

The earlier meta-analysis of the use of antibiotics for acute bacterial conjunctivitis mentioned in the original study [2] has been updated [8]. The later review includes five trials, three studies in hospital populations (which were covered in the earlier review), and two double-blind trials in primary care, including the study under discussion here. The results of the meta-analysis were that topical antibiotics improved clinical and microbiological remission at days 2–5, with relative risks of 1.24 for clinical remission and 1.77 for microbiological remission, both being statistically significant. The relative risks were reduced but still significant when based on assessments at 6–10 days, with relative risks for clinical remission of 1.11 and for microbiological cure of 1.56. The authors regarded this later day 6–10 benefit as marginal.

A further trial in primary care centres in The Netherlands assessing adults, randomized patients between fusidic acid, an alternative antibiotic to chloramphenicol, and placebo, and the results were rather similar to this study. Based on 73 subjects in the treatment group and 90 in the placebo group evaluated after 7 days, there was a small but not statistically significant increase in the clinical recovery rate, but also a significant increase in adverse effects. The authors' conclusion was the results did not support the routine use of fusidic acid [9].

## References

1. Rose PW, Harnden A, Brueggemann AB, *et al.* Chloramphenicol treatment for acute infective conjunctivitis in children in primary care: a randomised double-blind placebo-controlled trial. *Lancet* 2005; **366**: 37–43.

2. Sheikh A, Hurwitz B, Cave J. Antibiotics for acute bacterial conjunctivitis. *Cochrane Database Syst Rev* 2000; (2): CD001211.

3. Rose PW, Harnden A, Brueggemann AB, Perea R, Mant D. Antibiotics for acute infective conjunctivitis in children. *Lancet* 2005; **366**: 1431.

4. Altman DG, Schulz KF, Moher D, *et al.* The revised CONSORT statement for reporting randomized trials: explanation and elaboration. *Ann Intern Med* 2001; **134**: 663–694.

5. Medicines and Healthcare Products Regulatory Agency. Antibiotic eye drops available over the counter (OTC). 8-6-2005.

6. Saha N. Antibiotics for acute infective conjunctivitis in children. *Lancet* 2005; **366**: 1432.

7. Rose PW, Ziebland S, Harnden A, Mayon-White R, Mant D. Why do general practitioners prescribe antibiotics for acute infective conjunctivitis in children? Qualitative interviews with GPs and a questionnaire survey of parents and teachers. *Fam Pract* 2006; **23**: 226–232.

8. Sheikh A, Hurwitz B. Topical antibiotics for acute bacterial conjunctivitis: Cochrane systematic review and meta-analysis update. *Br J Gen Pract* 2005; **55**: 962–964.

9. Rietveld RP, ter Riet G, Bindels PJ, Bink D, Sloos JH, van Weert HC. The treatment of acute infectious conjunctivitis with fusidic acid: a randomised controlled trial. *Br J Gen Pract* 2005; **55**: 924–930.

Chapter 11

# Critical appraisal of a randomized trial of a preventive agent

In this chapter we will review an important randomized trial, published in *The Lancet*, 20 July 1991, **338**, 131–37 [1]. In contrast with the trial reviewed in Chapter 10, this concerned a preventive strategy. The summary and methods section are reproduced here, with permission from Elsevier, and the full paper can be accessed at www.thelancet.com.

## Prevention of neural tube defects: results of the Medical Research Council Vitamin Study

MRC Vitamin Study Research Group

### Summary

A randomized double-blind prevention trial with a factorial design was conducted at 33 centres in seven countries to determine whether supplementation with folic acid (one of the vitamins in the B group) or a mixture of seven other vitamins (A, D, $B_1$, $B_2$, $B_6$, C, and nicotinamide) around the time of conception can prevent neural tube defects (anencephaly, spina bifida, encephalocoele). A total of 1817 women at high risk of having a pregnancy with a neural tube defect, because of a previous affected pregnancy, were allocated at random to one of four groups—namely, folic acid, other vitamins, both, or neither. 1195 had a completed pregnancy in which the fetus or infant was known to have or not have a neural tube defect; 27 of these had a known neural tube defect, 6 in the folic-acid groups and 21 in the two other groups, a 72 per cent protective effect (relative risk 0.28, 95 per cent confidence interval 0.12–0.71). The other vitamins showed no significant protective effect (relative risk 0.80, 95 per cent CI 0.32–1.72). There was no demonstrable harm from the folic acid supplementation, though the ability of the study to detect rare or slight adverse effects was limited. Folic acid supplementation starting before pregnancy can now be firmly recommended for all women who have had an affected pregnancy, and public health measures should be taken to ensure that the diet of all women who may bear children contains an adequate amount of folic acid.

## Methods

The study was an international, multicentre, double-blind randomized trial involving 33 centres (17 in the UK and 16 in six other countries). Women with a previous pregnancy affected by a neural tube defect, not associated with the autosomal recessive disorder Meckel's syndrome, were eligible for the study if they were planning another pregnancy and were not already taking vitamin supplements. Women with epilepsy were excluded in case the folic acid supplementation adversely affected their treatment. Antenatal diagnosis of neural tube defects was available at all centres in the study. The effect of supplementation both with folic acid and with a selection of other vitamins was investigated by use of a factorial study design. Women were allocated at random to one of four supplementation groups, the supplements containing folic acid, other vitamins, both, or neither, in the following way:

| Group | Folic acid | Other vitamins |
|-------|------------|----------------|
| A | Yes | No |
| B | Yes | Yes |
| C | No | No |
| D | No | Yes |

Comparison of the outcome in groups A and B with those in groups C and D tested the effect of folic acid supplementation; comparison of the outcomes in groups B and D with those in groups A and C tested the effect of the other vitamins. Separate sets of random allocations were used for each centre to ensure that there would be approximately equal numbers of women in each supplementation group at each centre.

The capsules used in the study were prepared by the Boots Company and packaged in 2-week calendar 'blister' packs. Women in the trial were asked to take a single capsule each day from the date of randomization until 12 weeks of pregnancy (estimated from the first day of the last menstrual period). Capsules for those in the folic-acid groups contained 4 mg of folic acid—the larger of the two doses used in the previous studies being chosen because a negative result with the lower dose would have left the matter open. Capsules for those in the multivitamin groups contained vitamin A 4000 U, D 400 U, $B_1$ 1.5 mg, $B_2$ 1.5 mg, $B_6$ 1.0 mg, C 40 mg, and nicotinamide 15 mg. The control substance in the capsules was dried ferrous sulphate 120 mg and di-calcium phosphate 240 mg. The potency of the capsules was independently checked every three months by Hoffmann La Roche in Basel, Switzerland. The trial was double-blind, in that neither the doctor nor the patient knew which regimen had been allocated. It was agreed that the groups to which patients were allocated would normally be revealed only at the end of the trial. The randomization was carried out through the Clinical Trials Service Unit in Oxford.

Women invited to join the trial were given a week to decide if they wished to take part, so that they could consider the matter at leisure and discuss the matter further with others if they wished. All patients were given a printed information leaflet about the trial.

No special advice was specified regarding diet. On entry into the trial, samples of blood and urine were collected and sent to the central trial office in the Department of Environmental and Preventive Medicine at St Bartholomew's Hospital for folic acid analysis, performed by radioimmunoassay (Amersham International). Patients were then given capsules and requested to attend every three months so that a note could be made of their general health and how many capsules they had taken. Blood and urine samples were collected at each visit for dispatch to the trial office laboratory and a further supply of capsules was given. The last visit took place in the 12th week of pregnancy. The outcomes of all completed pregnancies were recorded, including details of any fetal malformation, sex, birthweight, and head circumference. In the event of a termination of pregnancy or miscarriage the fetus was examined if possible. A woman remained in the trial until she had a pregnancy in which the fetus could be classified as having a neural tube defect or not ('informative pregnancy'). If, for example, she had a miscarriage and the fetus was not examined, she remained in the study in the same randomization group until the end of the trial or until she had an informative pregnancy. In this way each woman contributed no more than one informative event to the study. The final results are based on the outcome of all informative pregnancies. Whenever a neural tube defect (anencephaly, spina bifida cystica, or encephalocoele) was reported, independent corroboration was sought, with a necropsy report if one was performed, or a description of the lesion for independent review at the trial centre in London (done without knowledge of the allocated group). To monitor possible toxicity associated with the supplementation, forms were provided for the notification of any medical event arising among the women in the trial irrespective of whether this was thought to be associated with the capsules. The health of each child born into the study was ascertained annually by sending a questionnaire to the mother on the infant's first, second and third birthday. This part of the study is continuing. The results of the study, available only to the principal investigator, the study administrator, and the data monitoring committee, were reviewed every six months to enable the study to be stopped early if, as indeed occurred, a clear result emerged.

## A. **Description of the evidence**

1. What was the exposure or intervention?
2. What was the outcome?
3. What was the study design?
4. What was the study population?
5. What was the main result?

The *objective* of this study was to test whether dietary supplementation with different types of vitamins could reduce the recurrence risk of neural tube defects in pregnancies in women who had already had at least one affected birth. The background, described in the introduction, notes that two intervention studies for such high-risk women had been done, with inconclusive results. One of the studies [2] was large, and showed a large and statistically significant decrease in recurrence risk in women taking a combination of folic acid with seven other vitamins, but as the study was not randomized, the difference might have been due to selection factors or other confounding factors. The second study was randomized and used only folic acid [3], but was too small and showed a non-significant benefit when analysed in an intention to treat manner, although the published results, analysed by compliance with treatment, showed a significant effect. Thus, from these trials, it was uncertain whether there was a true preventive action of dietary supplementation, and it was not clear if folic acid as a single agent or in combination with other vitamins was the more effective agent. As a result, a large randomized trial of high-risk women was designed.

The *intervention* was a dietary supplementation. Two types of supplement were tested; folic acid alone, 4 mg per day, and several vitamins other than folic acid. An efficient design to test two different interventions, a *2 × 2 factorial design*, was used, where the women were randomized into four groups, and then received folic acid, other vitamins, both folic acid and other vitamins, or neither. Four identical sets of capsules were prepared; three sets contained the three combinations of supplementation, and the capsules for the fourth group contained only ferrous sulphate and calcium phosphate, which were also included in all the other groups and are regarded as a placebo.

The *outcome* was the occurrence of a further neural tube defect. These defects comprise a set of congenital defects of the developing nervous system, and can usually be recognized easily in live births and still births, and in induced and spontaneous abortuses if appropriate examination is done. The expected frequency of such outcomes in pregnancies to women who have already had an affected baby is around 2–5 per cent.

The *study design* was a prospective double-blind randomized trial. A calculation of anticipated study size showed that approximately 2000 pregnancies would be needed, and therefore the study was international, involving 33 centres in seven countries. The *eligible population* comprised women with a previous pregnancy with an 'isolated' neural tube defect, i.e. excluding defects associated with Meckel's syndrome. This syndrome includes neural tube defects, but because it has an autosomal recessive inheritance pattern, it has a substantially higher recurrence risk than the more common situation of an isolated neural tube defect, which was the focus of this study. Because folic acid interacts with drugs used to control epilepsy, women with epilepsy were excluded from this study.

The main result (**Ex. 11.1**) consists of two comparisons. One is between all women randomized to take folic acid and all women randomized not to take folic acid. The second is between all women randomized to take other vitamins and all those randomized not to take other vitamins. The outcome variable is prevalence at birth, i.e. the number of affected babies over the total number of births. The results are shown in $2 \times 2$ tables, and the relative risk calculated as the ratio of the prevalence rates. A Mantel–Haenszel analysis is appropriate.

The main result is that six of the 593 births to mothers allocated folic acid were affected (1.0 per cent) compared with 21 of 602 births in those not receiving folic acid (3.5 per cent), giving a relative risk of 0.29 with 95 per cent

| TRIAL OF PREVENTION OF NEURAL TUBE DEFECT RECURRENCE: RESULTS | | | | |
|---|---|---|---|---|
| | Neural tube defects | Total pregnancies | Rate (%) | Relative risk | 95% CI |
| *Results in the four groups by supplement assigned in factorial design.* | | | | | |
| Folic acid and multivitamins | 4 | 295 | 1.36 | | |
| Folic acid, no multivitamins | 2 | 298 | 0.67 | | |
| No folic acid, multivitamins | 8 | 302 | 2.65 | | |
| No folic acid, no multivitamins | 13 | 300 | 4.33 | | |
| *Comparisons for each treatment contrast* | | | | | |
| Allocated folic acid | 6 | 593 | 1.01 | 0.29 | 0.12–0.71 |
| No folic acid | 21 | 602 | 3.49 | | |
| Relative risk for folic acid adjusted for stopping rule | | | | 0.33 | 0.06–0.80 |
| Allocated other vitamins | 12 | 597 | 2.01 | 0.80 | 0.37–1.72 |
| No other vitamins | 15 | 598 | 2.51 | | |

**Ex. 11.1.** Results of Medical Research Council trial: main treatment comparisons. From MRC Vitamin Study Research Group [1]

confidence limits of 0.12 to 0.71 (see Appendix Table 2 for the calculations). The prevalence in births to women receiving other vitamins was 2.0 per cent compared with 2.5 per cent in those not receiving other vitamins, giving a relative risk of 0.80. This modest reduction in risk is not statistically significant, with 95 per cent confidence limits of 0.37 to 1.72.

## B. **Internal validity: consideration of non-causal explanations**

### 6. **Are the results likely to be affected by observation bias?**

We must first assess if the recorded results in terms of pregnancy outcome are likely to be accurate, or whether they could be influenced by observation bias. There are two main issues. First, is the outcome of the pregnancy observable? A major problem with any study of birth defects is that what is observed is the net result of two processes: the occurrence of the birth defect, very early in pregnancy, and the survival of the affected fetus *in utero*. If affected fetuses do not survive, but are expelled as spontaneous abortuses early in the pregnancy, then the outcomes of pregnancy will not be measurable in a routine study. If they survive to present as later spontaneous abortions, as stillbirths, or as live births, then they can be observed. For these reasons the information on all pregnancies occurring, and whether these were 'informative', i.e. they could be examined to ascertain if a neural tube defect was present, is important (**Ex. 11.2**). Overall, 75 per cent of the women randomized had a pregnancy known to the study, and 88 per cent of these pregnancies were informative. The non-informative pregnancies could be different in terms of the occurrence of neural tube defects, and some pregnancies may have occurred without being recognized within the study. The important issue is whether there is any indication of differences between the mothers allocated folic acid and those not allocated folic acid; in fact, the two groups were extremely similar (Ex 11.2). There was a considerably higher number of terminations of informative pregnancies in mothers not receiving folic acid. This will include pregnancies terminated after recognition of a neural tube defect following antenatal diagnosis, as this service was available to all women in this study. There is also a somewhat higher number (three compared with none) of non-informative terminations, i.e. a termination of pregnancy for which information was not available to the study authors; these may include some neural tube defects. Overall, it seems unlikely that any differences in the ascertainment of pregnancy outcomes would influence the result.

The second issue is the completeness and accuracy of ascertainment of neural tube defects in informative pregnancies. In general, neural tube defects

TRIAL OF SUPPLEMENTATION: OUTCOMES

| | Allocated folic acid | | No folic acid | |
| --- | --- | --- | --- | --- |
| | Number | Per cent of total | Number | Per cent of total |
| Total women randomized | 910 | | 907 | |
| *Total outcomes* | | | | |
| Total pregnancies completed: | 677 | | 685 | |
| Ratio of pregnancies to women randomized | | 0.74 | | 0.76 |
| Miscarriage and ectopic pregnancies | 91 | 13.4 | 89 | 13.0 |
| Termination | 7 | 1.0 | 23 | 3.4 |
| Stillbirth | 4 | 0.6 | 3 | 0.4 |
| Live birth | 575 | 84.9 | 570 | 83.2 |
| *Non-informative pregnancies* | | | | |
| Total | 84 | 12.4 | 83 | 12.1 |
| Miscarriage | 80 | 11.8 | 74 | 10.8 |
| Ectopic | 4 | 0.6 | 6 | 0.9 |
| Termination | 0 | 0.0 | 3 | 0.4 |
| *Informative pregnancies* | | | | |
| Total | 593 | 87.6 | 602 | 87.9 |
| Live birth | 575 | 84.9 | 570 | 83.2 |
| Miscarriage | 7 | 1.0 | 9 | 1.3 |
| Stillbirth | 4 | 0.6 | 3 | 0.4 |
| Termination | 7 | 1.0 | 20 | 2.9 |
| *Abnormalities other than neural tube defects* | | | | |
| Total | 19 | 2.8 | 13 | 1.9 |

**Ex. 11.2.** Results of Medical Research Council trial: other outcomes of pregnancy. From MRC Vitamin Study Research Group [1]

are severe abnormalities that can be accurately recognized and classified if careful examination is performed, although this is more difficult for a termination than it is for a live birth. There are also minor and even subclinical forms of the condition, so that some biological occurrences of defects may not be recognized. The trial protocol called for independent corroboration of a report of the neural tube defect. The necropsy report or a description of the lesion was sent to the trial centre for independent review, and this was done without knowledge of the allocated group. A total of 27 neural tube defects were reported, and in the discussion the authors comment that in 23 cases the women had a termination of pregnancy after antenatal diagnosis, and in four there was a live birth, two of which survived. For 18 of the 25 dead cases there was a necropsy report, and there were confirmatory descriptions in the remaining seven. The authors state that they are confident about the reliability of the diagnoses. The reports of neural tube defects are likely to be valid. The main limitation is that it is difficult to be certain that all neural tube defects were counted; some may have occurred in non-informative pregnancies, some may not have been recognized at all, and some could have been missed in informative pregnancies, although that seems unlikely.

The main potential problem is less complete ascertainment in mothers allocated folic acid, as that direction of bias would contribute to the observed result. If the reported frequency of other abnormalities were also lower in pregnancies to women allocated folic acid, it would suggest general under-ascertainment or that folic acid prevents other abnormalities. In fact, the number of other abnormalities was slightly higher in the group allocated folic acid, suggesting that under-ascertainment did not occur (Ex. 11.2).

## 7. Are the results likely to be affected by confounding?

The primary strength of the randomized trial design is in protection against confounding. The previous large non-randomized trial of vitamin supplementation showed a statistically significant benefit [2], but because the women allocated the supplement were self-selected by their attendance at a specialized unit, that group may have had other features which put them at a lower risk of recurrence of neural tube defects. From the general epidemiology of these defects, factors such as higher social class, residence in low-risk geographical areas, lower parity, or age could reduce risk. In this study, randomization was used on a substantial number of mothers. In Table II of the paper the four groups resulting from the randomization are compared in terms of age, previous pregnancy history, and the number of previous pregnancies affected by neural tube defect, and information is also given on social class for the women within the UK; all of these show almost identical distributions between the four groups. The randomization was done within each centre, so that the distribution of mothers receiving or not receiving folic acid is similar over the different centres. This design provides good reassurance that the baseline characteristics of the different groups of mothers were the same.

Another major problem with the previous non-randomized study was that the women allocated the supplement were aware of it, and had probably received more information about the disease and their pregnancy than had the comparison women. Therefore the women receiving the supplement may have actively made other changes, such as improving their own diet in other ways, which may have confounded the effect of the supplement. The randomized trial used a double-blind design, so that all women involved were given the same information, and were given identical capsules. They were not given any special advice about diet. Many of the women involved in the trial may have taken other actions, such as modifying their diet, changing their consumption of substances such as alcohol, or changing their lifestyle in terms of exercise and occupation, and so on. The strength of the double-blind design is that all women received the same information, and therefore the extent to which they made other modifications should have been the same irrespective of the supplementation they received. The one danger that still remains, even with the double-blind design, is the possibility that all the women in the trial would make dramatic differences to other aspects of their diet, so that their total vitamin intake would increase to the point where the marginal effect of the supplementation would be irrelevant. Partially as a protection against this, and more directly to assess whether women actually took the allocated tablets, serum folic acid levels were assessed from blood samples at various times. These results (Table VII of the paper), show substantially higher serum folic acid levels in those allocated folic acid than in others, which both indicates compliance and shows that the folic acid levels were not increased in the whole group to the extent of removing the effect of the supplement.

## 8. Are the results likely to be affected by chance variation?

As noted above, the simple analysis of the results shows that the reduction in risk associated with folic acid supplementation is very unlikely to have recurred by chance, whereas the small reduction in risk associated with other vitamins is well within the likely range of chance variation. The results of this study were monitored by an independent review group, using a sequential method of analysis [4] which is described in the paper. The trial was terminated when the cumulative difference between the number of neural tube defects in the folic-acid group compared with the non-folic-acid group reached a preset boundary (Ex. 11.3). Because the trial was stopped at a point that depended on the results at that time, the relative risk estimate produced by standard methods is somewhat exaggerated. The relative risk needs to be calculated by a different method which allows for this early stopping; this gives a result of 0.33, with 95 per cent confidence limits of 0.06 to 0.80. This is not quite as extreme as the more simply calculated relative risk of 0.29. As the simpler estimate is very similar, it can be used to explore the results of this study further.

The relative risks and confidence limits shown in Ex. 11.1 can be reproduced by applying the formulae in Appendix Table 2, using the variance formulae in section 4A. The test-based confidence limits are very similar.

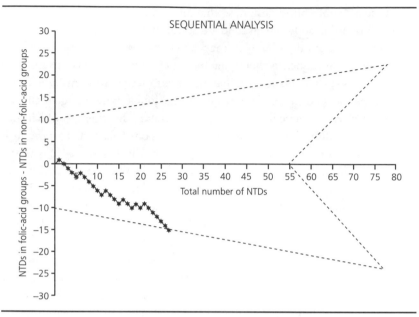

**Ex. 11.3.** Sequential analysis, showing cumulative difference between number of neural tube defects (NTDs) in the folic-acid and non-folic-acid groups plotted against total number of neural tube defects occurring in the trial. The boundaries of the diagram define the stopping points of the study. The methods used to determine the boundaries are described in the paper. From MRC Vitamin Study Research Group [1]

## C. **Internal validity: consideration of positive features of causation**

### 9. **Is there a correct time relationship?**

The time relationship is clear in this prospective intervention trial. It is stated that 7 per cent of women with informative pregnancies had stopped taking their capsules before they became pregnant, usually because they lost interest in participation. Specific results are not reported for these women; if the number were larger, some useful information on the effectiveness of the intervention if it is stopped before pregnancy would be given.

### 10. **Is the relationship strong?**

The overall relationship here is strong, with a 67 per cent reduction in risk. However, it is relevant that the result of the previous non-randomized trial was equally large, but that did not adequately deal with the possibility of uncontrolled confounding. Indeed, an even larger variation in risk was seen in an observational study comparing the recurrence risks in women grouped by the hospital which they had previously attended, and these large differences in risk remained unexplained by any known differences in supplementation, diet, or other factors [5]. Therefore, while the strength of the relationship is of critical importance in terms of the implementation and impact of these results, in terms of the interpretation of causality, it assists, but the main strength comes from the double-blind randomized design in reducing the possibility of confounding or observation bias.

## 11. Is there a dose–response relationship?

There is no opportunity here to assess any dose–response relationship, as only a single dose was used. The questions of whether a lower dose would be equally effective, or a higher dose would be more effective, are not resolved.

## 12. Are the results consistent within the study?

Consistency within the study can be looked at in a number of ways (**Ex. 11.4**). The geographical distribution breaks down primarily into centres within and outside the UK, and the results are virtually identical for each of these groups. There are two major categories of neural tube defect, anencephalus and spina bifida. The results show a protective effect for each defect, and although the relative risk is lower for spina bifida than it is for anencephalus, the confidence limits overlap. A major difference between the results for the two defects would raise a question of differences in ascertainment, or indicate a true biological difference. It would be possible to analyse the results by other characteristics such as maternal age or previous pregnancy history, but this is not done in this paper.

## 13. Is there any specificity within the study?

The most important specificity is that the protective effect was shown for folic acid, but not for the other set of vitamins. This distinction is based on a specific hypothesis set up in advance, and therefore can be accepted. The authors conclude that the result is specific to folic acid supplementation, a conclusion of considerable practical importance. However, the results did show some reduction in risk with the other vitamins, although it was not statistically significant, and so some benefit of the other vitamins cannot be ruled out. Although the numbers are insufficient for confident results, there is no evidence that the risk was lower in those who received both folic acid and other vitamins than in those who received folic acid alone (Ex. 11.1). There is no evidence of specificity in terms of the particular defect, as discussed above.

PREVENTION OF NEURAL TUBE DEFECT RECURRENCE: RESULTS IN SUBGROUPS

| | Neural tube defects | Total pregnancies | Rate(%) | Relative risk | 95% CI |
|---|---|---|---|---|---|
| *Comparison specific to anencephalus* | | | | | |
| Allocated folic acid | 3 | 593 | 0.51 | 0.44 | 0.11–1.67 |
| No folic acid | 7 | 602 | 1.16 | | |
| *Comparison specific to spina bifida and encephalocoele* | | | | | |
| Allocated folic acid | 3 | 593 | 0.51 | 0.22 | 0.06–0.75 |
| No folic acid | 14 | 602 | 2.33 | | |
| *Comparison specific to centres within the UK* | | | | | |
| Allocated folic acid | 3 | 261 | 1.15 | 0.38 | 0.11–1.40 |
| No folic acid | 8 | 262 | 3.05 | | |
| *Comparison specific to centres outside the UK* | | | | | |
| Allocated folic acid | 3 | 332 | 0.90 | 0.24 | 0.07–0.82 |
| No folic acid | 13 | 340 | 3.82 | | |

**Ex. 11.4.** Results of Medical Research Council trial: main treatment comparison within subgroups. From MRC Vitamin Study Research Group [1]

## Conclusions with regard to internal validity

The internal validity of this study is extremely high. It is difficult to make a good argument for any explanation of the main result other than that of causality. Because of the randomization, the groups of women being compared are very similar in several factors related to their risk. The occurrence of informative pregnancies, and the documentation of defects resulting from those pregnancies have been assessed consistently and in identical fashion for all women in this study. The main result is consistent with the pre-defined hypothesis and is strong, and the possibility of it occurring by chance variation is extremely remote. The results are consistent within different subgroups.

## D. **External validity: generalization of the results**

### 14. **Can the study results be applied to the eligible population?**

The eligible population consists of the next occurring pregnancy in each woman identified as eligible in the participating centres. The fact that a high proportion of pregnancies were informative is an important strength of the study. The study was designed to ensure that each woman contributed no more than one informative event, so that each informative pregnancy is an independent observation. Each woman remained in the trial until she had an informative pregnancy, or until the end of the trial; women who had an uninformative pregnancy remained in the study in the same randomization group until an informative pregnancy resulted or the trial ended.

The relationship between the participants and the total eligible population is not clear. Women invited to join the trial were given a week to decide if they wished to take part. There is no information given on how eligible women were identified, what proportion of them were invited to participate, or what proportion of those invited to participate did so. Therefore the participants were a selected subgroup of all eligible women. This is relevant only if the effect of the supplementation could be different in eligible women who did not participate; it is difficult to see how this would occur. We might expect that the participants would be more interested and more knowledgeable about the pregnancy and their risk state than non-participants, and so might be more active in making other changes such as other dietary alterations. Such an effect would apply to all the randomized groups, and its effect, if any, would be to reduce the effect of supplementation. Therefore the results should apply to the eligible population.

## 15. Can the study results be applied to the source population?

The source population consists of all women who had a previous affected pregnancy who were seen in any of the participating centres. The eligibility criteria were to be planning another pregnancy, not be already taking vitamin supplements, and not to have epilepsy. The first two criteria may exclude women who are both least and most prepared for a further pregnancy. As with the previous issue, the relevant question concerns the generalizability of the result of the study, and these exclusion criteria do not seem likely to limit that.

## 16. Can the study results be applied to other relevant populations?

The generalization of the result to appropriate target populations is a very important issue. The underlying biological hypothesis being tested was that vitamin supplementation reduces the *recurrence* risk of these defects in the reproductive population in general, i.e. on a worldwide basis. We have to ask to what extent are the women who had the opportunity to take part in the trial likely to be representative of all at-risk women, i.e. those who have had a previous affected child. Neural tube defects have a complex epidemiological pattern, and are much more common in some countries than others. This aetiology may differ in different societies. They are less common in Oriental, Asian, and African populations, and much more common in European populations, particularly those of British origin [6]. The centres participating were in Britain, Australia, and Canada, which have substantial British populations, and in Hungary and Israel, which have lower population risks of neural tube defects. It seems unlikely that there were many mothers of Asian or African origin in this study, and there could be differences in the aetiology of these defects in such women.

Therefore the results are likely to apply, on a worldwide basis, to mothers of European origin who have had a previous affected pregnancy. Direct information for non-European ethnic groups would be useful, but in its absence it is reasonable to generalize the results to such groups in addition. This is particularly so as the application of these results may have a high benefit-to-cost ratio. The results suggest that a dietary supplement, which does not appear to have any major toxic consequences and is readily available and cheap, can produce a substantial reduction in risk for high-risk mothers, but antenatal diagnosis where culturally and legally acceptable would still be offered as a further protection. It seems very reasonable to apply these results to high-risk mothers, on a worldwide basis.

The more challenging question is whether these results show that supplementation with folic acid will reduce the frequency of neural tube defects occurring for the first time in births to mothers without any previous history. A reasonable case is made in this paper that the results would apply. It is generally thought that neural tube defects have an environmental and a genetic component in their causation. We can consider these two factors as joint causes, under the simple models described in Chapter 3. If their joint effect is multiplicative, the relative risk for the environmental cause will be the same in recurrences as in first affected births, and the absolute effect (risk difference) will be greater. If the joint effect is additive, the absolute effect will be the same, and the relative risk for the environmental cause will be less in recurrences than in first affected births. Therefore on these models, the result from this study is either a valid estimate or an underestimate of the relative risk from folate supplementation for general population low-risk pregnancies. The situation in which it could be an overestimate is that of synergy, where the benefit of folate supplementation is particularly great, or even confined to, mothers with a genetic factor which also increases their overall risk. That would apply, for example, if high-risk mothers had a genetic defect hampering their folate metabolism, such that the supplement is beneficial even with normal dietary intakes.

However, the application of the result to the prevention of first occurrences of neural tube defects involves more than accepting the argument of causality. Even if the causal relationship applies, with the same relative risk, the balance of potential benefit to potential harm is dramatically different. These defects occur very early in embryological development, before the pregnancy is recognized, and so folic acid supplementation would have to be offered on a population basis to all women who could become pregnant, raising a unique public health challenge. While the risk without supplementation for women who have had a previous abnormal baby is around 2–5 per 100, the corresponding risk in mothers without such a history is around 1–2 per 1000. Therefore the number of women who would need supplementation to prevent one defect (the number needed to treat (NNT)) would rise from around 50 to 5000. Issues of cost, any possibility of side effects, and the social and ethical issues related to mass medication all become relevant.

## E. Comparison of these results with other evidence

### 17. Are the results consistent with other evidence, particularly evidence from studies of similar or more powerful study design?

This is the most powerful study design applied to this problem. The results are generally consistent with earlier studies using weaker designs. In the discussion the authors review the previous small randomized trial and the large non-randomized intervention study, which both showed a benefit, and also mention unpublished interim results of a further trial which will be discussed below. They also note six observational studies using cohort or case–control designs, of which all but one showed an association consistent with protection from increased folic acid consumption. However, the consistency question is not particularly relevant, as this study has the strongest design and is much more rigorous than any of the previous work. Therefore if the results of this trial had shown no benefit, the previous results from non-randomized trials or observation studies would not have offset that null result.

### 18. Does the total evidence suggest any specificity?

The specificity of the result with regard to folic acid alone is important. In the previous work, the large non-randomized study used several vitamins including folic acid. The observational studies are understandably very weak in separating the effects of different vitamins. Some are concerned with total dietary intakes, and women who consume high folate levels also tend to have high intakes of a wide range of other vitamins; others assess supplementation, which is rarely specific to particular preparations, or used and recalled consistently enough to assist. The previous randomized study used folic acid alone and suggested a benefit, but was too small to be conclusive. Therefore the factorial design of the trial, designed to evaluate this specificity, is very important.

19. **Are the results plausible in terms of the biological mechanism?**

There is no discussion of biological plausibility or the mechanisms of the effect in this paper. These defects had been produced in experimental animals by folic acid deficiency and by folate antagonists, but as the defects can be produced in animals by a wide range of dietary changes or external agents, these results did not appear particularly striking or important. When this trial was published in 1991 there was no accepted mechanism by which folic acid would protect against these defects. It seemed surprising to many that supplementation with a relatively low dose of a common vitamin could produce a dramatic reduction in the frequency of a common and severe congenital defect, whose occurrence had been studied intensively for several decades. However, this trial is a good example of an empirical advance preceding knowledge of mechanisms. These results stimulated a search for the mechanism by which the protective effect is produced, and considerable progress has been made, which will be reviewed briefly below.

20. **If a major effect is shown, is it coherent with the distribution of exposure and the outcome?**

The results show a major effect, and therefore coherence can be anticipated. However, coherence as it applies to the factors affecting the recurrence risk of these defects is difficult to establish, as there is little information available on factors, apart from the type of family history, that could relate to the degree of maternal folic acid deficiency as well as to any postulated genetic mechanism. But if, as the authors claim in the discussion, the results also apply to the primary prevention of defects, then the descriptive epidemiology of neural tube defects should fit with this new result. The epidemiology of these defects is complex, showing great variation in geography, time, season, maternal social circumstances, and so on, and the major limitation in judging coherence is that the variability in folic acid consumption is much less well documented. Folic acid is not a particularly easy dietary constituent to measure, and biologically available folic acid may differ considerably from the folate content of foods. There is little information on how the folic acid consumption or tissue levels in pregnant women vary by place, time, or personal or social factors. The demonstration that women in the lower social classes in Britain had low folate intakes was one of the factors leading to the use of supplementation, but this association was very non-specific, as such women have lower intakes of many nutrients. The authors note two issues of coherence.

The UK has one of the highest rates of neural tube defects in the world, and yet is not known to be particularly deficient in folic acid; the authors suggest that the UK population may indeed have low folic acid intakes, or that the types of folic acids in foods eaten there may be relatively poorly absorbed. They also suggest there could be an interaction with a genetically controlled disturbance of folic acid metabolism, a hypothesis which could of course explain much of the other variability of neural tube defect occurrence. They also note that studies of serum or red cell folate levels in women with affected and unaffected pregnancies have not in general shown substantial differences, and suggest that this may be because the range of values within a population is too narrow to demonstrate such differences easily.

## Summary of external validity

In summary, the primary result that folic acid reduces the recurrence rates of these defects can be applied on a worldwide basis. The size of the effect may vary, as the contribution of folic acid deficiency to aetiology may vary in different communities, because of differences in both the defect and the background level of folic intake.

The main issue in generalizability is whether these results on recurrences can be applied to first occurrences of these defects. A reasonable case on both biological and epidemiological grounds is made by the authors, but more direct evidence would be useful. The results are consistent with most observational studies of first occurrences of the defect. At the time of publication, the mechanism for the effect was basically unknown.

## Conclusions

This large individually randomized trial has produced a result which has extremely high internal validity, with observation bias and confounding being ruled out as alternative explanations (**Ex. 11.5**). The result for folic acid is very unlikely to be due to chance, although the precision of the result is still modest, as shown by the fairly wide confidence limits. The association has an appropriate time relationship, is strong, and is consistent by the type of defect and geographical area, and the benefit appears to be specific to folic acid rather than to other multivitamins. Generalization of the result to other high-risk women for the prevention of recurrence is reasonable. Generalization of the result to the situation of the first occurrence of these defects raises further questions, but is certainly strongly suggested by this study.

ASSESSMENT OF A RANDOMIZED TRIAL OF PREVENTION

A. *Description of the evidence*

| | | |
|---|---|---|
| 1 | Exposure | Folic acid 4 mg, or multivitamins, daily |
| 2 | Outcome | Recurrence of neural tube defects |
| 3 | Design | Individually randomized prospective double blind trial; 2 × 2 factorial design |
| 4 | Study population | Mothers with a previous neural tube defect; international, 33 centres |
| 5 | Main result | Reduction in recurrences after folic acid, relative risk 0.33; small reduction after multivitamins, *RR* 0.8 |

B. *Non-causal explanations*

| | | |
|---|---|---|
| 6 | Observation bias | Double-blind design, independent review of records on outcome, high proportion of informative pregnancies virtually rule out observation bias |
| 7 | Confounding | Randomized design on large numbers protects against confounding; data show comparability on several factors |
| 8 | Chance | Result for folic acid significant, 95% limits 0.12–0.71; result for multivitamins non-significant, limits 0.32–1.72 |

C. *Features consistent with causation*

| | | |
|---|---|---|
| 9 | Time relationship | Appropriate; controlled by prospective design |
| 10 | Strength | Folic acid result strong |
| 11 | Dose response | Not assessed; fixed dose |
| 12 | Consistency | Consistent by type of defect, geographical area |
| 13 | Specificity | Benefit specific to folic acid |

D. *External validity*

| | | |
|---|---|---|
| 14 | Eligible population | Participants represent eligible women |
| 15 | Source population | Selection factors for study entry undefined, but no reason not to generalize the result |
| 16 | Target populations | Application to high-risk mothers and recurrence clear, except perhaps non-European subjects. Extension to first occurrences likely but additional direct evidence would be desirable |

E. *Comparison with other evidence*

| | | |
|---|---|---|
| 17 | Consistency | Consistent with earlier intervention studies and with most observational studies |
| 18 | Specificity | No other studies can assess specificity to folic acid |
| 19 | Plausibility | Supported by animal evidence, but mechanism unknown |
| 20 | Coherence | Limited data on distribution of dietary folate; social class gradient coherent, but not specific to folic acid |

**Ex. 11.5.** Summary of assessment of the randomized trial of prevention of recurrence of neural tube defects (MRC Vitamin Study Research Group [1])

## Progress subsequent to this study

This is the strongest study of the six discussed in this section of the book. The study answered an important question and gave a definite result, which was accepted worldwide as relevant and important. This acceptance comes from the strengths of the study: a large international randomized double-blind trial of a feasible intervention.

The publication of this study in July 1991 led to rapid changes in clinical and public health practice. The primary result, that supplementation with 4 mg of folic acid per day would reduce the recurrence rate of these defects, was accepted quickly by health care authorities and professional associations worldwide as accepted clinical practice for high-risk women; for example, within a month, recommendations for high-risk women were issued by the US Centers for Disease Control (CDC) and by the Chief Medical Officer in England. The rapid acceptance of these results contrasts with the reception of the non-randomized trial by Smithells *et al.* in 1981 [2], although that study showed an even stronger protective effect with a relative risk of 0.15. Although that trial undoubtedly led to some clinical adoption of supplementation for high-risk women, most health authorities and professional associations did not advocate a clear policy because of the limitations of the study discussed in this chapter. The non-randomized study used a lower dose (0.36 mg folic acid per day) combined with other vitamins, and so the question of whether a lower-dose preparation would be effective was raised, but in the absence of evidence for toxicity, there was little enthusiasm to develop a trial on high-risk women to answer this question.

The more challenging issue was what action to take with regard to first occurrences of these defects. Could the results of this randomized trial, on recurrences of the defect, be applied to first occurrences? If not, another even larger trial would be needed to answer that question. Such a trial was being designed in China, and had reached the pilot study phase, but it was abandoned once the MRC trial results were known [7]. Observational studies continued in China [8]. The situation was considerably helped by the publication in 1992 of a study of primary prevention in Hungary, which used a randomized design with a multivitamin supplement including folic acid at a dose of 0.8 mg. This demonstrated a protective effect with regard to first occurrences [9,10]. This supportive result made subsequent public health decisions considerably easier. Before the end of 1992, both the CDC and the Chief Medical Officer in England issued recommendations that all women capable of becoming pregnant should take a supplement of 0.4 mg folic acid per day, in addition to ensuring a good diet. This lower dose was chosen as the Czech randomized study used 0.8 mg, the Smithells non-randomized study used 0.36 mg, and various observational studies showed benefits at similar low doses, and toxicity of the 4 mg dose recommended for high-risk women could not be excluded. Similar recommendations were made in many other countries.

Therefore the fact that folate supplementation reduces the risk of these defects was rapidly accepted. Discussion then concentrated on how best to apply this new knowledge, with the main challenge being that advice given once a woman knows she is pregnant is too late. The main approaches have been health education messages to encourage women in the reproductive age groups to take folic acid in anticipation of a possible pregnancy, and increasing the folic acid content of food stuffs, such as flour and cereals, by permissive or compulsory legislative moves, to increase the total folic acid consumption on a community basis [11,12]. For example, Canada and the USA introduced requirements to fortify flour and grain products in 1996 and 1998, respectively, giving about 70 µg extra folate per day, while Australia and the UK allow fortification but do not require it [13,14]. However, a review of trends in the occurrence of neural tube defects up to 1998 in 10 countries found no appreciable effect of recommendations made since 1992 [15]. In 2003, it was estimated that 40 countries had preventive programmes, but that fewer than 10 per cent of the 240 000 cases per year of preventable anencephalus and spina bifida were being prevented [16].

This trial also raises several general issues about the conduct of research. As pointed out in an editorial accompanying the trial result [17], Smithells and his colleagues wished to carry out a randomized trial in the 1970s, but permission to do so was refused by an ethics committee which insisted that all women at increased risk should be offered the supplement. This led to the non-randomized trial, giving results which, while strong and statistically significant, were not regarded as definitive by most authorities. Therefore this ethical committee decision delayed the development of fully randomized trial by some 10 years, and the considerable debate about it delayed recruitment into the MRC trial, so that it took 8 years to accumulate enough participating women to produce the results discussed above. This highlights the need for ethical committees to assess the scientific and ethical consequences of their decisions. On the other hand, the results of the non-randomized trial were correct; they demonstrated a large benefit for vitamin supplementation. Should this evidence from the non-randomized trial, in addition to the considerable number of observational studies, have been accepted as showing the preventive action of vitamin supplementation? By delaying public health policy until the results of the randomized trial came in 10 years later, many preventable defects must have occurred. This situation can be contrasted with the situations where randomized trials have produced results contradicting the conclusions from earlier studies, such as with beta-carotene, discussed in Chapter 6.

This trial also stimulated a great deal more work on the biochemistry of folic acid and the mechanisms of this preventive action. Much of this concentrated on the metabolic processes relating to folic acid, vitamin $B_{12}$, and DNA production. Specific genetic defects have been identified, such as a defect in the gene for 5,10 methylene-tetrahydrofolate reductase [18], which may make some women less able to utilize folic acid, so that they require a higher dietary intake for normal DNA synthesis [19,20]. Other research has shown that women with pregnancies with neural tube defects have autoantibodies to folate receptors [21].

Research has also been stimulated on whether folic acid supplementation can prevent other congenital abnormalities, such as cleft lip and palate [22], and the role of folic acid in chronic diseases such as heart disease and colon cancers. The evidence for the routine use of vitamin supplementation for such prevention is still uncertain [23,24]. However, Professor Wald, who led the MRC trial described in this chapter, is one of those proposing that the routine use of folic acid (0.8 mg daily), with a statin to lower cholesterol, drugs to reduce blood pressure, and aspirin, in a combined 'Polypill' for everyone over age 55 could prevent 80 per cent of cardiovascular disease, with adverse symptoms in 8–15 percent [25,26].

## References

1. **MRC (Medical Research Council) Vitamin Study Group.** Prevention of neural tube defects: results of the Medical Research Council Vitamin Study. *Lancet* 1991; **338**: 131–137.
2. **Smithells RW, Sheppard S, Schorah CJ, et al.** Apparent prevention of neural tube defects by periconceptional vitamin supplementation. *Arch Dis Child* 1981; **56**: 911–918.
3. **Laurence KM, James N, Miller MH, Tennant GB, Campbell H.** Double-blind randomised controlled trial of folate treatment before conception to prevent recurrence of neural-tube defects. *BMJ* 1981; **282**: 1509–1511.
4. **Armitage P.** *Sequential Medical Trials* (2nd edn). Oxford: Blackwell Scientific, 1975.
5. **MacCarthy PA, Dalrymple IJ, Duignan NM, et al.** Recurrence rates of neural tube defects in Dublin maternity hospitals. *Ir Med J* 1983; **76**: 78–79.
6. **Elwood JM, Little J, Elwood JH.** *Epidemiology and Control of Neural Tube Defects.* Oxford: Oxford University Press, 1992.
7. **Oakley GP, Jr., Erickson JD, James LM, Mulinare J, Cordero JF.** Prevention of folic acid-preventable spina bifida and anencephaly. *Ciba Found Symp* 1994; **181**: 212–231.
8. **Berry RJ, Li Z, Erickson JD, et al.** Prevention of neural-tube defects with folic acid in China. China–U.S. Collaborative Project for Neural Tube Defect Prevention. *N Engl J Med* 1999; **341**: 1485–1490.
9. **Czeizel AE, Dudas I.** Prevention of the first occurence of neural tube defects by periconceptional vitamin supplementation. *N Engl J Med* 1992; **327**: 1832–1835.

10. **Czeizel AE, Dudas I, Metneki J.** Pregnancy outcomes in a randomised controlled trial of periconceptional multivitamin supplementation. Final report. *Arch Gynecol Obstet* 1994; **255**: 131–139.

11. **Bentley JR, Ferrini RL, Hill LL.** American College of Preventive Medicine Public Policy Statement. Folic acid fortification of grain products in the U.S. to prevent neural tube defects. *Am J Prev Med* 1999; **16**: 264–267.

12. **Wald NJ, Bower C.** Folic acid and the prevention of neural tube defects. *BMJ* 1995; **310**: 1019–1020.

13. **Wald NJ.** Folic acid and the prevention of neural-tube defects. *N Engl J Med* 2004; **350**: 101–103.

14. **Bower C, de Klerk N, Milne E, et al.** Plenty of evidence on mandatory folate fortification. *Aust N Z J Public Health* 2006; **30**: 81–82.

15. **Botto LD, Lisi A, Robert-Gnansia E, et al.** International retrospective cohort study of neural tube defects in relation to folic acid recommendations: are the recommendations working? *BMJ* 2005; **330**: 571.

16. **Oakley GP Jr, Bell KN, Weber MB.** Recommendations for accelerating global action to prevent folic acid-preventable birth defects and other folate-deficiency diseases: meeting of experts on preventing folic acid-preventable neural tube defects. *Birth Defects Res A Clin Mol Teratol* 2004; **70**: 835–837.

17. Anonymous. Folic acid and neural tube defects. *Lancet* 1991; **338**: 153–154.

18. **Whitehead AJ, Gallagher P, Mills JL, et al.** A genetic defect in 5,10 methylenetetra-hydrofolate reductase in neural tube defects. *Q J Med* 1995; **88**: 763–766.

19. **Lucock M.** Folic acid: nutritional biochemistry, molecular biology, and role in disease processes. *Mol Genet Metab* 2000; **71**: 121–138.

20. **Mitchell LE, Adzick NS, Melchionne J, Pasquariello PS, Sutton LN, Whitehead AS.** Spina bifida. *Lancet* 2004; **364**: 1885–1895.

21. **Rothenberg SP, da Costa MP, Sequeira JM, et al.** Autoantibodies against folate receptors in women with a pregnancy complicated by a neural-tube defect. *N Engl J Med* 2004; **350**: 134–142.

22. **Botto LD, Olney RS, Erickson JD.** Vitamin supplements and the risk for congenital anomalies other than neural tube defects. *Am J Med Genet C Semin Med Genet* 2004; **125**: 12–21.

23. **US Preventive Services Task Force.** Routine vitamin supplementation to prevent cancer and cardiovascular disease. *Nutr Clin Care* 2003; **6**: 102–107.

24. **Strohle A, Wolters M, Hahn A.** Folic acid and colorectal cancer prevention: molecular mechanisms and epidemiological evidence (Review). *Int J Oncol* 2005; **26**: 1449–1464.

25. **Wald NJ, Law MR.** A strategy to reduce cardiovascular disease by more than 80%. *BMJ* 2003; **326**: 1419.

26. Anonymous. Combination pharmacotherapy for cardiovascular disease. *Ann Intern Med* 2005; **143**: 593–599.

# Chapter 12

# Critical appraisal of a prospective cohort study

This chapter deals with the assessment of an interesting prospective cohort study, published in *The Lancet*, 21 September 2002, **360**, 901–907, and available at www.thelancet.com [1]. The summary is reproduced here, with permission from Elsevier and the first author.

## Long-term relation between breastfeeding and development of atopy and asthma in children and young adults: a longitudinal study

Malcolm R Sears, Justina M Greene, Andrew R Willan, D Robin Taylor, Erin M Flannery, Jan O Cowan, G Peter Herbison, Richie Poulton

Summary

**Background.** Breastfeeding is widely advocated to reduce risk of atopy and asthma, but the evidence for such an effect is conflicting. We aimed to assess long-term outcomes of asthma and atopy related to breastfeeding in a New Zealand birth cohort.

**Methods.** Our cohort consisted of 1037 of 1139 children born in Dunedin, New Zealand, between April 1972, and March 1973, and residing in Otago province at age 3 years. Children were assessed every 2–5 years from ages 9 to 26 years with respiratory questionnaires, pulmonary function, bronchial challenge, and allergy skin tests. History of breastfeeding had been independently recorded in early childhood.

**Findings:** 504 (49%) of 1037 eligible children were breastfed (4 weeks or longer) and 533 (51%) were not. More children who were breastfed were atopic at all ages from 13 to 21 years to cats ($p = 0.0001$), house dust mites ($p = 0.0010$), and grass pollen ($p < 0.0001$) than those who were not. More children who were breastfed reported current asthma at each assessment between age 9 ($p = 0.0008$) and 26 years ($p = 0.0008$) than those who were not.

Breastfeeding effects were not affected by parental history of hayfever or asthma. Multifactor analysis controlling for socioeconomic status, parental smoking, birth order, and use of sheepskin bedding in infancy, showed odds ratios of 1.94 (95% CI 1.42–2.65, $p < 0.0001$) for any allergen positive at age 13 years, 2.40 (1.36–4.26, $p = 0.0003$) for current asthma at 9 years, and 1.83 (1.35–2.47, $p < 0.0001$) for current asthma at 9–26 years by repeated-measures analysis.

**Interpretation:** Breastfeeding does not protect children against atopy and asthma and may even increase the risk.

## A. Description of the evidence

1. What was the exposure or intervention?
2. What was the outcome?
3. What was the study design?
4. What was the study population?
5. What was the main result?

The exposed group comprises 504 children who had been breastfed for 4 weeks or longer and entered this prospective cohort study at age 3 years. The comparison group comprised 533 children who were not breastfed for as long as 4 weeks and entered the study at the same time.

This paper is one of many resulting from this prospective study, which incorporated detailed assessments of physical, psychological, and social factors for a cohort of children. An assessment of the results of skin prick tests to several allergens (with positive tests referred to as atopy) at age 13 years and at age 21, and to asthma ascertained at various examinations from the age of 9 years up to the age of 26 is presented. For the purpose of this chapter we will concentrate on the outcome of *current asthma at the age of 9*. This was the first age at which a comprehensive questionnaire on asthma was used. However, while concentrating on this result on asthma, we will consider the other results.

This is a classical prospective cohort study with active and intensive follow-up [2,3], and has produced over 900 scientific papers. As summarized in **Ex. 12.1**, it started as a study of all 1661 children born at the main maternity hospital in the small university city of Dunedin, New Zealand, between April 1972 and March 1973. All these children were included in a neonatal study. Later, a prospective cohort study was developed, and children eligible for this study were the members of that birth cohort who were still resident in the province of Otago, which includes Dunedin, at age 3 years; there were 1139 eligible children. These families were invited to participate and 91 per cent (1037 children) joined the study and so formed the study cohort. The study used very active

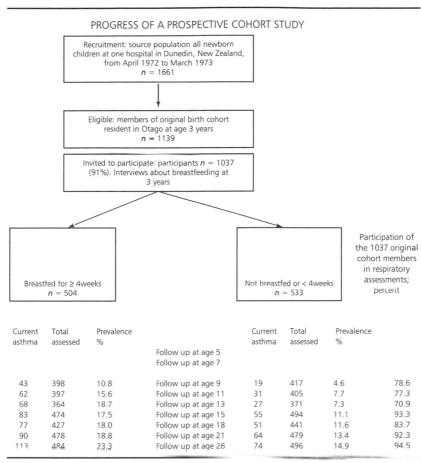

PROGRESS OF A PROSPECTIVE COHORT STUDY

Recruitment: source population all newborn children at one hospital in Dunedin, New Zealand, from April 1972 to March 1973
$n = 1661$

Eligible: members of original birth cohort resident in Otago at age 3 years
$n = 1139$

Invited to participate: participants $n = 1037$ (91%). Interviews about breastfeeding at 3 years

Breastfed for ≥ 4weeks
$n = 504$

Not breastfed or < 4weeks
$n = 533$

Participation of the 1037 original cohort members in respiratory assessments; percent

| Current asthma | Total assessed | Prevalence % | | Current asthma | Total assessed | Prevalence % | |
|---|---|---|---|---|---|---|---|
| | | | Follow up at age 5 | | | | |
| | | | Follow up at age 7 | | | | |
| 43 | 398 | 10.8 | Follow up at age 9 | 19 | 417 | 4.6 | 78.6 |
| 62 | 397 | 15.6 | Follow up at age 11 | 31 | 405 | 7.7 | 77.3 |
| 68 | 364 | 18.7 | Follow up at age 13 | 27 | 371 | 7.3 | 70.9 |
| 83 | 474 | 17.5 | Follow up at age 15 | 55 | 494 | 11.1 | 93.3 |
| 77 | 427 | 18.0 | Follow up at age 18 | 51 | 441 | 11.6 | 83.7 |
| 90 | 478 | 18.8 | Follow up at age 21 | 64 | 479 | 13.4 | 92.3 |
| 113 | 484 | 23.3 | Follow up at age 26 | 74 | 496 | 14.9 | 94.5 |

**Ex. 12.1.** Progress of a prospective cohort study of children in one city followed from age 3 years to age 26 years From Sears *et al.* [1]

assessment, with the subjects being asked to visit the study centre for a series of questionnaires and clinical and psychosocial assessments within a month of their birthday at ages 3, 5, 7, 9, 11, 13, 15, 18, 21, and 26 years. The study is still continuing, now with extension to the children of members of the original cohort. This prospective study, carried out in a community with a population of about 120 000, has become an interesting social phenomenon in its own right, with members of the group being actively involved and kept informed of the results of the study by newsletters and other means; information on the study can be found on the website at http://dunedinstudy.otago.ac.nz.

One of the main issues in a cohort study like this is retaining the members of the cohort as active participants in the assessments. The main value of such a study is the ability to compare the data for individuals as they are assessed at different ages. Exhibit 12.1 shows the participation in the assessments of asthma at the various ages (the total numbers participating in the study at various ages are slightly larger, as given on the website). Out of the 1037 study entrants at age 3 years, 815 (78.6 per cent) participated in the assessment at age 9. The numbers participating then decreased gradually to 735 participating at age 13. Then an increase in funding allowed larger numbers to participate in further assessments, with 980 (94.5 per cent) of the original cohort participating at age 26. This involved considerable effort, including providing airfares for subjects outside Dunedin and even outside New Zealand to participate, and carrying out some assessments in other centres.

We will concentrate on the assessment of asthma at the age of 9 years, which used a standardized comprehensive questionnaire and respiratory tests. The result is the prevalence of asthma at this age. These results are shown in **Ex. 12.2** in the format that has been used earlier in this book. Of those children who were breastfed, 43 (10.8 per cent) of the 398 assessed at age 9 had asthma, compared with 19 (4.6 per cent) of the 417 who were not breastfed. Therefore breastfeeding is associated with an increase in asthma, with an odds ratio of 2.54, 95 per cent confidence limits of 1.45 to 4.44, and a *P*-value of 0.0008.

A relative risk (the ratio of the prevalence rates) also can be calculated, which is 2.37, similar to the odds ratio as the frequency of the outcome is reasonably low. The risk difference is 6.2 per cent, and if we assume causality, the attributable proportion in the exposed is 58 per cent, i.e. the proportion of cases of asthma in breastfed children that are associated with breastfeeding. The attributable fraction in the population is 40 per cent; this is given by the alternative term of 'population attributable risk' in the paper. If this were an intervention study we would also calculate the number needed to treat, as the inverse of the risk difference. In an aetiological study, this calculation can also be used, but is better described as the number exposed for each additional case of asthma, which is 16. Exhibit 12.2 also shows the derivation of a Mantel–Haenszel statistical test following the methods described in Chapter 7, and the confidence limits for the results; these are identical to those published in this paper.

Errors can occur even in high-profile journals like *The Lancet*, and in this publication the summary and the text state that 504 eligible children were breastfed and 533 were not breastfed, whereas in the headings in Tables 1 and 2 of the paper these numbers are reversed. The numbers in the headings of the published tables are wrong, but the detailed results in these tables, including the numbers of children at later examinations, are correct.

## RESULTS OF A COHORT STUDY

*Result for primary outcome of asthma current at age 9 years*

|  | asthma | no asthma | total assessed | proportion affected | percentage affected |
|---|---|---|---|---|---|
| breastfed | 43 | 355 | 398 | 0.108 | 10.8 |
| not breastfed | 19 | 398 | 417 | 0.046 | 4.6 |
| Total | 62 | 753 | 815 | 0.076 | 7.6 |

prevalence of breastfed 0.49

*Risk calculations:*

| | | |
|---|---|---|
| relative risk | $= 0.108/0.046$ | 2.37 |
| odds ratio | $= 43 \times 398/(19 \times 355)$ | 2.54 |
| risk difference | $= (0.108 - 0.046) \times 100$ | 6.25 per cent |
| Number exposed per additional case $= 1/$(risk difference) | | 16.0 |

Assuming causality, attributable proportion in
exposed group $= 6.25/10.8$
Also $= (2.37 - 1)/2.37$        57.8 per cent
and attributable proportion in population
$= (7.6 - 4.6)/7.6$
Also $= 0.49 \times (2.37 - 1)/[0.49 \times (2.37 - 1) + 1]$    40.1 per cent

*Statistical test (Mantel–Haenszel):*

| | | |
|---|---|---|
| $a = 43$ | $E = 30.27730061$ | $V = 14.33066$ |
| $\chi^2 = 11.30$ | $\chi = 3.36$ | $P = 0.001$ |

*Confidence limits* are calculated based on the standard deviation of ln RR, ln OR, or RD, following Appendix Table 2

|  | value | ln | std dev | 95% confidence | limits |
|---|---|---|---|---|---|
| relative risk | 2.37 | 0.8634 | 0.2664 | 1.41 | 4.00 |
| odds ratio | 2.54 | 0.9311 | 0.2850 | 1.45 | 4.44 |
| risk difference (%) | 6.248 | | 1.861 | 2.6 | 9.9% |
| Number exposed per additional case $= 1/$ (risk difference) | | | | Infinity | 10.1 |

**Ex. 12.2.** Main outcome of cohort study comparing asthma at age 9 years in breastfed and non-breastfed children from Table 1 in Sears *et al.* [1]

# B. **Internal validity: consideration of non-causal explanations**

## 6. **Are the results likely to be affected by observation bias?**

One simple issue to be checked is: Is there any possibility of miscoding of data? The general care and quality control of this study would seem to make such an explanation untenable, and the authors did check this thoroughly (M. Sears, personal communication).

The study shows a higher recorded prevalence of asthma in children who were breastfed than in those who were not. As in any study, there are questions of non-differential error and of bias. Neither the classification of children as breastfed or not, nor the classification of children as having asthma at age 9, will be totally accurate. Some degree of error is likely with both these assessments. If this error is substantial, but non-differential, it will act to reduce the association towards the null value.

Is there observation bias? The extreme case would be that the excess prevalence observed is not a true excess, but an artefact. The issue is whether there is systematic bias in the observations made, rather than merely non-differential variation. Such observation bias could only occur if the validity of the assessment of asthma at age 9 is different in children who were breastfed and in those who were not, or if the validity of the assessment of breastfeeding was different in those children who later developed asthma compared with those who did not.

The protection is that the two assessments, of breastfeeding and of asthma, were made independently, and were both made in standardized ways. The history of breastfeeding was documented by interviews with the parents when the children were aged 3 years, and this information was validated by comparison with the records maintained by child health nurses. In New Zealand these are known as 'Plunket' nurses after an eminent early twentieth century doctor, and parents usually keep the 'Plunket books' recording their children's assessments. Therefore the breastfeeding history was documented long before the assessment of asthma at age 9. Some children who later had asthma may have had related conditions earlier in life, but these would only influence the history taken on breastfeeding if they were generally accepted as being related to breastfeeding at the time of the assessment at age 3.

In the assessment at age 9, a trained interviewer used a comprehensive standardized questionnaire and respiratory function tests were performed, including spirometry and a methacholine challenge test, which assesses airway hyper-responsiveness. The definition of current asthma used in the study was 'a positive response to the question "Do you (does your child) have asthma?" together with symptoms reported within the previous 12 months'. This is somewhat unclear, as it is not stated what symptoms or how many symptoms were required. It is stated that the definition was not dependent on whether treatment was prescribed or used. As we will see later, the association between breastfeeding and asthma is very controversial, and studies vary in their definitions of both breastfeeding and asthma, so that variations in definitions are important in interpretation.

Because the assessment of the exposure was made several years before the assessment of the outcome, and both were made by standardized methods, observation bias can be reasonably dismissed as contributing to these results. The issue of random error in the assessment of both outcome and exposure having an effect on the results of the study needs to be kept in mind. The details of the definitions of outcome and exposure may affect the generalizability of the study and comparisons with other studies.

## 7. Are the results likely to be affected by confounding?

From the definition of confounding, we need to consider if breastfed and non-breastfed children differ in terms of factors that could affect the occurrence of asthma. In the results section of the paper, it is noted that several factors were more common in the children who were breastfed: being first born, having parents of higher socio-economic status, having non-smoking mothers, and having had a sheepskin on their bed in infancy. These factors are potential confounding factors, and whether they are confounding will depend on whether they are independently associated with asthma. Girls and boys had similar proportions of being breastfed, and a history of hayfever or asthma in either mother or father was not related to breastfeeding, so these factors will not be confounding. The parental history of asthma or hayfever is of general interest, and so a cross-tabulation is given, which is reproduced in **Ex. 12.3**, applying the Mantel–Haenszel stratified analysis shown in Chapter 6. This shows that compared with the crude odds ratio of 2.54 relating asthma to breastfeeding, the Mantel–Haenszel odds ratio corrected for confounding by parental history is very similar at 2.43, and its confidence limits are also similar. This cross-tabulation assesses both confounding and effect modification. The association between breastfeeding and asthma might be expected to differ in children with a family history of asthma or hayfever, but this is not so; the odds ratio is 2.26 where the family history is positive and 2.66 where the family history is negative, and this variation is well within the range of the confidence limits. A statistical test of heterogeneity shows a chi-square statistic of only 0.02, and a very high $P$-value.

Confounding is addressed in this paper by a multivariate analysis. The precise multivariate model is not described, but is likely to be similar to the logistic regression model described in Chapter 7. **Exhibit 12.4** shows the univariate odds ratio for factors which had statistically significant associations with asthma, compared with the associations seen after fitting a multivariate model including all these variables. Breastfeeding shows an odds ratio of 2.54, as has already been noted, and with control for family history, father's smoking, and cat ownership, this shows very little change, being 2.40 with similar confidence limits. The other associations were also little changed by the multivariate analysis, showing that these factors, while associated with asthma, were not strongly

ASSOCIATION OF ASTHMA WITH BREASTFEEDING, STRATIFIED BY FAMILY HISTORY
OF ASTHMA OR ATOPY

*Overall association*

| | asthma at 9 years | not affected | total cohort | prevalence rate | prevalence per cent | % by exposure | odds ratio |
|---|---|---|---|---|---|---|---|
| breastfed > 4 weeks | **43** | 355 | **398** | 0.108 | 10.8 | 48.8 | 2.54 |
| not breastfed | **19** | 398 | **417** | 0.046 | 4.6 | 51.2 | |
| Total | 62 | 753 | 815 | 0.076 | 7.6 | 100.0 | |

*Stratum 1: family history positive*

| | asthma at 9 years | not affected | total cohort | prevalence rate | prevalence per cent | % by exposure | odds ratio |
|---|---|---|---|---|---|---|---|
| breastfed > 4 weeks | **23** | 151 | **174** | 0.132 | 13.2 | 50.0 | 2.26 |
| not breastfed | **11** | 163 | **174** | 0.063 | 6.3 | 50.0 | |
| Total | 34 | 314 | 348 | 0.098 | 9.8 | 100.0 | |

*Stratum 2: family history negative*

| | asthma at 9 years | not affected | total cohort | prevalence rate | prevalence per cent | % by exposure | odds ratio |
|---|---|---|---|---|---|---|---|
| breastfed > 4 weeks | **19** | 197 | **216** | 0.088 | 8.8 | 48.5 | 2.66 |
| not breastfed | **8** | 221 | **229** | 0.035 | 3.5 | 51.5 | |
| Total | 27 | 418 | 445 | 0.061 | 6.1 | 100.0 | |

*Crude and stratified analyses*

| | | 95% confidence limits | | | ln OR | dev OR |
|---|---|---|---|---|---|---|
| Overall crude odds ratio | | 2.54 | 1.45 | 4.44 | 0.9311 | 0.2850 |
| Mantel–Haenszel odds ratio | | 2.43 | 1.39 | 4.26 | 0.8881 | 0.2869 |
| Heterogeneity $\chi^2$ | 0.0217 | d.f. = 1 | $P = 0.9$ | | | |

| *Missing data* | asthma at 9 years | not affected | total cohort |
|---|---|---|---|
| breastfed > 4 weeks | 1 | 7 | 8 |
| not breastfed | 0 | 14 | 14 |
| Total | 1 | 21 | 22 |

**Ex. 12.3.** Analysis of association between asthma and breastfeeding, stratified for family history of asthma or atopy. Data from Table 4 of Sears *et al.* [1]

associated with breastfeeding and therefore were not confounding. The largest change is a strengthening of the association with father's smoking from an odds ratio of 1.34 to 1.60 in the multivariate analysis. This shows that father's smoking must be either negatively associated with breastfeeding or with a positive family history, or positively associated with cat ownership.

ASSOCIATIONS WITH ASTHMA IN UNIVARIATE AND MULTIVARIATE ANALYSIS

| Factor | Univariate analysis odds ratio | 95% confidence limits | Multivariate analysis odds ratio | 95% confidence limits | Change in odds ratio, % |
|---|---|---|---|---|---|
| Breastfed > 4 weeks | 2.54 | 1.45–4.44 | 2.40 | 1.36–4.26 | –5.5 |
| Family history positive | 1.68 | 0.99–2.84 | 1.60 | 0.93–2.74 | –4.8 |
| Cat ownership to 9 years | 0.54 | 0.31–0.95 | 0.56 | 0.32–1.01 | 3.7 |
| Father smoked | 1.34 | 0.79–2.28 | 1.60 | 0.93–2.77 | 19.4 |
| Father's history positive | 1.36 | 0.76–2.45 | | | |
| Mother's history positive | 1.57 | 0.92–2.70 | | | |
| Male sex | 1.47 | 0.87–2.51 | | | |
| Socio-economic status | 0.95 | 0.78–1.15 | | | |
| Mother smoked | 1.04 | 0.61–1.77 | | | |
| First born | 1.17 | 0.69–1.98 | | | |
| Use of sheepskin in infancy | 1.42 | 0.82–2.47 | | | |

**Ex. 12.4.** Univariate and multivariate analyses of associations with asthma. Data from Table 5 of Sears et al. [1]

A question can be raised regarding the inclusion of the variable on cat owner-ship. This is referred to as 'cat ownership to 9 years', which presumably means the family ownership of a cat at any time before the child's ninth birthday, and it shows a strong negative association, with an odds ratio for asthma of 0.56 after control for other factors. If this is causal, it means that cat ownership pre-vents asthma, and this could be a useful and practical method of prevention! However, given the lack of information on the time relationships, it is likely that some families with a child with asthma would avoid owning a cat because of the generally held belief that contact with cats can produce allergies and respiratory effects. Therefore this association may be due to reverse causation: the child's asthma may prevent cat ownership. If that is true, it is not an inde-pendent risk factor for asthma, and should not be included in the multivariate model. However, it was probably anticipated that cat ownership could be an independent risk factor, associated with an expected *increase* in risk, in which case its inclusion in the model would be important. As its inclusion does not affect the association between breastfeeding and asthma, this is an intriguing issue but one that does not affect the interpretation of this study.

The relationship between asthma and breastfeeding has an odds ratio of 2.54. This association is stronger than the other associations seen in the study, with odds ratios of 1.6 for family history in relationship to asthma and also for father's smoking in relationship to asthma, and weaker relationships for the other variables assessed. This makes it unlikely that more careful control for any of the factors already included in the study would change the results.

Our answer to question 7 is that the result is unlikely to be affected by con-founding by any of the factors considered in this study. The main limitation is that there could be other factors associated with both asthma and breast-feeding that have not been assessed in this study. In any observational study, an assessment needs to be made of whether there are other factors likely to be confounding. This requires expert knowledge or a literature review, and is often the source of considerable debate, particularly if various studies give inconsistent results. This will be discussed later.

## 8. Are the results likely to be affected by chance variation?

The association shown here is quite strong, with the lower 95 per cent confi-dence limit being 1.45 and the upper limit 4.44. The association and its confi-dence limits change very little after multivariate control for confounding factors, and we have dismissed any substantial issue with observation bias. The statistical methods used are appropriate, and we can conclude that chance variation is a very unlikely explanation for the results seen.

In summary, the study is acceptable in terms of observation bias and chance variation being unlikely explanations of the results, and we proceed with the knowledge that both a causal association, or an association due to confounding by factors not addressed in the study, are viable hypotheses to explain the results seen.

## C. Internal validity: consideration of positive features of causation

### 9. Is there a correct time relationship?

The time relationship is consistent with causation, as the exposure is time limited and substantially before the assessment of outcome. Information on the age at first occurrence of asthma would be of interest, but it appears that respiratory assessments were not made at the 3-, 5-, and 7-year assessments, and retrospective assessment would be less certain. Information on current asthma in subsequent years from 11 through to 26 is presented in the paper, and shows a slowly increasing prevalence in both breastfed and non-breastfed individuals (Ex. 12.1); the association strengthens until age 13 when the odds ratio is 2.93, and then diminishes somewhat, but remains increased and statistically significant at all ages. In this study with repeated time-dependent measurements on individuals, more specialized statistical methods were also used to take this regular testing into account, and these gave consistent results.

Could children who develop asthma have earlier related conditions, for example due to the same immunological mechanism? There is a theoretical issue that if children who were later diagnosed with their asthma had allergic conditions in very early life which might have led to the avoidance or early discontinuation of breastfeeding, we could have protopathic bias, where an earlier related condition could influence the exposure. This was mentioned in Chapter 6. However, no evidence is given to suggest this.

### 10. Is the relationship strong?

The relationship is reasonably strong with an odds ratio of 2.54. As noted, this association is stronger than the other associations seen in the study, with odds ratios of 1.6 for both family history and father's smoking in relationship to asthma, and weaker relationships for the other variables assessed. Whether there is another unmeasured factor which could produce confounding is still an open question, but such a factor would have to have at least as strong an association with asthma to explain the association seen. As the exposure—being breastfed— was very common, the attributable risk in the population is high.

## 11. **Is there a dose–response relationship?**

On simple logic, if breastfeeding increases asthma, a dose–response relationship might be expected with the duration of breastfeeding representing the
dose. Data are given on the numbers of children with durations of breastfeeding recorded from 1 to 3 weeks up to over 26 weeks (6 months). However, in
**Ex. 12.5** the confidence limits for the prevalence of asthma are shown, which
were not shown in the original table, and this makes it clear that the numbers
available are insufficient to judge whether the frequency of asthma varies with
different durations of breastfeeding beyond 4 weeks. These results are not very
helpful in assessing dose–response. They could show if there is a minimum
duration of breastfeeding necessary to produce the increase in asthma, i.e. a
threshold effect. On the results given, the frequency of asthma is increased
with all durations above 4 weeks. There is no indication of any increase in
children breastfed from 1 to 3 weeks compared with never being breastfed, but
this is based on very small numbers and is insecure.

Aspects of dose–response can also apply to the severity of outcome. There
are some further details given on the asthma, whether it was accompanied by
airway hyper-responsiveness, and whether there was current significant
wheeze. These results were consistent with the main association shown
between breastfeeding and asthma.

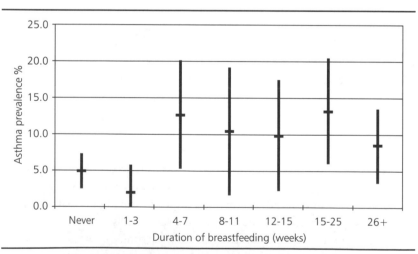

**Ex. 12.5.** Prevalence of asthma at age 9 years, by duration of breastfeeding (weeks):
data show the point estimate and 95 per cent confidence limits. Derived from data
in Table 3 of Sears *et al.* [1]

12. **Are the results consistent within the study?**

**and**

13. **Is there any specificity within the study?**

The key result, the relationship of breastfeeding to asthma at age 9 years, is consistent with similar increased risks being observed subsequently in the study from the ages of 11 to 26, and is consistent with increased risks of atopy assessed at age 13 and age 21 by allergen testing to five different exposures. The elevated odds ratios for current asthma are consistent with increased risks of current wheeze with airways hyper-responsiveness. The association with asthma was similar in both children with a family history of hayfever or asthma and those without such a history, and as discussed below no variation with duration of breastfeeding was seen.

The factors included as confounders in the multivariate analysis are listed. Results to assess if the main association varied with any of these factors (effect modification rather than confounding) are not given. Given the relatively small number of cases of asthma, subdividing the data into numerous subgroups is not a reliable form of analysis, as has been discussed in Chapter 7.

## Conclusions with regard to internal validity

The prospective study design used here has great strength. The information on the exposure was collected independently from the assessment of outcome. The results at this assessment, at age 9 years, were consistent with outcomes assessed at later up to age 26, and the internal consistency of the findings adds to the strength of these results.

There are two reasonable explanations for the results seen: (i) they reflect a causal relationship between being breastfed and asthma, and (ii) the observed results are due to confounding by some unidentified factor or factors. A general problem with observational studies is whether further confounding factors can be excluded with confidence. Breastfeeding is a complex social behaviour, and whether a child is breastfed or not, and for how long, is related to a large number of factors. A reasonable number of these have been explored in this study, but it would not be difficult to postulate other factors that could be related to breastfeeding. Is there any empirical evidence, or a strong case based on reasonable likelihood, that any of these factors related to breastfeeding would also be related to asthma? To contribute to these results, the direction of this association would need to be positive, i.e. a factor would need to be more common in breastfed children and also more common in asthmatic children, or less common in breastfed children and less common in asthmatic children.

We now proceed, with that conclusion in mind, to consider the external validity of the study.

## D. **External validity: generalization of the results**

### 14. **Can the study results be applied to the eligible population?**

These results apply to the 815 children assessed for asthma at the age of 9 years, who comprised 79 per cent of the 1037 children who joined the cohort at age 3 years. The proportions participating were 398/504 (79 per cent) in breastfed and 417/533 (78 per cent) in non-breastfed children, so there is no variation in follow-up by exposure. These 1037 cohort entrants were 91 per cent of the eligible population of 1139 children at that age (Ex. 12.1), and it is stated in the results that the childhood characteristics of the participants (based presumably on medical records) did not differ significantly from the 102 children who did not participate. The children in the eligible population who were available for assessment at age 9 might differ from the rest in ways which could influence the prevalence of asthma, and so the overall prevalence of asthma in those assessed could be different than in the entire eligible group. However, the fact that this selection effect was similar in breastfed and non-breastfed children makes it unlikely that it would influence the association between breastfeeding and asthma. Therefore the result can be applied to the eligible population.

### 15. **Can the study results be applied to the source population?**

The difference between the eligible population and the source population relates to the cohort study being based on 3-year-old children, the 1139 eligible, i.e. those who were resident in the region at age 3 years, who comprised 69 per cent of the originally identified birth cohort of 1661 newborns. This is a reasonable criterion, although inclusion from birth would be better and is used in some other studies. Selection factors would have to be related to both breastfeeding and asthma to alter the associations seen. Therefore, although the participants in the asthma assessment represent only 815/1661, i.e. 49 per cent of the original neonatal source population, it is reasonable to apply the results to the source population.

### 16. **Can the study results be applied to other relevant populations?**

The application of these results to other relevant populations is much more difficult. As will be discussed further, the major factor in this consideration is the consistency or otherwise of these results compared with those of other studies. The factors related to breastfeeding may well differ in different communities and at different time periods. Asthma is a multifactorial disease, which shows considerable variations between different populations, and can be associated with a multitude of environmental factors including climatically related factors. It is also a complex disease, which may have a number of subtypes with differing aetiological components. Thus whether the results of this study are likely to apply to other centres in New Zealand, to children in other countries, or to different time periods (these children were born in the early 1970s) are all issues open to discussion. It is pointed out in the paper that the families represented the full range of socio-economic status in New Zealand, but they were predominately of European ancestry. The application of these results to the Maori population of New Zealand would be questionable without further evidence.

## Summary of external validity

Our conclusions on external validity must be cautious. Within the study, generalization of the key result to the eligible population and to the entire source population is appropriate. The source population is essentially a whole community, and there seems no reason why the results would not be applicable to other generally similar communities. However, the results are different from those of a number of other studies based in other countries and other time periods, and so the wider applicability of these results is unclear. The essential issue is whether these differences in results of different studies are due to true differences in the association, or differences in what has been assessed, or other differences in the methods used in the studies.

## E. Comparison of the results with other evidence

We have gone about as far as we can in assessing this particular paper. Further discussion will take into account other relevant information, and will require an up-to-date review of the literature. It is not appropriate to consider such issues in detail here. We will consider the other evidence available at the time of publication of this paper. We can also use our assessment of the paper to identify the particular questions that need to be answered by other work.

As noted above, this prospective cohort study has high internal validity for an observational study, but we have identified confounding by other unidentified factors as the main issue in interpretation. The fact that the study results may not be generalizable to other populations has been noted.

Both the discussion in this paper, and an assessment of subsequent studies shows that this is indeed a controversial topic. There are many other studies, including other prospective cohort studies and meta-analyses.

## 17. Are the results consistent with other evidence, particularly evidence from studies of similar or more powerful study design?

The only more powerful study design would be an intervention trial. Clearly, an intervention trial of breastfeeding on a large representative general population of newborns would be difficult to perform and would be regarded as unethical, as there are many other reasons to support breastfeeding as superior. There have been intervention trials in high-risk groups, such as children born to parents with strong histories of allergic conditions, but based understandably on shorter-term endpoints. For example, the first such trial compared low-birthweight infants randomized to human breast milk or cows' milk, assessing allergic reactions (including asthma and wheezing) at 9 and 18 months of age. There was no difference in the prevalence of allergic reactions at 18 months in the whole trial, although in the subgroup of infants with a positive family history of allergy, those fed with cows' milk had a higher frequency of allergies, mainly eczema [4]. The results of such intervention studies are not necessarily applicable to the general population.

The other relevant method of investigation is a case–control study comparing children with asthma with unaffected controls, gathering information on breastfeeding and other factors retrospectively. This is a weaker design, as there is potential recall bias, although this might be alleviated if previous records were available to document breastfeeding. The advantage of such a case–control study is that further consideration could be given to a wider range of potential confounders, and to other clinical and laboratory aspects. Several case–control studies have been done; some give results consistent with this study, but others provide contrasting results. For example, a Canadian study of children aged 3–4 years and a Brazilian study of children aged 7–14 years showed protective effects of breastfeeding [5,6], but a Japanese study of 6- to 15-year-olds showed increased asthma with breastfeeding [7]. A case–control analysis within a large national examination survey in the USA of children aged 2 months to 6 years showed no association with breastfeeding [8].

Thus the major issue is consistency between this and other prospective cohort studies. In the discussion in the paper, there is consideration of other studies published before this one. The authors state that when the study was done breastfeeding was widely advocated to reduce the risk of asthma, and they note that these results surprised them, as their working hypothesis was that breastfeeding would protect against asthma in childhood. For example, based on a review of the literature up to 2001 a Scandinavian multidisciplinary group concluded that exclusive breastfeeding reduced atopic disease [9].

To compare this study with all others on the topic is a very large task, and is not appropriate here. The current results appear inconsistent with some other large and carefully performed studies, using similar cohort designs, for example [10–12]. A meta-analysis of 12 prospective studies in developing countries published up to 1999, including over 8000 children with a mean follow-up of 4 years, concluded that exclusive breastfeeding in the first 3 months of life gave protection against the development of asthma (odds ratio 0.70, 95 per cent limits 0.60 to 0.81), and greater protection in children with a family history of atopy (odds ratio 0.52) [13]. A similar result was found for atopic dermatitis [14].

In their discussion, the authors suggest that the explanation may be that breastfeeding may be protective against asthma and similar conditions in early childhood, while increasing the risk of asthma in later childhood. Few of the cohort studies went beyond 6 years. An increased risk of asthma in later childhood is shown by some other cohort studies [15]. Thus the apparent discrepancies between studies may relate to variation in the age at assessment.

## 18. Does the total evidence suggest any specificity?

As mentioned, the authors propose that the association between breastfeeding and asthma may be different at different ages. Other factors that have been suggested as modifiers of the association between breastfeeding and asthma are that the duration of the breastfeeding may be critical, exclusive breastfeeding with no exposure to cows' milk products may be critical, and the association with asthma may differ depending on the family history of atopy or the personal history of atopy in the child. This study did assess length of time of breastfeeding and family history, without showing variations, but the breastfeeding used cannot be assumed to be exclusive.

## 19. Are the results plausible in terms of a biological mechanism?

This study shows the weakness of plausibility as a criterion in the assessment of the likely validity of findings. The authors point out that the most accepted belief before their study was that breastfeeding reduced asthma. A great deal has been written on the biological mechanisms behind this, related to protection against the development of inappropriate immune reactions [16]. Indeed there is the impression that belief in this underlying mechanism is very strong amongst certain authorities, and this belief might be very little influenced by the results of this or other studies that throw it into question. However, the possible mechanisms behind the associations seen in this study are sufficiently complex that it is not difficult to come up with a plausible biological mechanism that would explain an *increase* in asthma related to breastfeeding, and the authors consider several such mechanisms in their discussion.

## 20. **If a major effect is shown, is it coherent with the distribution of the exposure and the outcome?**

This study does show a major effect. Because breastfeeding is a common exposure, applying to about half the children in this cohort, and its association with asthma is quite strong, if the association is causal there must be a major effect on the frequency of asthma. If causal, and if the risk estimate is correct, in this population 40 per cent of all cases of asthma at the age of 9 years are caused by breastfeeding for more than 4 weeks. This is based on the attributable proportion in the population, as shown in Ex. 12.2. This is high, and so there should be some coherence between the prevalence of breastfeeding and the prevalence of asthma 9 years later. The authors state that in the early 1970s, when these children were born, the rate of breastfeeding, at around 50 per cent, was relatively low; by 1980 it had increased to over 80 per cent. We can calculate approximately what effect this would have on asthma prevalence. With an odds ratio of 2.5 and prevalence of exposure of 0.5, the frequency of asthma in the whole population, compared with the frequency in the low risk group, is $(0.5 \times 2.5) + (0.5 \times 1) = 1.75$. If the prevalence of exposure rises to 0.8, this becomes $(0.8 \times 2.5) + (0.2 \times 1) = 2.2$. Since $2.2/1.75 = 1.25$, the frequency of asthma at age 9 would be increased by 25 per cent, which should be measurable. (This result is only approximate, and assumes both causality for this association and that all other aetiological factors and diagnostic criteria stay constant). Also, if the result from this study does apply to different populations, there should be a positive association, comparing populations, between the prevalence of breastfeeding and the prevalence of asthma 9 years later. In more general terms, there seems no doubt that the frequency of breastfeeding, at least for a few weeks, has increased in most developed countries from the 1970s, but the incidence of asthma in childhood has also greatly increased, at least to the 1990s [17,18]. This is consistent with the current study, but inconsistent with the general opinion that breastfeeding reduces asthma, so either this study is correct, or other factors are dominant, or the trends reflect changes in classification or recording.

## Conclusions

Working through this critical appraisal shows that this is a substantial and carefully performed prospective cohort study, in which the information on outcome, asthma at the age of 9 years, is very clear, and the information on breastfeeding is almost equally clear. The results show a substantial association, which is highly statistically significant. Observation bias and chance variation are very unlikely explanations for the results seen. Although several major factors were adequately controlled, the possibility of uncontrolled confounding remains, as there are many factors which could be confounding in this situation.

The external validity in terms of the application of the results to the source population is also high. The major question is: If these results are valid, why are they not consistently seen in other studies from different places in the world? Could the difference be in relationship to the age at onset of asthma, as these authors have suggested, or to some specificity in the type of asthma, or to some confounding factor or cofactor which is involved in the causal process and which varies in different places?

So we are left with two reasonable hypotheses to explain the observations seen (**Ex. 12.6**). One is that they do show a causal relationship. This may be specific to asthma at age 9 years (or close to it), and may not apply to asthma assessed at younger ages. The other is that the association is due to confounding, most likely by factors not measured in this study.

## Subsequent development

This study generated considerable controversy, because the results were in the opposite direction to those expected. As is usual in these circumstances, there was considerable debate. Such debates can show bias, in that a study with a result in conflict with the common preconception is often subject to extremely rigorous cross-examination, whereas a study which might be methodologically much weaker but which produces results in accordance with the common viewpoint is often accepted in the literature and quoted extensively without such critical appraisal.

Among the criticisms of this study [19] were that in this cohort exclusive breastfeeding was unusual, and so the breastfed children could have had some exposure to cows' milk. However, that should only produce a bias towards a null result by misclassification of the exposure, and does not explain the clear positive association seen. The absence of dose–response was also noted as a weakness, as was the lack of interaction with a family history of atopy, but these are not essential elements of causation and their absence does not show any fault in the methodology. A more serious criticism was that the information on feeding patterns in infancy could be biased because the information was collected only at age 3 years. However, the authors showed that the maternal recall at that age was supported in more than 98 per cent of instances by the records of infant care nurses, which were completed concurrently with

ASSESSMENT OF A PROSPECTIVE COHORT STUDY

Breastfeeding and asthma: Sears *et al.* [1]

A. *Description of evidence*

| | | |
|---|---|---|
| 1 | Exposure | Breastfeeding for at least 4 weeks; controls less than 4 weeks' breastfeeding or none. |
| 2 | Outcome | Asthma, from history and clinical assessment at age 9 years. |
| 3 | Design | Cohort study, prospective from age 3 years. |
| 4 | Study population | Children born in one hospital in Dunedin, New Zealand, from April 1972 to March 1973 and resident in the area at age 3 years. |
| 5 | Main result | Current prevalence of asthma 10.8% if breastfed; 4.6% controls. Odds ratio 2.54, 95% confidence limits 1.45 to 4.44. |

B. *Non-causal explanations*

| | | |
|---|---|---|
| 6 | Observation bias | Outcome assessment based on combination of clinical histories and respiratory tests. Breastfeeding data recorded at age 3 years, consistent with nurses' records made throughout infancy. Observation bias unlikely. |
| 7 | Confounding | Several factors, including sex, birth order, socio-economic status, parental smoking, cat ownership, family history of atopy, have been controlled, but other confounders are possible. |
| 8 | Chance | Unlikely to be due to chance: main result has $P$-value less than 0.001. |

C. *Positive features of causation*

| | | |
|---|---|---|
| 9 | Time relationship | Compatible with causation; no data on time of onset of asthma prior to age 9 years; data at later ages consistent. |
| 10 | Strength | Main result strong; large enough to be clinically important. |
| 11 | Dose response | Data insufficient to assess a relationship with number of months of breastfeeding; no clear variation with severity of asthma. |
| 12 | Consistency | Association with asthma consistent with later assessments at ages 11–26, and with associations with atopy. |
| 13 | Specificity | No variation seen with family history or duration of breastfeeding. |

Summary of internal validity: result shows substantial effect, unlikely to be due to chance; observation bias unlikely; but there may be effects of unknown confounders.

D. *External validity*

| | | |
|---|---|---|
| 14 | To the eligible population | Participants represent 79% of cohort participants at age 3, and 72% of eligible population. Loss to follow-up is independent of exposure. Main result applies to eligible population. |

**Ex. 12.6. cont'd**

15 To the source population | Eligible population was 62% of the original birth cohort, but eligibility depends on place of residence only. Result should apply to source population.

16 To other populations | Source population is births in one community in southern New Zealand in 1972–1973. Applicability of results to other communities and time periods unknown. Extension of results to other age groups unknown.

*E. Other evidence*

17 Consistency | Several other large prospective cohort studies, and meta-analyses. Several studies support opposite association, with lower asthma risk if breastfed. Effect may vary with age at assessment of asthma; some support from other studies of an increased risk in later childhood.

18 Specificity | Association for asthma may be shared with other atopy outcomes. Variation in length of breastfeeding, whether breastfeeding is exclusive, and with family history of asthma or atopy may be relevant. Association may change with age.

19 Plausibility | Despite general view that breastfeeding may protect against atopy, mechanisms are complex and any effect can be supported.

20 Coherence | Population attributable risk is high because prevalence of breastfeeding is high, so if causal and generalizable should show coherence in time and place. Asthma and breastfeeding both increasing in time. Geographical coherence not assessed.

Summary of external validity: study is done in one community, and other data from different places often seem conflicting, so external validity is limited and depends on the emergence of supporting data from other studies. Age at assessment may be critical.

**Ex. 12.6.** Assessment of causality in a prospective cohort study. Study of breastfeeding and asthma and atopy in later childhood, by Sears *et al.* [1]

early childhood [20]. The fact that only 69 per cent of the original cohort of neonates were included in this cohort has also been given as a criticism, and while it is a limitation in comparison with other cohorts starting from birth, it would only affect the results if the selection into the prospective cohort was related to both breastfeeding and the prevalence of asthma much later at age 9, which seems unlikely. The same review [19] made some other clearly inaccurate comments, for example in claiming that some confounding factors were ignored when they were in fact included in the analysis.

A useful review [21] brings together studies of breastfeeding and outcomes considered in two groups, atopy including eczema and other allergies, and asthma; one of the general issues is whether these outcomes should be treated separately or considered together. This review emphasizes prospective cohort studies in developed countries, and shows that some show protective effects against asthma, others show no effect, and others show an increased risk in asthma, such as the current study. This review concludes that 'one can still not make a definite statement that breastfeeding will help prevent sensitisation to allergens in infants or later respiratory illness such as asthma', although the authors also say 'the preponderance of evidence does suggest that, overall, exclusive breastfeeding for at least four months seems to protect against the development of atopic dermatitis in infants and early childhood wheezing'. Other recent reviews also show the complex findings of various studies [22].

Of course, the use of breastfeeding goes much beyond this topic, and even the present authors do not use their data to suggest that the current approach of encouraging breastfeeding should be changed. A major Cochrane systematic review of the optimal duration of exclusive breastfeeding, with an emphasis on developing countries, led to a World Health Assembly resolution to recommend exclusive breastfeeding for 6 months, based mainly on a reduction in gastrointestinal tract infections, although noting that no reduction in atopic outcomes or asthma had been demonstrated in studies from Finland, Australia, and Belarus [23].

The authors of the study discussed in this chapter have emphasized their finding of an increase in the prevalence of asthma at 9 years, and their results are supported by several other studies that assess asthma or similar outcomes in later childhood [15,20], but are not supported by some others [24]. They have proposed that breastfeeding may protect against asthma and other allergic conditions in younger childhood, but that the association in later childhood and adolescence may be quite different. More information will come from larger studies or meta-analyses; for example, an international project is under way to combine the analysis of 18 European birth cohorts [25].

# References

1. Sears MR, Greene JM, Willan AR, *et al.* Long-term relation between breastfeeding and development of atopy and asthma in children and young adults: a longitudinal study. *Lancet* 2002; **360**: 901–907.

2. **Silva PA, Stanton W.** *From Child to Adult: The Dunedin Multidisciplinary Health and Development Study.* New York: Oxford University Press, 1997.

3. **Poulton R, Hancox RJ, Moffitt TE.** The Dunedin Multidisciplinary Health and Development Study: 1972–2006. *Int J Epidemiol* 2006; in press.

4. **Lucas A, Brooke OG, Morley R, Cole TJ, Bamford MF.** Early diet of preterm infants and development of allergic or atopic disease: randomised prospective study. *BMJ* 1990; **300**: 837–840.

5. **Infante-Rivard C, Amre D, Gautrin D, Malo JL.** Family size, day-care attendance, and breastfeeding in relation to the incidence of childhood asthma. *Am J Epidemiol* 2001; **153**: 653–658.

6. **Romieu I, Werneck G, Ruiz VS, White M, Hernandez M.** Breastfeeding and asthma among Brazilian children. *J Asthma* 2000; **37**: 575–583.

7. **Takemura Y, Sakurai Y, Honjo S,** *et al.* Relation between breastfeeding and the prevalence of asthma : the Tokorozawa Childhood Asthma and Pollinosis Study. *Am J Epidemiol* 2001; **154**: 115–119.

8. **Rust GS, Thompson CJ, Minor P, vis-Mitchell W, Holloway K, Murray V.** Does breastfeeding protect children from asthma? Analysis of NHANES III survey data. *J Natl Med Assoc* 2001; **93**: 139–148.

9. **van Odijk J., Kull I, Borres MP,** *et al.* Breastfeeding and allergic disease: a multidisciplinary review of the literature (1966–2001) on the mode of early feeding in infancy and its impact on later atopic manifestations. *Allergy* 2003; **58**: 833–843.

10. **Oddy WH, de Klerk NH, Sly PD, Holt PG.** The effects of respiratory infections, atopy, and breastfeeding on childhood asthma. *Eur Respir J* 2002, **19**: 899–905.

11. **Oddy WH, Sherriff JL, de Klerk NH,** *et al.* The relation of breastfeeding and body mass index to asthma and atopy in children: a prospective cohort study to age 6 years. *Am J Public Health* 2004; **94**: 1531–1537.

12. **Rothenbacher D, Weyermann M, Beermann C, Brenner H.** Breastfeeding, soluble CD14 concentration in breast milk and risk of atopic dermatitis and asthma in early childhood: birth cohort study. *Clin Exp Allergy* 2005; **35**: 1014–1021.

13. **Gdalevich M, Mimouni D, Mimouni M.** Breast-feeding and the risk of bronchial asthma in childhood: a systematic review with meta-analysis of prospective studies. *J Pediatr* 2001; **139**: 261–266.

14. **Gdalevich M, Mimouni D, David M, Mimouni M.** Breast-feeding and the onset of atopic dermatitis in childhood: a systematic review and meta-analysis of prospective studies. *J Am Acad Dermatol* 2001; **45**: 520–527.

15. **Wright AL, Holberg CJ, Taussig LM, Martinez FD.** Factors influencing the relation of infant feeding to asthma and recurrent wheeze in childhood. *Thorax* 2001; **56**: 192–197.

16. **Halken S.** Prevention of allergic disease in childhood: clinical and epidemiological aspects of primary and secondary allergy prevention. *Pediatr Allergy Immunol* 2004; **15** (Suppl 16): 4–32.

17. **Akinbami LJ, Schoendorf KC.** Trends in childhood asthma: prevalence, health care utilization, and mortality. *Pediatrics* 2002; **110**: 315–322.

18. **Pearce N, Douwes J.** The global epidemiology of asthma in children. *Int J Tuberc Lung Dis* 2006; **10**: 125–132.

19. **Peat JK, Allen J, Oddy W, Webb K.** Breastfeeding and asthma: appraising the controversy. *Pediatr Pulmonol* 2003; **35**: 331–334.

20. **Sears MR, Taylor DR, Poulton R.** Breastfeeding and asthma: appraising the controversy–a rebuttal. *Pediatr Pulmonol* 2003; **36**: 366–368.

21. **Friedman NJ, Zeiger RS.** The role of breast-feeding in the development of allergies and asthma. *J Allergy Clin Immunol* 2005; **115**: 1238–1248.

22. **Wills-Karp M, Brandt D, Morrow AL.** Understanding the origin of asthma and its relationship to breastfeeding. *Adv Exp Med Biol* 2004; **554**: 171–191.

23. **Kramer MS, Kakuma R.** The optimal duration of exclusive breastfeeding: a systematic review. *Adv Exp Med Biol* 2004; **554**: 63–77.

24. **Burgess SW, Dakin CJ, O'Callaghan MJ.** Breastfeeding does not increase the risk of asthma at 14 years. *Pediatrics* 2006; **117**: e787–e792.

25. **Keil T, Kulig M, Simpson A,** *et al.* European birth cohort studies on asthma and atopic diseases. I: Comparison of study designs—a GALEN initiative. *Allergy* 2006; **61**: 221–228.

Chapter 13

# Critical appraisal of a retrospective cohort study

This study was published in *The Lancet*, 26 October 1991, **338**, 1027–1032 [1], and is available at www.thelancet.com. The abstract, introduction, and part of the methods section of the paper are reproduced here, with permission from Elsevier and the first author.

## Cancer mortality in workers exposed to chlorophenoxy herbicides and chlorophenols

Rodolfo Saracci, Manolis Kogevinas, Pier-Alberto Bertazzi, Bas H. Bueno de Mesquita, David Coggon, Lois M Green, Timo Kauppinen, Kristan A. L'Abbé, Margareta Littorin, Elsebeth Lynge, John D Mathews, Manfred Neuberger, John Osman, Neil Pearce, Regina Winkelman.

## Abstract

Epidemiological studies have revealed an increased risk of cancer, notably soft-tissue sarcomas and non-Hodgkin's lymphomas, in people occupationally exposed to chlorophenoxy herbicides, including those contaminated by 2,3,7,8-tetrachlorodibenzo-$p$-dioxin (TCDD). We report here a historical cohort study of mortality in an international register of 18 910 production workers or sprayers from ten countries.

Exposure was reconstructed through questionnaires, factory or spraying records, and job histories. Cause-specific national death rates were used as reference. No excess was observed in all-cause mortality, for all neoplasms, for the most common epithelial cancers, or for lymphomas. A statistically non-significant two-fold excess risk, based on 4 observed deaths, was noted for soft-tissue sarcoma with a standardised mortality ratio (SMR) of 196 and 95% confidence interval (CI) 53–502; this was concentrated as a six-fold statistically significant excess, occurring 10–19 years from first exposure in the cohort as a whole (SMR = 606 [165–1552]) and, for the same time period, as a nine-fold excess among sprayers (SMR = 882 [182–2579]). Risks appeared to be increased for cancers of the testicle, thyroid, other endocrine glands, and nose and nasal cavity, based on small numbers of deaths.

The excess of soft-tissue sarcomas among sprayers is compatible with a causal role of chlorophenoxy herbicides but the excess does not seem to be specifically associated with those herbicides probably contaminated by TCDD.

## Introduction

Chlorophenoxy herbicides have been used extensively since the mid-1950s for control of weeds and for removing unwanted brush on non-crop land. In the 1960s an equal mixture of 2,4-dichloro and 2,4,5-trichloro phenoxyacetic acids (agent orange) was heavily used in South Vietnam and Cambodia for defoliation by the US armed forces. Since 1969 in several industrialised countries, production and use of some compounds, and especially of 2,4,5-trichlorophenoxy acetic acid (2,4,5-T) and it derivatives have been reduced or banned. Chlorinated phenols are intermediates in the production of those chlorophenoxy herbicides and are also used directly for wood preservation. Both groups of compounds may be contaminated during the production process with polychlorinated dioxins and furans, including tetrachlorodibenzo-$p$-dioxin (dioxin, TCDD), which is a widespread contaminant of the general environment.

Studies of cancer risks have revealed excesses for soft-tissue sarcoma and non-Hodgkin's lymphoma in populations exposed to chlorophenoxy herbicides, chlorinated phenols, dioxins, and furans during manufacture and spraying or after accidents. In 1987 an International Agency for Research on Cancer (IARC) working group concluded that there was 'limited' evidence of human carcinogenicity for chlorophenoxy herbicides and chlorinated phenols. A recent paper, focussing on exposure in chemical plants to 'dioxin', reported excesses for cancer of the respiratory tract and soft-tissue sarcoma, but could not exclude the contribution of smoking and other exposures in the workplace. We present here the first detailed mortality analysis of a large international cohort of workers (the International Register of Workers Exposed to Phenoxy Herbicides and their Contaminants) set up by the IARC in association with the US National Institute of Environmental Health Sciences (NIEHS). Results for some cohorts in the register have been reported earlier but for different follow-up periods.

## Materials and methods
### Study population

The register incorporates information on 17 372 male workers, 1537 female workers, and 1 of unknown sex, distributed among twenty cohorts from ten countries. Since publication of the register population minor corrections have led to the exclusion of 62 workers found to be ineligible. Workers from one

British company which both produced and sprayed herbicides have been separated here into two cohorts (14 and 20).

The register includes workers ever employed in production or spraying, except in the cohorts from Australia, Canada, and New Zealand, in which minimum employment periods of 1 year, 6 months, and 1 month, respectively, were specified. Eligibility of cohorts depended on the completeness at company level of records identifying workers and on the ability to ensure tracing rates of 95% or more. Follow-up for mortality was based either on computerised national record systems or on active follow-up procedures. Additional information on cases of soft-tissue sarcoma and non-Hodgkin's lymphoma cases was sought from medical records and cancer registries. Denmark, New Zealand, Finland and Sweden provided incidence data from population-based cancer registries. Person-years at risk were calculated from 1955 onwards since only from that year were cancer-specific mortality rates available for all participating countries. Excluded from the analysis were 220 workers who either died or were lost to follow-up before 1955, 105 workers with unknown year of first exposure, 131 with unknown year of birth, 1 with unknown sex, and 63 with other missing information. The 18 390 workers included comprise 16 863 males and 1527 females, and 307 488 person-years at risk were accumulated, with an average follow-up of 17 years. Workers lost to follow-up constituted 5% of the total cohort, and in no individual cohort did this proportion exceed 10%.

## Exposure assessment

Questionnaires were constructed for factories producing chlorophenoxy herbicides or chlorinated phenols and for spraying cohorts. These were completed with the assistance of industrial hygienists, workers, and/or factory personnel. Industry and other production records were also used. Job histories were examined when available. Workers were classified as exposed, probably exposed, exposure unknown, or non-exposed.

*Exposed workers* ($n = 13\ 482$) comprise all known to have sprayed chlorophenoxy herbicides and all who had worked in any of the following departments at factories producing chlorophenoxy herbicides or chlorinated phenols: synthesis, finishing, formulation, packing, maintenance/repair, laboratory, chemical effluent/waste, cleaning, shipping/transportation/stores/warehouse, plant supervision, cleaning during accident, and other and unclassified exposure.

*Probably exposed workers* ($n = 416$) comprise all workers in cohorts 15 and 18; no job titles were available but it was judged that most workers would have been exposed. Exposed and probably exposed are aggregated for some analyses.

*Workers with unknown exposure* ($n = 541$) had no information on exposure status.

*Non-exposed workers* ($n = 3951$) were those never employed in the parts of factories which produced chlorophenoxy herbicides or chlorinated phenols and who never sprayed chlorophenoxy herbicides came mainly from Australia, Denmark, Netherlands, New Zealand, and UK (224, 1966, 1283, 214, and 180, respectively). Although not exposed to chlorophenoxy herbicides they were exposed to other chemicals, such as dyes and rodenticides.

Workers were also categorised as producers (12,492) and sprayers (5898). Exposed and probably exposed workers were also classified by groups of chemicals produced or sprayed (9377 chlorophenoxy herbicides, 408 chlorinated phenols, and 4113 both) and within the manufacturing cohorts by department (3034 main production, 1522 maintenance and cleaning, 1665 other, 1907 unclassifiable). A substantial number of workers producing chlorophenoxy herbicides may also have exposed to chlorophenols (e.g. *p*-chloro-*o*-cresol) which are used as raw materials in the synthesis of chlorophenoxy acids. Exposure to the most toxic dioxin congener (2,3,7,8-TCDD) may occur during production of 2,4,5-TCP and 2,4,5-T, and during spraying of herbicides containing 2,4,5-T or its derivatives. Ten factories ($n = 6845$) had either not produced 2,4,5-T or had produced very little of it (around 10 tonnes per year during the study period). Workers in these factories were exposed to various chlorophenoxy herbicides, chlorinated phenols, polychlorinated dibenzodioxins, and furans but were probably not exposed to TCDD. Thus within the register population it was possible to differentiate workers probably exposed to TCDD and workers probably not exposed to TCDD.

## Statistical analysis

The person-years method was used to derive standardised mortality ratios (SMR) with 95% confidence intervals (CI) based on the Poisson distribution. An excess or deficit of an SMR is regarded as statistically significant at $p < 0.05$ (two-tail) when the CI does not include 100. The WHO Mortality Data Bank was used to compute national mortality reference rates for sex, age (in 5-year age groups), and calendar period (in 5-year periods, except when such a period coincides with an ICD revision). Duration of exposure was treated as a time-dependent variable in the allocation of person-years at risk. Poisson regression analysis was applied for selected sites.

## Coding

Coding of underlying cause of death was done nationally. A conversion table has been prepared in IARC to allow the pooling of results over different ICD revisions. About 40% of soft-tissue sarcomas (one of the a priori neoplasms of interest) develop in parenchymal organs and are not coded under ICD 171 (8th and

9th revision, 'malignant neoplasms of connective and other soft tissue'). Histological diagnoses were not generally available for sarcomas not coded as ICD 171. SMRs for soft-tissue sarcoma therefore relate only to sarcomas coded as ICD 171. Information on other sarcomas, identified from medical records and cancer registration, is presented but no statistical analysis was done.

## A. **Description of the evidence**

1. What was the exposure or intervention?

2. What was the outcome?

3. What was the study design?

4. What was the study population?

5. What was the main result?

The objective was to assess various possible effects of a specific exposure: *chlorophenoxy herbicides*. These chemicals have been widely used since the 1950s for controlling unwanted plant growth, and formed a component of the notorious 'agent orange' used in the Vietnam War for defoliation. The closely related *chlorinated phenol* compounds are intermediates in the production of these herbicides, and are also used themselves for wood preservation. Both sets of compounds may be contaminated during production by a range of other compounds, including tetrachlorodibenzo-dioxin (TCDD). This information is given in the introduction to the paper, which also gives more detailed references. This study is based on exposure to these compounds, defined through holding an occupation likely to involve such exposure.

The outcome was mortality, from all causes, with particular attention given to mortality from specified types of cancer.

Being exposure based, this is a cohort study, and is a retrospective (historical) cohort study. The study population was identified through current and past employment records, which were linked to mortality records to give outcome information.

The study population were workers identified through the 'International Register of Workers Exposed to Phenoxy Herbicides and their Contaminants', which was set up by an international and a US group. This consisted of 20 separate cohorts representing different employers, workplaces, and countries, involving in total 18 390 workers (16 863 male, 1527 female) from 10 countries. The derivation of the study participants is shown in **Ex. 13.1**.

Information on where each employee in the register worked and when, and a more detailed job history for most workers, was available. Job histories were categorized by levels of exposure, using the experience of industrial hygienists and workers. The employees were grouped into '*exposed*' workers, who had jobs

DESIGN OF A RETROSPECTIVE COHORT STUDY

| | Total group | | |
|---|---|---|---|
| | In study | Excluded | |
| *Source population, from Register (SP)* | 18972 | | % of source |
| Found ineligible | | 62 | 0.3 |
| Died or lost to follow up before 1955 | | 220 | 1.2 |
| Total excluded | | 282 | 1.5 |
| *Eligible population (EP)* | 18690 | | % of eligible |
| Unknown year of birth | | 131 | 0.7 |
| Unknown year of first exposure | | 105 | 0.6 |
| Unknown sex | | 1 | 0.0 |
| Other missing information | | 63 | 0.3 |
| Total not approached | | 300 | 1.6 |
| *Included in study cohort* | 18390 | | |
| Participants in study | 18390 | | |
| Loss to follow-up* | | unknown | "<5%" |
| *Participants in analysis (PA)* | 18390 | | |
| Voluntary response rate | not applicable | | |
| Participation rate | =PA/EP | | 98.4% |
| Eligible/source population | =EP/SP | | 98.5% |
| Participants/source population | =PA/SP | | 96.9% |

*subjects lost to follow up contribute to the analysis until their follow-up ends

*Distribution of participants by exposure category*

| | |
|---|---|
| Exposed | 13482 |
| Probably exposed | 416 |
| Unknown exposure | 541 |
| Non-exposed | 3951 |

**Ex. 13.1.** Derivation of the cohort of workers contributing to the analysis of Saracci *et al.* [1]

regarded as very likely to involve exposure to chlorophenoxy herbicides or chlorinated phenols, '*probably exposed*' workers, which included all workers in two cohorts where no detailed job information was available, a group of workers with '*unknown exposure*', where there was no information, and a group of '*non-exposed*' workers. The last group comprised workers who had been employed in workplaces within the registry, but who had never been employed in the parts of the factories which produced the chemicals, and had never sprayed them; these workers are regarded as being non-exposed to the chemicals in question, although they were exposed to other chemicals. Therefore the study has an *external* control group, shown by the comparison of observed mortality with the mortality expected on the basis of national data, and also an *internal* comparison, comparing different categories of exposure.

Results for total mortality, major causes of mortality, and cancer mortality are presented. For this review, we will concentrate on the result that is emphasized by the authors, which is *mortality from soft-tissue sarcoma*. This is emphasized because previous studies had demonstrated excesses of incidence or mortality of soft-tissue sarcoma in relationship to exposure to these chemicals, so that the hypothesis of an increased mortality rate was established a priori, and the study is testing that hypothesis. For many of the other results, the study is a hypothesis generation study, as the findings are unanticipated.

The mortality of the identified cohorts is compared with the expected mortality based on national mortality statistics by sex, age, and calendar period for the country relating to the individual cohort. For each cause of mortality the observed number of deaths is compared with the expected number, the ratio being the standardized mortality ratio (SMR). This is expressed in percentage terms, the null value being 100 and higher values showing an excess mortality. Ninety-five per cent two sided confidence intervals are calculated.

The main result with regard to soft-tissue sarcoma (**Ex. 13.2**) is that for exposed and probably exposed workers combined; four deaths were observed compared with 2.04 expected, giving an SMR of 196, with 95 per cent confidence limits of 53 to 502. For the non-exposed workers, there were no observed deaths, compared with 0.42 expected; the SMR of zero has confidence limits of 0 to 878. Therefore the main result is an excess mortality rate from soft-tissue sarcoma in workers exposed to chlorophenoxy herbicides or chlorinated phenols. We need to assess whether this association is likely to be due to a causal relationship.

## B. Internal validity: consideration of non-causal explanations

### 6. Are the results likely to be affected by observation bias?

As the key result with regard to soft-tissue sarcomas is dependent on the observation of four deaths, observation bias and observation error are both relevant. If even one or two true occurrences of death from this disease have been missed, or if some of the deaths recorded are erroneous, the results could be greatly affected.

In terms of *bias*, the essential issue is whether the recognition and recording, which includes the classification of the death using the International Classification of Diseases, was done in an identical manner in these workers as in the general population (with reference to the external control comparison), and

MORTALITY FROM SOFT TISSUE SARCOMA

| Subgroups | Observed number of cases | Expected number of cases | SMR | 95% confidence limits |
|---|---|---|---|---|
| *Exposure* | | | | |
| exposed or probably exposed | 4 | 2.04 | 196 | 53–502 |
| non-exposed | 0 | 0.42 | 0 | 0–878 |
| *Type of work* | | | | |
| production workers | 1 | 1.03 | 97 | 3–541 |
| sprayers | 3 | 1.01 | 297 | 61–868 |
| *Chemicals used* | | | | |
| both | 1 | 0.48 | 208 | 5–1161 |
| phenoxy | 3 | 1.50 | 200 | 41–585 |
| chlorophenols | 0 | 0.06 | 0 | 0–6148 |
| *Exposure to TCDD* | | | | |
| probable | 2 | 1.00 | 200 | 24–723 |
| unlikely | 2 | 1.04 | 193 | 23–695 |
| *Years since first exposure* | | | | |
| 30+ | 0 | 0.24 | 0 | 0–1537 |
| 20–29 | 0 | 0.52 | 0 | 0–709 |
| 10–19 | 4 | 0.66 | 606 | 165–1552 |
| 0–9 | 0 | 0.50 | 0 | 0–738 |
| *Duration of exposure* | | | | |
| 20+ | 0 | 0.15 | 0 | 0–2459 |
| 10–19 | 2 | 0.29 | 690 | 84–2491 |
| 1–9 | 0 | 0.89 | 0 | 0–415 |
| <1 | 2 | 0.59 | 339 | 41–1125 |

**Ex. 13.2.** Main results for deaths from soft-tissue sarcoma: from the retrospective cohort study of Saracci *et al.* [1]. Results taken from Table III of the paper, SMR = standardized mortality ratio (100 = null result); TCCD = 2,3,7,8-tetra chlorodibenzo-*p*-dioxin

whether it was done in an identical fashion in groups defined with different levels of exposure (for the internal comparison). Bias compared with the general population could arise if this disease or others like it were thought to be more common in such workers: if so, there could be greater clinical awareness for this condition, specific diagnostic procedures might be more likely to be done, if it did occur it could be more likely to be recorded on the clinical record or on a death certificate, and an ambiguous record might be more likely to be coded to sarcoma. A study of this issue done now would need to take account of such potential biases, as the possible association between herbicide exposure and soft-tissue sarcomas is now widely recognized. However, the observation period for mortality in this study largely preceded such interest. The period of observation varies with the different cohorts: the starting dates range from 1955 to 1975, and the cut-off dates range from 1982 to 1988. The earliest suspicion of a link, which can be judged from the extensive list of references given in this paper, appears to be from a case–control study published in 1979. It seems unlikely that this suspicion would have affected clinical practice or death certification until some years after that. The potential bias could be addressed by seeing if the excess mortality was confined to deaths occurring in the later years, when knowledge of the potential hypothesis would be more widespread. An analysis by calendar year of death would of course have to be appropriately adjusted for the associations between year of death, duration of exposure, and year since first exposure; no such analysis is presented here. Therefore while observation bias remains a theoretical possibility, it is unlikely to be a major issue.

The question of the *error* in the reported mortality from soft-tissue sarcomas is of greater significance. These cancers are not particularly easy to diagnose, and they are not very clearly defined in clinical or pathological terms; therefore some deaths from soft-tissue sarcomas could have been inadequately described on a death certificate and coded to some other category. It is less likely that any of the deaths recorded as being from soft-tissue sarcomas were in fact from something else. This type of inaccuracy, occurring without bias, would produce some misclassification of the outcome, and would weaken the power of the study to detect a real effect; this could mean that the observed result is an underestimate of the true relationship.

## 7. Are the results likely to be affected by confounding?

In assessing potential confounders, we need to ask the two general questions. Apart from these herbicides, what factors are known to increase or decrease the risk of death from soft-tissue sarcoma? What other exposures are likely to be associated with exposure to these chemicals? The first question is not addressed in the paper, and so further review of the literature is necessary. This is rather unproductive. Apart from the general confounders of age, sex, and country (which are controlled in this study because the expected numbers of deaths are based on analyses specific to those factors), little is known about causal factors for soft-tissue sarcoma. The disease is not known to be related to smoking, which is often a confounding factor in occupational studies. In terms of factors associated with the exposure, the most obvious are other chemical exposures. The study participants have worked in jobs which involve using or manufacturing chemicals, and are very likely to have been exposed to many chemicals. This is discussed in the paper, and the authors indeed conclude that their attempt to relate risks to specific agents was 'only partially successful' (discussion, paragraph 1). They argue that the most specific exposure to chlorophenoxy herbicides would be in sprayers, rather than production workers. The results show that the excess mortality was confined to sprayers, with an SMR of 297 based on three deaths, whereas the SMR in production workers was not increased, being 97 based on one death.

There is information, based on the job history, with regard to whether exposure was likely to have been to phenoxy compounds, chlorophenols, or both, and whether exposure to TCDD was likely. There were no deaths in those exposed only to chlorophenols, with the excess mortality being seen both in those exposed to phenoxy compounds (three deaths, SMR 200) and in those exposed to both (one death, SMR 208). There was no difference in the SMR by likely exposure to TCDD (Ex. 13.2).

The information with regard to spraying versus production work, and the information on likely individual chemical exposure, suggest that the association is primarily with phenoxy herbicides, rather than with chlorophenols or TCDD. Given the limitations of the classification of exposure and the very small numbers, this conclusion can only be tentative.

Potential confounding factors can also be identified by examining other mortality outcomes. For example, if the exposed workers had increased mortality from cancers related to smoking, it would suggest that they smoked more than the general population. If, in addition, soft-tissue sarcoma were related to smoking, smoking would be a confounder. In fact, neither of these relationships is supported. In this study, the SMR for lung cancer in exposed workers was not increased, being 102, and review of the literature shows that sarcomas are not known to be related to smoking, The pattern of other mortality is difficult to interpret because of the small numbers. Results are presented for 29 different cancer sites, of which 17 have SMRs above 100 and 12 below; there is nothing in the pattern which suggests any other causal agent which could be a confounder in the association with soft-tissue sarcomas.

## 8. Are the results likely to be affected by chance variation?

The increased SMR in exposed and probably exposed workers is not statistically significant, being 196, with a 95 per cent confidence interval of 53 to 502. In other words, the result is compatible with a mortality rate from soft-tissue sarcomas of approximately half that of the general population, up to a rate of five times. This demonstrates the weakness of cohort studies in dealing with rare outcomes; this study involved nearly 19 000 workers and was a major logistic effort, but for this particular outcome it is a very weak study. The effective sample size depends on the four observed deaths. Therefore we need to keep chance variation as a quite likely explanation of the overall result.

The SMR is the ratio of the observed to expected numbers of deaths from a particular cause, as noted in Chapter 6. The statistical assessment is based on the Poisson distribution, which is appropriate for rare events. The variance of the number of events on this distribution is equal to the expected number, so a chi-squared statistic (one degree of freedom) testing the difference in an SMR from the null value of 1 or 100 is given by $(Obs - Exp)^2/Exp$; for the data on sarcoma $\chi^2 = (4 - 2.04)^2/2.04 = 1.88$ ; $P = 0.17$ from Appendix Table 15. Confidence limits are much more useful, and formulae for them are given, with a useful discussion, by Checkoway et al. [2]. These formulae will produce the confidence limits published in this paper. The test-based method of calculating confidence limits is not advisable on such small numbers.

## C. Internal validity: consideration of positive features of causation

### 9. Is there a correct time relationship?

The first criterion for the time relationship is that exposure to these chemicals must have occurred before the onset of the sarcoma. Workers were included in the register and classified as exposed from the first year of the study or from the time they began a job falling into that exposure classification; in three of the cohorts minimum employment periods of 1 month, 6 months, and 1 year were specified. Once enrolled, their time experience contributed to the person-years at risk denominator, continuing until death or the end of the follow-up period. The relevant biological effect, causing the sarcoma, could predate death from the sarcoma by several years. Therefore, in those workers who develop a sarcoma, exposure after causation has been added erroneously to the denominator, and this gives an error. However, the number of workers to whom this applies is so small that it would make no difference to the results. Some of the sarcomas may indeed have originated prior to first chemical exposure, or prior to the date of entry into the cohort. These issues are addressed in analyses which look at the time dimensions of the study. If the association is causal, we would not expect death to occur within a few years of first exposure; it would happen after a time interval representing the induction time of the cancer plus the interval from cancer development to death. We might expect risk to rise steadily with time since first exposure or, as an alternative, postulate that risk would peak at a certain time after exposure and then subsequently decrease. In fact, there were no deaths within 0–9 years after first exposure, and all four deaths occurred between 10–19 years, with no deaths in the categories of 20–29 years and over 30 years since first exposure. The expected numbers show that there were substantial person-years of follow-up in these categories. The 10–19 years time-frame is compatible with a causal relationship, although the very small number of observed deaths prevents any firm conclusion about the time-specificity of the risk relationship.

## 10. Is the relationship strong?

This relationship is not particularly strong; the overall effect is a doubling of risk, four observed deaths compared with two expected. Of course, it is likely that the observed SMR, if there is a true causal effect, is an underestimate, because the categorization of exposure must have a great deal of error. The exposure is based on a job history, and for some of the groups of workers is simply employment as no specific job history was available. Within those categorized as exposed there are probably many workers with minimal exposure, and perhaps only a small group with very high levels of exposure. The SMR relates to the average exposure of this overall group. The fact that it is not particularly large means that such a result could occur through a modest amount of error or bias in the observation of death from soft-tissue sarcoma, the effect on an unidentified confounding factor, or, of course, chance variation. As all four deaths occurred in one particular category of year since first exposure, 10–19 years, for this interval there were four observed deaths and 0.66 expected, giving an SMR of 606. This is statistically significant, with a lower 95% confidence interval of 165, but as this is a post hoc choice of category, undue emphasis should not be put on this result.

## 11. Is there a dose–response relationship?

Dose–response relationships have been assessed in a number of ways in this study. First, results are presented for workers regarded as exposed or probably exposed (combined), and also for those regarded as non-exposed, with the relevant SMRs being 196 and zero. All four deaths in the combined exposure group were in exposed workers. Although this difference could be due to chance, it is consistent with causality. Similarly, those classified as sprayers have an increased SMR, with no increase being seen in production workers. This is consistent with causality if the level of exposure to these chemicals was higher in sprayers than in production workers. It is not clear whether this is true. The authors argue that the sprayers were more likely to be exposed *specifically* to these chemicals rather than to other chemicals, but they do not comment on the relative *intensity* of exposure of sprayers and production workers.

The other measure of dose–response is duration of exposure, and we would expect that the risk would increase with duration of exposure. In particular, those workers who had a very modest time of exposure might show little increase in risk. Duration of exposure was categorized into four groups, from less than 1 year up to 20 or more years. Two of the deaths occurred in workers with 10–19 years of exposure, giving an SMR of 690, and the other two deaths occurred in workers with less than 1 year of exposure, giving an SMR of 339. Thus these data do not show a dose–response relationship; indeed, the occurrence of two of the four deaths in workers with less than 1 year of exposure tends to argue against these chemicals being the cause of all four deaths.

## 12. Are the results consistent within the study?

Consistency in this study is assessed by the factors regarded as indicating high levels of exposure; these have been discussed. The number of outcome events is too small to assess other relevant aspects of consistency, for example by country, or in men and women.

## 13. Is there any specificity within the study?

A particular association with soft-tissue sarcomas would be more convincing if it were strong, and if there were no other excesses from other causes of death. In the workers categorized as exposed, there are several causes of death with SMRs higher than 200, and they are a mixed group. They include cancers of unspecified digestive organs, nose or nasal cavities, the male breast, the testes, the thyroid gland, and other endocrine glands, and there is a high SMR for benign and unspecified neoplasms. There are high SMRs for several other cancer sites in workers classified as probably exposed. Therefore the association with sarcoma is not specific in terms of the outcome. Specificity in terms of the exposure has been discussed; it appears to be specific to phenoxy herbicides.

## Conclusions with regard to internal validity

So what can we conclude about the internal validity of this study with regard to the association with sarcoma? The study seems unlikely to be open to systematic observation bias, but unsystematic error in the outcome could influence the study results. The classification of exposure is open to considerable error, reducing the power of the study to show a real association. Confounding by exposures to other chemicals seems a possible explanation of the results, and so little is known about the causation of this disease that unrecognized confounding factors cannot be ruled out. Chance variation is a quite likely alternative explanation of the results seen, as the overall result is not significant at conventional levels. Certain subcategorizations of the results are significant, and the authors put considerable stress on the SMR of 606 obtained by only assessing 10–19 years from first exposure, and the SMR of 882 by using the same criterion plus restricting to sprayers rather than production workers. While both of these examples of specificity can be justified, these justifications are essentially after the fact. Specific associations at this time period and in this particular group of workers were not clearly specified as a priori hypotheses to be tested, and so the statistical significance of these selected results has to be viewed with caution. In general, therefore, this study on its own cannot be regarded as pointing unequivocally towards a causal explanation, as the possibilities of observation bias, confounding, and chance variation all remain.

## D. **External validity: generalization of the results**

### 14. **Can the study results be applied to the eligible population?**

Generalization of the results from the participant population, those who were followed up so that mortality could be determined, to the eligible population, those employees in workplaces cooperating with the international registry, seems without problems; the participation rate was 98.4 per cent (Ex. 13.1). The main issue is whether large numbers of workers within these cohorts were lost to follow-up, and so did not contribute to the results for the whole time period. In the methods section, the loss to follow-up overall is given as about 5 per cent of the total cohort, and did not exceed 10 per cent in any particular constituent cohort. This is a very high follow-up rate.

### 15. **Can the study results be applied to the source population?**

In this study the source and eligible populations are basically the same, if we can accept that all eligible male workers in the work forces in the study were enrolled in the documented cohorts. Problems would have arisen if workers for whom exposure could not be categorized were excluded, but this was not done; such workers were maintained in the study, and results for this 'unknown exposure category' are also shown.

### 16. **Can the study results be applied to other relevant populations?**

The generalization of the results to other target populations is more difficult. We need to review the objective of the study, and we can consider it as either pragmatic or explanatory. A pragmatic objective is to assess if occupational exposure to these chemicals is associated with an increase in the mortality from soft-tissue sarcoma, which clearly has implications for management, control, and industrial compensation. The relevant issue is whether these exposed workers are representative of a wider population of exposed workers. If the workplaces contributing to this international register had particularly high levels of exposure, the association seen, even if true, might not apply to workers in other workplaces with considerably lower levels of exposure. If the workplaces studied had particularly low exposures, perhaps by having particularly good industrial hygiene standards and practices, the results could underestimate the problem. As production of these compounds has been restricted or banned in recent years (as stated in the introduction) current industrial exposures may be more stringently controlled and exposure levels may be lower than they were in the workplaces studied here.

We could argue that the purpose of the study is explanatory—to assess whether there is a causal relationship between these chemicals and soft-tissue sarcoma in general scientific terms. In this argument, we view these occupational groups not as representing occupationally exposed subjects in general, but as a natural experiment to observe the results of in human subjects. Whereas the pragmatic objective would be best fulfilled if the exposures of these workers were typical of a wider workforce, this is not relevant to an explanatory objective; indeed, selection of workplaces with the highest exposure levels would maximize the power of the study.

The other limitations, applying to both interpretations, are in gender and geography. The participants were mainly men, and so the association, if valid, might not apply to women. The workforces represented are predominantly of European ethnic backgrounds; the results might not apply to other ethnic groups. These issues would need to be explored if the results from this study were much more striking.

## E. Comparison of the results with other evidence

On its own, this study is rather unconvincing. Its generalizability, at least to adult males and with regard to the levels of exposure experienced in workplaces, are probably quite reasonable. The great weakness is the internal validity of the study. The association found is of modest size and could well occur through observational bias or error, confounding, or chance variation; none of these non-causal explanations can be ruled out confidently. Therefore the consistency with other evidence is critical.

### 17. Are the results consistent with other evidence, particularly evidence from studies of similar or more powerful study design?

We would expect any individual study of this question to be weak, because of the difficulties of studying a rare disease and a particular chemical exposure which is usually accompanied by other chemical exposures. Therefore the consistency of a large number of studies of different designs and different situations is crucial. Indeed, a meta-analysis of all available studies would give the best guidance on the topic. In the introduction to this paper it is stated that several studies had shown excesses of soft-tissue sarcoma linked to these or closely related chemicals. Given the rarity of soft-tissue sarcoma, a major problem with all studies will be small numbers, and because of this there could be a major problem of publication bias. A small study showing an excess may be published, but a small study showing no excess might not be published or even submitted for publication.

## 18. Does the total evidence suggest any specificity?

This total evidence does suggest a specific relationship between exposure to these chemicals and soft-tissue sarcoma, although associations with other diseases such as non-Hodgkin's lymphoma, which is also a tumour of non-epithelial tissue, have been suggested. Of course, a small increase in other more common diseases, such as lung cancer, would be even more difficult to detect.

## 19. Are the results plausible in terms of a biological mechanism?

Plausibility is quite important. It is relevant to know if these chemicals have carcinogenic actions, as tested on cell systems or animal models. The authors state that this evidence has been considered by the International Agency for Research in Cancer, which has a system of assessing evidence for carcinogenicity, which concluded that there was 'limited' evidence of human carcinogenicity. In other words, the relationship is regarded as plausible by a well-respected international multidisciplinary group.

## 20. If a major effect is shown, is it coherent with the distribution of the exposure and the outcome?

The argument of coherence is relevant only if the exposure in question is a major cause of the outcome, so that the occurrence of exposure and outcome would be linked, and this link would be detectable. A relative risk of the order of 2, as suggested here, means that this is not likely, although of course if real, this risk is likely to be an underestimate. A coherence argument predicts that the mortality from this disease would have increased since the 1950s when these herbicides were introduced. However, a time trend analysis of a rare condition which is difficult to classify is open to changes in diagnostic classification patterns, as well as to the influences of unidentified causal factors. It could also be argued that these sarcomas should be more common in populations with heavier exposures, which might include rural or agricultural populations, or specific workforces, and these issues could be explored in descriptive data sets looking at mortality by occupation or place of residence. It is unlikely that any of these types of analyses would add greatly to the arguments for and against causality, and they are much weaker methods than the cohort study presented here.

## Conclusions

Assessed on its own, this study has produced results which are consistent with causality, but are not convincing, as other explanations cannot be excluded (**Ex. 13.3**). Taken with the background of several other studies which also suggest an increase in this rare condition with this particular exposure, the overall evidence becomes much more persuasive. It appears from the literature reviewed in this paper that there are a considerable number of studies supporting this association. However, the balance of these reports may be influenced by publication bias. The association is plausible on the grounds of the potential carcinogenicity of these chemicals in non-human systems. Further consideration would have to assess the other published studies with a similar critical appraisal approach. The best method to assess the human evidence would be a systematic meta-analysis, in which considerable efforts would have to be made to identify relevant sets of data which might not have been published in easily accessible sources.

## Subsequent development

When published, this study was the most powerful human study of exposure to these chemicals. Even before this study, in 1986, the International Agency for Research on Cancer (IARC) had classified chlorophenoxy herbicides as having 'limited evidence of carcinogenicity in humans', group 2B in their classification, on the basis of case–control studies and limited cohort studies, together with strong animal and laboratory evidence of carcinogenicity of these compounds and the frequent contaminant TCDD [3]. This ruling still applies.

The cohort study has been expanded and continued, and a further report shows an SMR of 2.0 for soft-tissue sarcoma, based on six deaths, and of 1.12 for all cancers, both significantly increased, and also shows increases, although not significant, in mortality from non-Hodgkin's lymphoma and lung cancer [4]. The major new finding was that these increased risks appeared to be restricted to workers who were exposed to TCDD or similar contaminants; those exposed to phenoxy herbicides with minimal or no contamination showed only a small excess of soft-tissue sarcoma (SMR 1.35) and no excess of

ASSESSMENT OF A RETROSPECTIVE COHORT STUDY

A. *Description of the evidence*

| | | |
|---|---|---|
| 1 | Exposure | Occupational exposure to chlorophenoxy herbicides or chlorophenols |
| 2 | Outcome | Cancer mortality, by site |
| 3 | Design | Retrospective cohort study, average follow-up 17 years |
| 4 | Study population | 20 employee groups in 10 countries since 1955, Europe, Australia, Canada, New Zealand; over 90% male |
| 5 | Main result | Increased mortality from soft tissue sarcoma |

B. *Non-causal explanations*

| | | |
|---|---|---|
| 6 | Observation bias | Cancer deaths ascertained through routine methods; unlikely to be biased; may be incomplete ascertainment |
| 7 | Confounding | Confounding by other chemical exposures, smoking, other factors possible, but few other causal agents known for these cancers |
| 8 | Chance | Overall result non-significant, based on 4 observed deaths, SMR 196, 95% limits 53–502. For sprayers, also non-significant. Significant excesses at 10–19 years from first exposure; but this is a post hoc category |

C. *Features consistent with causation*

| | | |
|---|---|---|
| 9 | Time relationship | All 4 deaths occurred 10–19 years from first exposure; time relationship reasonable |
| 10 | Strength | Not strong: relative risk about 2; in sprayers 3 |
| 11 | Dose response | Not clear: 2 cases with duration of exposure less than 1 year |
| 12 | Consistency | Numbers too small to assess usefully |
| 13 | Specificity | Disease excess may be specific; no overall cancer excess; non-significant excesses of some other cancers |

D. *External validity*

| | | |
|---|---|---|
| 14 | Eligible population | Participants represent eligible employees |
| 15 | Source population | May represent major exposed workers internationally; no data on how exposure levels compare with workplaces not included in the source population |
| 16 | Target populations | Past exposures from 1955; current industrial exposures may be lower. Data may not apply to women |

E. *Comparison with other evidence*

| | | |
|---|---|---|
| 17 | Consistency | Consistent with some earlier small studies, which created the hypothesis in relation to soft-tissue sarcomas |
| 18 | Specificity | Association with this type of cancer may be specific |
| 19 | Plausibility | These chemicals are accepted as carcinogens; unclear why this cancer type should be affected particularly |
| 20 | Coherence | Too little known about this disease to assess coherence |

**Ex. 13.3.** Summary of assessment of the retrospective cohort study of workers exposed to chlorophenoxy herbicides and chlorophenols [1].

other cancers. However, these results are based on small numbers, with only two deaths from soft-tissue sarcomas.

A study of the female workers in this international cohort population has also been carried out [5], which is of particular interest because the animal experimental work on TCDD has suggested that it is a much more potent carcinogen in female than in male rats. No overall excess cancer risk was found in the 701 female workers followed up, but there was a significantly increased incidence (standardized incidence ratio 222) for total cancer in the subgroup exposed to herbicides contaminated with TCDD. There were no cases of soft-tissue sarcoma or non-Hodgkin's lymphoma in the female workers. Noncancer mortality has also been studied in this international cohort of workers, finding an increased rate of ischaemic heart disease in workers exposed to TCDD and similar contaminants [6].

Another study used record linkage methods to assess cancer in the children of workers at Canadian sawmills who may have been exposed to chlorophenol fungicides [7]. Over 19 000 children were identified, but there were only 40 cases of cancer, and no significant increased risk was shown.

Case–control studies have shown associations between chlorophenol exposure and cancers of the nasal sinuses [8] and nasopharynx [9], and have suggested some specificity in subtypes of sarcomas associated with chlorophenols [10].

## References

1. Saracci R, Kogevinas M, Bertazzi P-A, *et al.* Cancer mortality in workers exposed to chlorophenoxy herbicides and chlorophenols. *Lancet* 1991; **338**: 1027–1032.

2. Checkoway H, Pearce NP, Kriebel D, *Research Methods in Occupational Epidemiology* (2nd edn). Oxford: Oxford University Press, 2004.

3. International Agency for Research on Cancer. Occupational exposures to chlorophenoxy herbicides. *IARC Monogr Eval Carcinog Risk Chem Hum* 1986; **41**: 357–406.

4. Kogevinas M, Becher H, Benn T, *et al.* Cancer mortality in workers exposed to phenoxy herbicides, chlorophenols, and dioxins. An expanded and updated international cohort study. *Am J Epidemiol* 1997; **145**: 1061–1075.

5. Kogevinas M, Saracci R, Winkelmann R, *et al.* Cancer incidence and mortality in women occupationally exposed to chlorophenoxy herbicides, chlorophenols, and dioxins. *Cancer Causes Control* 1993; **4**: 547–553.

6. Vena J, Boffetta P, Becher H, *et al.* Exposure to dioxin and nonneoplastic mortality in the expanded IARC international cohort study of phenoxy herbicide and chlorophenol production workers and sprayers. *Environ Health Perspect* 1998; **106** (Suppl 2): 645–653.

7. Heacock H, Hertzman C, Demers PA, *et al.* Childhood cancer in the offspring of male sawmill workers occupationally exposed to chlorophenate fungicides. *Environ Health Perspect* 2000; **108**: 499–503.

8. Zhu K, Levine RS, Brann EA, Hall HI, Caplan LS, Gnepp DR. Case–control study evaluating the homogeneity and heterogeneity of risk factors between sinonasal and nasopharyngeal cancers. *Int J Cancer* 2002; **99**: 119–123.

9. Mirabelli MC, Hoppin JA, Tolbert PE, Herrick RF, Gnepp DR, Brann EA. Occupational exposure to chlorophenol and the risk of nasal and nasopharyngeal cancers among U.S. men aged 30 to 60. *Am J Ind Med* 2000; **37**: 532–541.

10. Hoppin JA, Tolbert PE, Flanders WD, *et al.* Occupational risk factors for sarcoma subtypes. *Epidemiology* 1999; **10**: 300–306.

Chapter 14

# Critical appraisal of a matched case–control study

In this chapter, we review a small matched case–control study, which was the first publication showing an important relationship between a disease and a widely used drug. It has been chosen because it is now of historical importance, and is a good example of an individually matched study with several issues of interpretation. In addition, it shows an interesting way of assessing confounding, which is valid although not usually used in current studies. The abstract, methods, and results are reproduced here, with the permission of the first author and the journal (excerpted with permission from the publishers from the *New England Journal of Medicine*, 4 December 1975, **293**, 1167–1170. Copyright 1975 Massachusetts Medical Society. All rights reserved).

## Increased risk of endometrial carcinoma among users of conjugated estrogens

Harry K Ziel, William D Finkle

## Abstract

The possibility that the use of conjugated estrogens increases the risk of endometrial carcinoma was investigated in patients and a twofold age-matched control series from the same population. Conjugated estrogens (principally sodium estrone sulfate) use was recorded for 57 per cent of 94 patients with endometrial carcinoma, and for 15 per cent of controls. The corresponding point estimate of the (instantaneous) risk ratio was 7.6 with a one-sided 95 per cent lower confidence limit of 4.7. The risk-ratio estimate increased with duration of exposure: from 5.6 for 1 to 4.9 years' exposure to 13.9 for seven or more years. The estimated proportion of cases related to conjugated estrogens, the etiologic fraction, was 50 per cent with a one-sided 95 per cent lower confidence limit of 41 per cent. These data suggest that conjugated estrogens have an etiologic role in endometrial carcinoma.

## Subjects and Methods

### Patients

Between July 1, 1970, and December 31, 1974, the diagnosis of endometrial cancer was made in 94 patients at the Kaiser Permanente Medical Center, Los Angeles, and reported to its tumour registry. The criterion for the definition of endometrial cancer was a pathological diagnosis of endometrial adenocarcinoma or adenocanthoma; mixed Müllerian sarcoma and choriocarcinoma were excluded.

### Control subjects

Control subjects were selected in the following way. The membership files of the Southern Californian Kaiser Foundation Health Plan population were reviewed, and all members in the vicinity of the Los Angeles facility whose record designations ended in arbitrarily selected numbers were identified and listed. From the list, two control subjects were selected for each patient and matched for birth date within one year, area of residence by postal zip code, duration of Health Plan membership (each control subject had been a member at least as long as the associated patient), and potential for the development of endometrial cancer by the control subject's having an intact uterus. The patient and the two control subjects thus constituted a matched triple.

### Record review

The data source for the 94 matched triples was the clinic record. To avoid information bias that could result from the more probing clinical history taken after identification of the cancer, the following procedure was employed for each matched triple. A medical-records clerk requested all three records from the record room and reviewed those of the control subjects to determine whether they had an intact uterus. Subjects without an intact uterus were replaced by selection of others from the original list. The clerk determined the date of diagnosis for each patient, and then the date one year before that diagnosis (the reference date). The clerk concealed all information in the record after the reference date. For control subjects, information recorded during the same period was similarly concealed. The record was then given to an abstractor, who filled out the abstract form without knowing whether the record was that of a patient or a control.

### Results

For any given triple, there were six possible combinations of conjugated-estrogen use; all three were users; the patient and one of the control subjects were users; and so forth. The observed frequencies for each of the six possible combinations for each of the 94 triples are shown in Table 1. These data were used to estimate the risk ratio associated with the use of conjugated estrogens and the etiologic fraction (the proportion of cases due to conjugated estrogens). The (maximum-likelihood) point estimate of the relative risk ($\hat{RR}$) is 7.6. The significance test statistic ($\chi_1^2$) is 49 ($P \ll 10^{-8}$). The approximate 95 per cent one-sided lower confidence limit of the risk ratio (RR) is 4.7. The point estimate of the etiologic fraction ($\hat{EF}$) is 50 per cent. For this parameter, Miettinen's proposed (test-based) computation of the 95 per cent one-sided lower confidence limit (EF) yields 41 per cent.

Data on the relative risk ratio to duration of exposure are given in Table 2. Even with only 1.0 to 4.9 years of use, the point estimate is 5.6, with a corresponding 95 per cent one-sided confidence limit of 2.7. For uses of less than one year's duration, the data are too scanty to be informative.

## A. **Description of the evidence**

1. What was the exposure or intervention?
2. What was the outcome?
3. What was the study design?
4. What was the study population?
5. What was the main result?

The exposure is the use of conjugated estrogenic drugs, as recorded in medical records up to 1 year before the date of diagnosis of the cases, or the equivalent time for the controls (we will use the American spelling in this chapter). The outcome is the pathologically confirmed diagnosis of endometrial adenocarcinoma or adenocanthoma. The design is an individually matched retrospective case–control study. The case subjects were diagnosed at the Kaiser Permanente Medical Centre between 1970 and 1974, and were reported to its tumour registry. For each case, two controls were chosen from the membership files of the health plan which operates this hospital, matched for birth date within 1 year, area of residence by postal code, duration of health plan membership, and possession of an intact uterus. The main result of the study was that estrogen use was recorded in 57 per cent of cases and in 15 per cent of controls, giving an odds ratio of 7.6 for 'ever use' (**Ex. 14.1**). The note at the end of this chapter explains how this is calculated.

## B. **Internal validity – consideration of non-causal explanations**

### 6. **Are the results likely to be affected by observation bias?**

Since this is a case–control study, the major problems relate to the assessment of exposure. Assessment of disease status is straightforward. For the cases, this was

ESTROGENS AND ENDOMETRIAL CANCER - RESULTS

Distribution of triples by use of conjugated estrogens

| Patients' use of conjugated estrogens | Controls' use of conjugated estrogens | | | |
|---|---|---|---|---|
| | Both | One | Neither | Totals |
| Used | 1 | 16 | 37 | 54 |
| Did not use | 0 | 11 | 29 | 40 |
| Totals | 1 | 27 | 66 | 94 |

| | Used conjugated estrogens | | Did not use conjugated estrogens | | Totals |
|---|---|---|---|---|---|
| Exposure rates: | No. | % | No | % | |
| Patients | 54 | (57) | 40 | (43) | 94 |
| Controls | 29 | (15) | 159 | (85) | 188 |

**Ex. 14.1.** History of conjugated estrogen use among 94 patients with endometrial cancer and 188 matched control subjects: the matching criteria were age, area of residence, duration of Health Plan membership, and intact uterus. Data shown as presented in Table 1 in the original paper. From Ziel and Finkle [1]

a pathologically confirmed diagnosis with little chance of inaccuracy. It is possible that some of the control subjects had undiagnosed endometrial adenocarcinoma, but this would result only in a reduction of the observed risk ratio.

The information on estrogen use is based on a medical record review done in a blind fashion. One clerk obtained the records for each set of cases and controls, and concealed all information recorded after a reference date 1 year before the date of diagnosis for the case, and a corresponding date for the controls. A different clerk abstracted the information from each record, without knowing whether the record belonged to a case or a control. Further information on the quality of the medical records would be helpful, in particular any independent assessment of the completeness and accuracy of drug recording. There could be substantial under-reporting of drug usage, as drugs might have been used that were not prescribed within this particular health plan, or were not recorded; also, some drugs prescribed may not have been used. Such errors, if randomly distributed amongst all subjects, would serve only to reduce the observed association. The crucial question is whether there is any likelihood of estrogen use being more completely recorded in those subjects who were later diagnosed as have endometrial cancer than in the control subjects. The blindness of the abstraction, and the exclusion of any material relating to the period 1 year before diagnosis provides some protection. Could other factors affect this? Endometrial cancer is more common in the higher socio-economic groups. Might such patients have more completely recorded drug histories? This seems unlikely as all the study participants used the same health care system. Is it possible that patients who eventually were diagnosed with endometrial cancer had a more frequent history of gynaecological and related problems, resulting not only in a greater prescribing of these drugs but also a greater recording of such prescribing? For parity, obesity, and age at menopause, the data were more complete for the cases than for the controls. Could the information on estrogens also be more complete? Counter-arguments are that no excess was seen for several other drugs, an indication for the use of estrogens was recorded more frequently in the controls, and that the association was very strong (see below). It seems unwise to accept totally results based on review of one medical record, without independent verification, and the issue of observation bias cannot be dismissed.

## 7. Are the results likely to be affected by confounding?

The subjects were matched by age, area of residence (which probably gives some measure of socio-economic matching), and duration of health plan membership; a matched analysis has been performed. Potential confounding factors are those related both to the incidence of endometrial cancer and to the use of estrogenic drugs. The literature on endometrial cancer was reviewed in the paper; at that time there were several recognized risk factors such as high parity, obesity, and late age at menopause. For each of these, the authors used information from the medical records to assess the confounding effect by stratified analysis. Substantial data were missing on each of these topics. Rather than presenting unconfounded odds ratio estimates obtained from the stratified analysis, the authors have used a less familiar technique in calculating the 'confounding risk ratio', which is a measure of the extent to which the association is produced by confounding. An explanation of this method is given at the end of this chapter. The confounding effect for each of the three factors of parity, obesity, and age at menopause is very minor, but the analysis is limited by the missing data. No other confounding factors had been shown to have major associations. Some protection against the observed association being due to confounding is given by the strength of the association; the odds ratio is high compared with the odds ratio of 1.5–3 usually quoted for factors such as parity or obesity.

At the time this paper was published there was little written on the factors related to estrogen use. Of prime importance is the indication for estrogen usage, as the observed association with the drug could be disguising a true association with the indication for the drug. The indications for the use of conjugated estrogens are unclear, and must reflect psychological and social as well as medical factors. The most frequently recorded indication was hot flashes. If the case patients used more estrogenic drugs, and if the indications for use of estrogens were the same in cases and controls, this implies that the case subjects suffered from hot flashes more frequently than did the controls, suffered from them more severely, sought treatment more readily, or for some other reason were given these drugs as treatment more readily. Thus there is a competing hypothesis that endometrial cancer could be related to hot flashes. A further possibility is that cases might have a high usage of drugs in general; this can be dismissed as the cases were recorded as using diazepam, reserpine, and thyroid drugs less commonly than were the controls. Thus there is protection against confounding by most of the major known risk factors for endometrial carcinoma. However, there is a viable alternative hypothesis to causation—that the disease is related not to the use of estrogens but to the indications for their use.

## 8. Are the results likely to be affected by chance variation?

The estimated odds ratio is 7.6, and the associated $P$-value is less than $10^{-8}$, giving 95 per cent two-sided confidence limits of 4.3 and 13.4. Thus chance variation can be excluded. The methods used in the statistical analysis are a little different from those presented in this text; a note on them is given at the end of this chapter. Some publications will use more complex methods than those described in this book, which may have particular advantages for that study. However, the results should differ greatly from those obtained by the methods described here. The reader might like to apply the methods for analysis of a matched case–control study that are presented in Appendix Table 6. These give an odds ratio of 8.2, and an associated $\chi^2$ statistic of 48.8.

## Summary: non-causal explanations

Thus of the three non-causal explanations, we can effectively exclude chance, but must keep in mind the possibilities of observation bias and of confounding, particularly by the indication for drug usage.

## C. Internal validity: consideration of positive features of causation

### 9. Is there a correct time relationship?

This study, as is common with case–control studies, is fairly weak with regard to time relationships. The method of data collection has the important feature of excluding any information recorded in the year before clinical diagnosis, and therefore we can conclude that the drugs assessed were prescribed before the endometrial cancer was diagnosed. But could the disease or its precursor have been present even earlier, and have produced symptoms which led to the prescription for the drugs? We do not know if any of the case subjects had previous tests (e.g. a curettage) that would have detected the disease or a related state such as hyperplasia. The time relationship is not clear; no data for risk by time since first use of estrogens are given. As it is unlikely that the records go back many years, we assume that the risk is seen only a few years from first exposure. This appears inconsistent with a cancer initiator action, which typically takes decades; if the risk is causal, it shows a short-term action.

## 10. Is the association strong?

The relationship is strong, with a high odds ratio of 7.6. This odds ratio is greater than those associated with even extremes of parity, obesity, late menopause, and other recognized risk factors for endometrial carcinoma, making it unlikely that this association could be produced by confounding by such factors. However, it is no protection against the association being due to the indication for the drug rather than the usage of the drug, as the association between these two may be very close. To assess its relevance for observation bias, it is useful to go to the raw data, which show that estrogen use was recorded for 57 per cent of the case subjects compared with 15 per cent of the controls. Thus for the association to be totally due to observation bias would require, for example, that estrogen use was always recorded for the case subjects, but recorded on only about 25 per cent of occasions for the controls; this seems implausible. Thus the strength of the association protects against some aspects of confounding and against observation bias, but not against what is emerging as the chief competing hypothesis—an association with the indication rather than with the drug prescribed.

## 11. Is there a dose–response relationship?

Information on this is limited by the completeness of the records, but the data in **Ex. 14.2** show the odds ratio increasing from shorter to longer exposures. While the odds ratios for each exposure category are significantly different from the unexposed, a test for trend is not included. This dose–response is not very helpful; it could occur if the relationship were produced by confounding by the indication for the drug, or even from observation bias. Information on the relationship between risk and time since first use or since last use might be of more help, but is not given.

| Group | RELATIONSHIP WITH DURATION OF EXPOSURE | | | | | | |
|---|---|---|---|---|---|---|---|
| | Duration of exposure (yr) | | | | | | |
| | Unknown | ≥7 | 5.0–6.9 | 1.0–4.9 | <1 | Non-exposed | Totals |
| Patients (No.) | 14 | 14 | 9 | 14 | 3 | 40 | 94 |
| Controls (No.) | 6 | 4 | 5 | 10 | 4 | 159 | 188 |
| RR | 9.3 | 13.9 | 7.2 | 5.6 | | (1.0)[†] | |
| (RR) | 4.2 | 6.0 | 2.8 | 2.7 | | | |
| $\chi_1^2$ | 22 | 26 | 12 | 15 | | | |
| P | $<10^{-5}$ | $<10^{-5}$ | <.01 | <.01 | | | |

**Ex. 14.2.** Duration of use of conjugated estrogens by patients with endometrial cancer and by control subjects with risk-ratio analysis: point estimate (RR), 95 per cent one-sided lower confidence bound (RR), and chi-square test statistic ($\chi_1^2$). [†]Reference group. Data shown as presented in Table 2 of the original paper. From Ziel and Finkle [1]

## 12. Are the results consistent within the study? and
## 13. Is there any specificity within the study?

The association shows some specificity, as no increased risks were seen with diazepam, reserpine, and thyroid drugs. This protects mainly against gross observation bias, i.e. the possibility that all drugs would be recorded more frequently for the cases. Beyond that, a separation of patients with different indications for the use of the estrogen drugs would be helpful, but this would probably need a special study rather than one using routine medical records. Separation of different estrogenic preparations would also help, but there is no information on the precise preparations used. An association with a particular drug is more convincing if no association is seen with other drugs used for the same indications.

## Conclusions with regard to internal validity

The second part of our assessment of internal validity has not been particularly helpful, and this is often the situation in assessing a relatively small study. Larger studies give more opportunity to assess consistency between subgroups, dose–response relationships, and so on. Therefore the assessment of internal validity depends on the comparison of the causal hypothesis with the alternatives of bias and confounding. The main alternative hypothesis is that the association is not due to the drug itself, but to the symptoms for which the drug has been prescribed, which might be caused by the developing carcinoma, or be indications of an altered physiological state produced by mechanisms akin to those producing the tumour. To assess this alternative we need information from other studies, as will be seen.

## D. External validity: generalization of the results

### 14. Can the study results to applied to the eligible population?

The eligible population comprises the members of the Kaiser Foundation Health Plan, and there is little problem applying the results to them. If we accept that they would all attend this medical centre and that the tumour registry is efficient, all patients with a histological diagnosis during the stated time period were included, and medical records on all of them were obtained. The control subjects, apart from the appropriate matching criteria, should be representative of unaffected members of the plan, with the limitation that they include only women with an intact uterus. This is an appropriate criterion, both on the argument that women without a uterus are not at risk of developing endometrial cancer and therefore are not eligible as cases, and also because women who have had their uterus removed may be different in terms of estrogen usage.

### 15. Can the study results be applied to the source population?

The source and eligible populations in this study are essentially the same.

### 16. Can the study results be applied to other relevant populations?

The study was done on members of the Kaiser Foundation Health Plan diagnosed between 1970 and 1974 in Los Angeles. Are members of this health plan different from women in Los Angeles in general? Further information would be required, but we might assume that plan members are likely to be fairly affluent stable subjects, who can afford a comprehensive prepaid health plan. No information is given on racial origin. However, the representativeness of the subjects in the study is not the most important issue. The main question is: Is the *association* seen likely to apply to other women? If the true relationship is between the drug and the disease, the finding is likely to be widely applicable. In other populations, the value of the odds ratio may be considerably different, depending on the usual dosage and length of time the drugs are used. If the true association is with a specific type of drug, the association may not be seen in societies where other types are used. Even if the association is consistent, its importance will depend on the type, frequency, and dosage of the drugs used, and on the level of background incidence of endometrial cancer, produced by other factors. In this study population, a strong association is seen with a drug used frequently—in 15 per cent of controls; the attributable proportion is 87 per cent in those exposed and 50 per cent in the population—if causal, estrogens are the main cause of the disease. (These calculations are shown at the end of this chapter.)

## E. **Comparison of the results with other evidence**

### 17. **Are the results consistent with other evidence, particularly evidence from studies of similar or more powerful study design?**

This study was chosen because it was one of the first to suggest this association. In the same issue of the same journal another case–control study, from Seattle, was published, showing a similar association, and this strengthens the credibility of these results [2]. However, if this other study is assessed, bearing in mind the conclusion we have reached on the present study, i.e. that the association is likely to be either causal or due to an association between the indication for the drug and endometrial cancer, we find that the same limitation applies to its interpretation. Because of the importance of the association suggested, these two papers were followed reasonably rapidly by several other case–control studies and some cohort studies. There have been randomized trials of estrogen use, but these have been too small to assess the outcome of endometrial cancer.

### 18. **Does the total evidence suggest any specificity?**

At the time this paper was published there was no relevant information. However, several later studies confirmed the association in the USA, where conjugated estrogens were used widely, whereas studies in some other countries showed no risk because the use of conjugated estrogens was much less. It appears that patients who would be treated with conjugated estrogens in the USA would be treated with a mixture of estrogens and progestogens in Europe, and this combination did not appear to confer a marked increased risk of endometrial cancer.

### 19. **Are the results plausible in terms of a biological mechanism?**

The authors review epidemiological and experimental evidence that estrogens may produce endometrial cancer, and the association seems biologically acceptable. The time issue is relevant. Cancer-initiating factors produce tumours only many years after exposure, but this association does not fit this pattern. Hormones in general are not initiators of cancer, but act as cancer promoters, and this action would be consistent with a short-term effect.

20. **If a major effect is shown, is it coherent with the distribution of the exposure and the outcome?**

This study does show a major effect, and the authors calculated that in this population approximately 50 per cent of endometrial cancer was caused by these drugs, if the association they have shown is causal. They also noted that the usage of these drugs quadrupled between 1962 and 1973, and therefore a noticeable increase in the incidence of endometrial carcinoma in the USA would be expected. They reviewed the literature available at that time, which did not show any such increase, but pointed out that an increase might be disguised by an increase in the prevalence of hysterectomy for non-cancer reasons. Subsequent work published some months later, using better information, did show a substantial rise in the incidence of endometrial cancer in the USA. Strong evidence of causality is given by the trends in the years after the publication of this and other studies; there was a reduction in the prescribing of these drugs, and a fairly rapid reduction in the incidence of this tumour [3,4]. As well as the time relationship, we would expect the excess incidence to occur in geographical areas, and in social groups, in which the usage of these estrogenic drugs was maximum, and the difference between American and European experience in this regard has already been mentioned.

Coherence is the item on which the two major hypotheses can be separated. If the association with the drug is merely indicating a true association with symptoms, the rapid rise in use of the drugs will not affect the incidence rate, while a direct effect of the magnitude given will have doubled the previous incidence in this population. Thus, given the size of the effect, there should be a close association between the use of these drugs and the incidence of endometrial cancer in terms of time, place, and person. If the real relationship is with the indication, no such associations will be found. Therefore the concordance of drug usage and disease subsequently shown between countries, social groups, and over time is crucial.

## Conclusions

The study shows a large and important association, which is most likely to be due to one of two mechanisms; either a causal relationship between the use of these particular drugs and the development of endometrial cancer, or an association between the indications for those drugs and an increased risk of endometrial cancer (**Ex. 14.3**). There are other possibilities, that the result reflects other confounding factors, or that it is produced by observation bias with regard to the medical records on which the data on estrogen exposure were based, but these seem less likely. If the association is real, it is likely to

---

ASSESSMENT OF A CASE-CONTROL STUDY

A. *Description of evidence*

| | | |
|---|---|---|
| 1 | Exposure | Conjugated estrogens; use in period up to 1 year before diagnosis; assessed from medical records |
| 2 | Outcome | Endometrial cancer; adenocarcinoma, adenoacanthoma |
| 3 | Design | Case–control study |
| 4 | Study population | Cases—all those diagnosed at Kaiser Permanante Medical Center, Los Angeles, July 1970-Dec. l974; $n = 94$<br>Controls—from LA members of Kaiser plan, matched for age, residence, length of membership; two per case |
| 5 | Main result | Odds ratio = 7.6; 95 per cent confidence limits = 4.3 to 13.4; strong positive association of estrogen use with endometrial cancer |

B. *Non-causal explanations*

| | | |
|---|---|---|
| 6 | Observation bias | Possible—recording of drug use might be more complete on cases, despite protection of blind abstraction and avoiding period immediately before diagnosis |
| 7 | Confounding | Major risk factors for endometrial cancer controlled by matching or stratification. Most likely non-causal hypothesis is an association with the indications for drug usage |
| 8 | Chance | Can be excluded |

C. *Features consistent with causation*

| | | |
|---|---|---|
| 9 | Time relationship | Drug usage at least 1 year before clinical diagnosis, but it is possible that preclinical or precursor state might have existed prior to then |
| 10 | Strength | Strong association—protects against many alternative hypotheses but not helpful if the true association is with the indication for the drug |
| 11 | Dose response | Seen with total duration of exposure |
| 12 | Consistency | Information not available |
| 13 | Specificity | Information not available |

D. *External validity*

| | | |
|---|---|---|
| 14 | Eligible population | No difficulties in applying results |
| 15 | Source population | Same as eligible |
| 16 | Other populations | While frequency and mode of usage may vary, association, if causal, is likely to be widely applicable. Studies in other populations may help distinguish causal hypothesis from hypothesis of an association with the indication for the drug, and indicate which particular drugs are involved |

E. *Comparison with other evidence*

| | | |
|---|---|---|
| 17 | Consistency | One other case-control study at time of publication. Further support later. No strong support for competing hypothesis of the association being with indications for the drug |

**Ex. 14.3. cont'd**

| | |
|---|---|
| 18 Specificity | Evidence for specificity to unconjugated estrogens used alone emerged later |
| 19 Plausibility | Time relationship makes a long-term cancer initiator action unlikely. A short-term promoter action is plausible and supported by some experimental work |
| 20 Coherence | Shown by later work. Evidence of incidence rate of endometrial cancer rising with use of estrogenic drugs and later falling is strong evidence against the competing hypothesis of the association being with the indication |

**Ex. 14.3.** Summary of assessment of the case-control study of endometrial cancer by Ziel and Finkle [1]

apply to other women who are exposed to these same agents, and therefore is of substantial practical importance.

Thus, in assessing priorities for further investigation and for critical reading of subsequent results, we shall look particularly for studies that can differentiate between a direct effect of the drug and an effect of the indications for the drug. One piece of evidence that has already been noted is the secular variation in the incidence of the disease. Studies in other countries, where women presumably have the same sort of symptoms but may be treated differently, are helpful. Other than that, we look for studies using more reliable methods of assessing drug exposure, perhaps medical records supplemented by independent reviews or direct interviews, even though recall bias may then become an issue. Prospective studies of users of these drugs would be useful, and the ultimate would be a trial in which women regarded as eligible for treatment with conjugated estrogens were randomized either to receive such treatment or to receive a non-estrogen alternative. However, to mount such a study would be extremely difficult in terms of the number of women required, and also might be regarded as unethical. Randomized trials have been set up to look at the short-term effects of estrogens, such as the relief of symptoms, but are not large enough to look at cancer incidence.

## Subsequent development

This paper, and the other case–control study published simultaneously [2], provided the first information on an important relationship between estrogenic drugs and endometrial cancer. The studies raised much controversy and were vigorously criticized, primarily by gynaecologists who had used the drugs clinically for many years and were reluctant to accept epidemiological evidence of a major hazard. In arguments reminiscent of the debate concerning smoking and lung cancer in the 1950s, some of the criticisms were along the lines that case–control studies could not demonstrate causation. One anonymous editorialist in a prominent journal (*The Lancet*) criticized the studies on the grounds that they were not prospective and randomized, without discussing the reality that a prospective randomized trial to answer this question would be logistically extremely difficult because of the numbers required, and of course ethically dubious [5]. In response to this, the authors of one of the observational studies commented that if such rules of evidence were applied generally, even the cause of pregnancy could not be regarded as established [6].

The main more serious controversy related to the difficulty of separating an association with the drug itself from an association with the indications for the drug. Studies comparing patients with endometrial cancer with other patients attending the same gynaecological services who had had similar presenting symptoms, such as uterine bleeding, showed similar rates of estrogen usage and therefore no association. However, subsequent studies demonstrated that the most reasonable explanation for these results was that estrogenic drugs caused both benign hyperplasia leading to bleeding, and also endometrial cancer [7]. Further work also established that if estrogenic preparations were used together with progestogens, the risk of endometrial cancer was no longer increased, thus providing a management plan that could avoid this problem. Endometrial cancer risk is increased approximately 10-fold after prolonged estrogen use. However, the tumours produced tend to be diagnosed earlier because they bleed easily, and are usually of low grade and stage with an excellent prognosis [8]. With the benefit of hindsight, this association between endometrial cancer and estrogenic drugs represents an example of an important aetiological relationship being first demonstrated in retrospective case–control studies.

Thirty years on, the association of estrogen drugs with endometrial cancer is accepted, and use of estrogenic drugs alone is regarded as contraindicated in women with an intact uterus [9]. A meta-analysis of 30 observational studies showed an overall relative risk estimate of 2.3 comparing users with non-users, rising to 9.5 after 10 years of use [10]. A Cochrane systematic review of 15 randomized trials and a further meta-analysis of both trials and observational studies have been done [11,12], which showed that combined estrogen and progesterone therapy does not increase endometrial cancer risk. Although these drugs do control menopausal symptoms, their longer-term risks and benefits are still controversial.

The US Preventive Services Task Force has assessed the risks and benefits of this therapy. They concluded that, while both unopposed estrogen and estrogen–progesterone combined therapy reduced the risk of fractures, both may increase the risk of stroke, dementia, and impaired cognitive function (all with 'fair' evidence using the Task Force's classification, described in Chapter 9), and venous thromboembolism (good evidence for combined therapy, fair for estrogen alone). In addition, combined therapy increased breast cancer (good evidence) and may decrease colorectal cancer (fair evidence). Neither therapy confers any reduction in the risk of heart disease, despite earlier evidence. On the basis of all the evidence, the US Preventive Services Task Force recommends against the use of either combined or unopposed estrogen for the prevention of chronic conditions, at grade D ('at least fair evidence that the intervention is ineffective or that harms outweigh benefits') [13].

# The analysis used in the paper by Ziel and Finkle

## Main analysis

The basic data for this matched case–control study with two controls per case are given in Ex. 14.1. The formula shown in Appendix Table 6 gives an odds ratio of 8.2. This is rather different from the maximum likelihood point estimate calculated by the authors by a more complicated iterative procedure, which is 7.6, and such disparity is to be expected with these relatively small numbers. The chi-squared statistic, calculated by the variant of the Mantel–Haenszel procedure given in Appendix Table 6 is 48.8, identical with that given in the paper. A chi statistic of 6.98 ($\sqrt{48.8}$) is out of the range of most conventional tables; but using the function shown in Appendix Table 16 gives the corresponding two-sided $P$-value as $<10^{-9}$.

The odds ratio calculated from an unmatched analysis can also be derived from Ex. 14.1, which gives a value of 7.4; the difference between this and the result of the matched paired analysis is small. In Ex. 14.2, where small numbers are subdivided by duration of exposure, unmatched analyses are used, and the appropriate chi-squared statistic can be derived by the usual formula for case–control studies given in Appendix Table 1; an exact test (Appendix Table 4) and a test for trend (Appendix Table 7) can also be applied.

The test-based confidence limits calculated in the paper use the test-based method shown in Ex. 7.7, incorporating the maximum likelihood point estimate of odds ratio derived by the authors and the chi statistic of 6.98.

## Control of confounding

Briefly, the confounding risk ratio [14] is the odds ratio linking exposure to outcome, which is produced by the confounder; it can be thought of as the risk ratio which would be observed in the absence of any direct association. If there is no confounding, it will be 1.0; if the crude association is totally due to confounding, the confounding risk ratio will equal the crude risk ratio. The crude risk ratio $OR_c$, the confounding risk ratio $OR_f$, and the unconfounded or standardized risk ratio $OR_s$ are simply related as follows:

$$OR_c = OR_f \times OR_s.$$

Thus controlling for parity gives a crude odds ratio ($OR_c$) for estrogens and endometrial cancer of 6.71 (different from the risk for the whole study because of the missing data), and a confounding odds ratio $OR_f$ of 1.18 (showing very little confounding). The unconfounded odds ratio $OR_s$ is given by 6.71/1.18 = 5.69. The authors also calculate a 'confounding effect' relating the extent of confounding to the size of the unconfounded risk ratio, giving $(1.18 - 1)/(5.69 - 1) = 4$ per cent.

## Attributable proportion

Using the formulae shown in Ex. 3.6, the overall odds ratio is 7.6 and the proportion $p$ of controls exposed is 15 per cent (Ex. 14.1). The attributable proportion (= 'aetiological fraction') in those exposed is

$$(OR - 1)/OR = 87 \text{ per cent}$$

and the attributable proportion in the population is

$$p(OR - 1)/(p(OR - 1) + 1) = 50 \text{ per cent}.$$

## References

1. **Ziel HK, Finkle WD.** Increased risk of endometrial carcinoma among users of conjugated estrogens. *N Engl J Med* 1975; **293**: 1167–1170.
2. **Smith DC, Prentice R, Thompson DJ, Herrmann WL.** Association of exogenous estrogen and endometrial carcinoma. *N Engl J Med* 1975; **293**: 1164–1167.
3. **Weiss NS, Szekely DR, Austin DF.** Increasing incidence of endometrial cancer in the United States. *N Engl J Med* 1976; **294**: 1259–1262.
4. **Austin DF, Roe KM.** The decreasing incidence of endometrial cancer: public health implications. *Am J Public Health* 1982; **72**: 65–68.
5. Anonymous. Hormone replacement therapy and endometrial carcinoma. *Lancet* 1977; **i**: 577–578.
6. **Mack TM, Pike MC.** Hormone replacement therapy and endometrial carcinoma. *Lancet* 1977; **i**: 1358.
7. **Hulka BS, Grimson RC, Greenberg BG, et al.** 'Alternative' controls in a case–control study of endometrial cancer and exogenous estrogen. *Am J Epidemiol* 1980; **112**: 376–387.
8. **Hulka BS.** Links between hormone replacement therapy and neoplasia. *Fertil Steril* 1994; **62**(6 Suppl 2): 168S–175S.

9. **The North American Menopause Society.** Role of progestogen in hormone therapy for postmenopausal women: position statement of The North American Menopause Society. *Menopause* 2003; **10**: 113–132.

10. **Grady D, Gebretsadik T, Kerlikowske K, Ernster V, Petitti D.** Hormone replacement therapy and endometrial cancer risk: a meta-analysis. *Obstet Gynecol* 1995; **85**: 304–313.

11. **Farquhar CM, Marjoribanks J, Lethaby A, Lamberts Q, Suckling JA.** Long term hormone therapy for perimenopausal and postmenopausal women. *Cochrane Database Syst Rev* 2005; Jul 20 (3): CD004143.

12. **Nelson HD, Humphrey LL, Nygren P, Teutsch SM, Allan JD.** Postmenopausal hormone replacement therapy: scientific review. *JAMA* 2002; **288**: 872–881.

13. **U.S. Preventive Services Task Force.** Hormone therapy for the prevention of chronic conditions in postmenopausal women: recommendations from the U.S. Preventive Services Task Force. *Ann Intern Med* 2005; **142**: 855–860.

14. **Miettinen OS.** Components of the crude risk ratio. *Am J Epidemiol* 1972; **96**: 168–172.

# Chapter 15

# Critical appraisal of a large population-based case–control study

We will now discuss a large population-based case–control study, published in the *Journal of the National Cancer Institute*, June 21 1995, **87**, 923–929 [1], and available at http://jncicancerspectrum.oxfordjournals.org. The abstract is reproduced here, courtesy of Oxford University Press and the first author.

## Risk of breast cancer in relation to lifetime alcohol consumption

Matthew P Longnecker, Polly A Newcomb, Robert Mittendorf, E Robert Greenberg, Richard W Clapp, Gregory F Bogdan, John Baron, Brian MacMahon, Walter C Willett

## Abstract

**Background**. Although an association between alcohol consumption and risk of breast cancer has been observed in many studies, questions of major importance remain, including the nature of the dose–response relationship and the effects of drinking at various periods in life.

**Purpose**. Our goal was to address the issues listed above with a large case–control study.

**Methods**. We conducted a population-based case–control study in Maine, Massachusetts (excluding the four counties that include metropolitan Boston), New Hampshire, and Wisconsin. Case patients were eligible if their diagnosis of invasive breast cancer was first reported to one of the four statewide cancer registries during the period of 1988 through 1991. During the accrual period, 11 879 potentially eligible case patients and 16 217 control subjects were identified. After excluding ineligible women from the study, telephone interviews were obtained from 6888 case patients and 9424 control subjects. Complete data for recent alcohol consumption, and thus final eligibility for study participation, were determined for 6662 case patients and 9163 control subjects. The average age at time of interview was 58.7 years. The questions on alcohol use addressed average consumption during five periods of the subjects' lives: ages 16–19, 20–29, 30–39, 40–59, and 60–74 years. Similar responses from 211 control subjects upon reinterview 6–12 months later were taken to be indicative of the reliability of the questionnaire used in this study.

**Results.** Lifetime average alcohol consumption (measured as the average grams per day consumed from age 16 to the recent past) and recent alcohol consumption (average grams per day consumed in the previous age interval) were associated with risk of developing breast cancer. The multivariate relative risk of breast cancer, in those who drink compared with abstainers, associated with average lifetime consumption of 12–18 g/day of alcohol (about one drink) was 1.39 (95% confidence interval [CI] = 1.16–1.67), of 19–32 g/day (about two drinks) was 1.69 (95% CI = 1.36–2.10), of 33–45 g/day (about three drinks) was 2.30 (95% CI = 1.51–3.51), and of greater than or equal to 46 g/day (four or more drinks) was 1.75 (95% CI = 1.65–2.64) (*P* for trend <.0001). The multivariate relative risk per 13 g/day (about one drink) of alcohol consumed before 30 years of age was 1.09 (95% CI = 0.95–1.24), whereas the relative risk associated with recent consumption of 13 g/day was 1.21 (95% CI = 1.09–1.34).

**Conclusions.** In these data, alcohol consumption was clearly related to breast cancer risk. Risk appeared to increase even at moderate levels of consumption. For women of all ages combined, consumption before 30 years of age was not an important determinant of risk.


A. **Description of the evidence**

1. What was the exposure or intervention?
2. What was the outcome?
3. What was the study design?
4. What was the study population?
5. What was the main result?

The exposure in this study is previous alcohol consumption, and the outcome is breast cancer; this is a case–control study. The association between alcohol consumption and breast cancer was already well established [2], as noted in the introduction, and so the objective of this study was to measure the association more precisely, particularly with regard to the dose–response relationship and the effects of alcohol consumption at different ages. Cases were obtained from population-based cancer registries, and controls from the corresponding general populations. The study population was women resident in four defined areas of the USA, who had cancer diagnosed and reported to the corresponding registries between 1988 and 1991, and were aged under 75 years. Controls were selected from the general population within that age range from the same four areas. A prime issue in any case–control study is finding an appropriate listing of population members from which controls can be chosen. In this study the listings chosen were the drivers' licence lists held at state level for subjects aged under 65, and the list of Medicare beneficiaries for subjects aged between 65 and 74. The interviews were carried out by telephone. For these reasons, the controls, if aged under 65, had to have a driving licence and a listed telephone number, and therefore similar restrictions were made for the cases. For the age range 65–74, all subjects should be on Medicare files, and therefore the restriction was only in terms of telephone listings. The full methods section as published is detailed and worth reading.

The main result was a positive association between increasing risk of breast cancer and increasing lifetime alcohol intake. **Ex. 15.1** shows the results for lifetime average daily alcohol consumption, showing the ability of this large study to explore the dose relationship. Average daily alcohol consumption was divided into seven categories, and relative risks were calculated for each category with reference to the zero consumption category. The numbers of case and control subjects in each group, and the crude odds ratios (which in this study are equivalent to relative risks) are shown; these are calculated from the raw data by the methods shown in Chapter 3 and Appendix Table 1. These crude relative risks are not presented in the published paper as they do not take any of the confounding factors into account, but calculating the crude risks when appraising a paper is useful in understanding the data and may illustrate any major discrepancies. The published results show the relative risks adjusted for age and state by the Mantel–Haenszel method, as these are the chief demographic variables on which comparability is required. The 'multivariate adjusted' relative risks, adjusted for the range of variables described in the methods section, are also shown; these will be discussed under 'confounding' below. These three sets of results are generally quite similar. The most appropriate results to use for interpretation are the multivariate adjusted risk ratios, and these are given in the summary. There is a steadily increasing risk with increasing alcohol consumption except in the highest category, where the relative risk is lower than would be expected from a simple linear trend. The association can also be expressed as the relative risk per 13 g/day intake; this unit is used because it is equivalent to one drink of most types of alcoholic beverage. This is a useful parameter for making comparisons between subgroups, as will be shown. The statistical tests will be discussed in due course.

BREAST CANCER AND ALCOHOL CONSUMPTION: RESULTS

*All subjects, by lifetime average alcohol consumption*

| Alcohol g/day | Numbers of cases | Numbers of controls | *Crude odds ratio* | RR: age and state adjusted | RR: multivariate adjusted risk ratio |
|---|---|---|---|---|---|
| 0 | 698 | 1165 | *1 (Ref)* | 1 (Ref) | 1 (Ref) |
| >0–5 | 4080 | 5864 | *1.16* | 1.11 | 1.13 |
| 6–11 | 900 | 1141 | *1.32* | 1.23 | 1.24 |
| 12–18 | 351 | 409 | *1.43* | 1.45 | 1.39 |
| 19–32 | 248 | 233 | *1.78* | 1.76 | 1.69 |
| 33–45 | 63 | 40 | *2.63* | 2.58 | 2.30 |
| >=46 | 59 | 55 | *1.79* | 1.95 | 1.75 |

RR = relative risk (odds ratio)
Ref = referent group

**Ex. 15.1.** Format of the results of the large case–control study showing the ability to explore dose–response relationships and confounder control. The crude odds ratios (not in the published table) are calculated directly from the data given; the published data were the relative risks (odds ratios) after adjustment for age and state only, and after adjustment for several confounders using a logistic regression model (see text). Data from Table 4 of Longnecker *et al.* [1]

## B. **Internal validity: consideration of non-causal explanations**

### 6. **Are the results likely to be affected by observation bias?**

The hypothesis is that breast cancer occurrence is increased by alcohol intake in the years prior to that occurrence. Therefore the issue of observation bias concerns the relationship of the recorded information on alcohol intake to the biologically relevant level of alcohol intake. Non-differential error will reduce the observed relative risk towards the null value. Bias, i.e. a different relationship between recorded and true relevant alcohol use in the case compared with the control series, could have any type of effect on the result. The information was collected by a standardized telephone interview taking on average less than 25 minutes. The questions were quite detailed, addressing five different time periods, and consumption of beer, wine, and liquor separately. A typical question was 'On average, how often did you drink one bottle, glass, or can of beer when you were in your twenties?' The questionnaire instrument also included questions on lactation, hormone use, physical activity in adolescence and early adulthood, vitamin A intake, established breast cancer risk factors, and other characteristics. The data collected related to the time period prior to diagnosis or to the 'reference date' for control subjects, defined as the date of interview minus the median time between diagnosis and interview for case patients in that state. This is to produce the same time interval between interview and the last relevant time of alcohol consumption for the controls as for the cases.

The main protection against bias is the standardization of methods, and so the questions were identical, and were presented in an identical fashion to both cases and controls. An important protection was that the interviewers were blind to the status of the interviewee at the start of the interview. Of course, many subjects would directly or indirectly make it clear to the interviewer whether they were breast cancer patients or not. The interview began with a request that participants not discuss their medical history until the end of the interview, and the interviewers were asked to record if they were still unaware of the case or control status of the interviewee by the end of the interview; this was so for 74 per cent of cases and 90 per cent of controls.

To assess the reproducibility of the questionnaire, 211 control subjects were re-interviewed after an interval of 6–12 months. The rank correlation coefficients between the average amount of alcohol consumed daily reported in the two interviews are presented for four different time periods; these range from 0.75 to 0.84. This re-test reliability is quite reasonable, although even a correlation of 0.8 suggests that an observed relative risk of 2.0 will relate to a true odds ratio of 2.4, based on the formula described in Chapter 5. However, this correlation of 0.8 is high compared with similar assessments of questionnaires or of clinical history items.

The critical issue is whether there could be bias. In the absence of a true difference, is there any reason why women who have had breast cancer would tend to report higher, or lower, alcohol consumption than comparison women from the general population? The authors note two studies which looked at re-test consistency of alcohol consumption assessed for both breast cancer cases and controls; they showed similar results for the two groups, suggesting that bias is unlikely. A useful extension of the study would have been to assess re-test reliability on a sample of cases as well as on controls. The literature reviewed in this publication suggests that reporting is generally reasonable, although some under-reporting is more likely amongst those who have very high alcohol intake. Such bias could affect the dose–response results seen in Ex 15.1; assuming there is a true relationship, if cases with the highest alcohol consumption tended to under-report this, the risks in the highest categories may be underestimated.

Some of the interviews were carried out a considerable time after diagnosis, and it could be argued that differential recall bias might be particularly strong either a considerable time after diagnosis, or (perhaps more likely) shortly after diagnosis. Results are given for cases interviewed within 14 months of diagnosis, and these were not substantially different from those based on all case patients. An analysis restricted to subjects where the interviewer was still blind to their status at the end of their interview would also be helpful, but is not reported. Thus some non-differential misclassification is inevitable, and so the reported relative risks are likely to underestimate the true relationship. Observation bias cannot be totally excluded, but it seems unlikely that the bias would be substantial enough to account for the main result, or to make a very large difference to it.

## 7. **Are the results likely to be affected by confounding?**

The issue of confounding is complex. There are a large number of factors which are known to alter the risk of breast cancer, including age, ethnic origin, social class, many aspects of reproductive history, diet, and obesity. A large number of factors would be expected to differ between women with different levels of alcohol consumption, including many of these same factors. Therefore the potential for confounding is very considerable. Individual matching for more than the general demographic factors would be difficult. Some matching on a frequency basis was used to make the ratio of controls to case subjects at least one in each 5-year group, and the groups were frequency matched by state. The main method of confounder control was to obtain information on other established risk factors for breast cancer, and use this in a multivariate analysis. Therefore the results are expressed in two ways. Relative risks adjusted simply for age in 5-year categories and state, by the Mantel–Haenszel method, are given, and in addition multivariate adjusted relative risks are shown. These relative risks are from a logistic regression model (of the type described in Chapter 6) with 6390 case patients and 8794 control subjects. As well as alcohol consumption, terms were included for age, state, age at first term pregnancy, parity, body mass index (an index of obesity), age at menarche, education, previous history of benign breast disease, and family history of breast cancer. The number of categories of each of these is given in the methods section. The use of oral contraceptives and replacement oestrogens were also considered as potential confounding factors, but in these data they were not correlated with alcohol consumption and therefore were not retained. As 98 per cent of the cases were white, race is not further considered. This multivariate adjustment did not make much difference to the results as shown in Ex. 15.1; the multivariate adjusted relative risks are not greatly different from the results adjusted only for age and state.

There are two main issues with regard to confounding. One is whether the potential confounding factors that have been identified have been adequately dealt with. The ability to control their confounding depends on obtaining accurate information on them, and using this information in an appropriate multivariate model. If the data on confounders have a high degree of error, this could compromise the ability to deal with confounding. While it is impossible to conclude that all confounding by these known factors has been totally removed, given that the approach used did not produce major differences in the association of alcohol intake and breast cancer, it is unlikely that further attempts to improve on confounder control by these variables would produce any greater difference.

The second issue is whether there could be confounding by other factors that have not been studied. This cannot be excluded. We need to consider whether any established risk factors for breast cancer, which could also be related to alcohol consumption, have not been considered in this study. One possibility is diet. No dietary information was collected, although aspects of diet have been considered as risk factors for breast cancer and could well be associated with alcohol consumption. However, the relationship of breast cancer was not very clear when this study was done; for example, a major meta-analysis of cohort studies showed no association with fat intake [3]. The evidence for an association with obesity, for example with weight gain in middle life, has become stronger since [4]. The associations seen with aspects of diet have not in general been stronger than that seen here with alcohol consumption; it is possible that the relationship with diet is confounded by alcohol consumption, rather than the other way round. There could also be some further as yet unrecognized factors, which would be important if they were true confounders, being a risk factor for breast cancer and also being independently association with alcohol consumption. There will also be factors which are intermediates in the association between alcohol consumption and breast cancer; indeed, it is very unlikely that the association, if causal, is direct in biochemical terms, and alcohol consumption may produce some metabolic or hormonal change which in turn increases the breast cancer risk. Such a factor would not be a confounder, as it would be an intermediate on the causal pathway, as discussed in Chapter 6.

## 8. Are the results likely to be affected by chance variation?

Chance variation is appropriately assessed by looking at the results after multivariate adjustment, as in Ex. 15.1. For all women, the relative risk for lifetime average consumption rises from the referent value of 1 in those with no alcohol consumption up to 1.75 in the highest category, and the values in all six categories used are individually statistically significant, with the lower 95 per cent confidence limit being greater than 1 (Table 4 in the original paper).

An appropriate overall statistical test is a test for trend; this is highly significant, with $P < 0.0001$. The statistical model used the square root of the alcohol consumption as this gave a better fit to the data, as described in the methods section. The overall association can also be expressed as the relative risk per 13 g/day, which is 1.31, with 95 per cent confidence limits of 1.20 to 1.43. The same format and statistical tests are applied to the results for more specific groups, as will be discussed. One of the objectives of this study was to compare the effects of alcohol consumption at different ages, as this should elucidate the mechanism of the association. We will discuss this further under the heading of specificity.

## Summary: non-causal explanations

To summarize, observation bias has been as well controlled as is feasible in a retrospective study, but the possibility of biased responses from the subjects cannot be totally excluded. There will be some non-differential misclassification, although the re-test reliability of the methods used has been shown to be high. Confounding by most potential confounding factors has been adequately controlled by multivariate methods, but there remains the possibility of confounding by other factors not included in the study. Chance variation can be confidently excluded because the size of the study gives narrow confidence limits for the estimates of effect, and there is a regular dose–response relationship.

## C. Internal validity: consideration of positive features of causation

### 9. Is there a correct time relationship?

Alcohol consumption after the recognition of cancer is clearly irrelevant to the causal hypothesis. Case patients were interviewed at a median of 14 months after diagnosis, and the interviews were restricted to asking about intakes up to the time of diagnosis, or a corresponding date for the controls. The accuracy of this cut-off might be less good where the interval from diagnosis to interview was longer, and no detailed information (e.g. the maximum time interval) is given. However, as noted before, the results were similar in those interviewed within 14 months of diagnosis to those in all subjects. The relevant time of alcohol intake depends on whether the relevant process is the first initiation phase of cancer development, or a later stage such as promotion, and so could be from a few to many years before clinical diagnosis.

### 10. Is the association strong?

The relationship is only moderately strong. For all women, the relative risks reach approximately 2.0 at the highest alcohol intake level measured.

Given that the range of alcohol consumption measured is quite wide, zero to approximately three to four alcoholic drinks per day, this size of relative risk is not particularly impressive. It is consistent with causality, and could arise if alcohol is a relatively minor contributor to breast cancer risk compared with other factors. Because of the high prevalence of alcohol consumption in the population, a relative risk of 2 or even less is important in clinical and public health terms. However, it does raise the question of whether alcohol intake is merely a rather inaccurate estimator of a more fundamental causal factor which, if identified, might show a much stronger association.

## 11. Is there a dose–response relationship?

The dose–response relationship is one of the main features of this study, as average daily consumption can be categorized over a considerable range. The dose–response relationship is shown for lifetime consumption in Ex 15.1, and data are also given for recent consumption, for consumption before age 30, and for pre-menopausal and post-menopausal women separately. In each of these groups there is a regular positive dose–response relationship. The study is large enough for the relative risks at moderate levels of consumption to have narrow confidence limits, and therefore they can be interpreted with some assurance. One of the objectives was to assess the risks related to moderate alcohol consumption, and so these results are given in the abstract; for example, for consumption of about one alcoholic drink per day, the relative risk is 1.39 with a 95 per cent confidence level of 1.16 to 1.67, a quite precise measure of effect. The regular dose–response relationships give considerable protection against the association being due to observation bias, as observation bias would be unlikely to be consistently related to the amount of alcohol consumption; we might expect observation bias to apply particularly to those with very heavy consumption, giving a rather erratic dose–response relationship. It is less protection against confounding, as if a confounding factor were regularly and systematically related to alcohol consumption, it could be consistent with a regular dose–response relationship.

## 12. Are the results consistent within the study?
## and
## 13. Is there any specificity within the study?

In this study, specificity and consistency are assessed with respect to three factors: the consumption of alcohol at different ages, the occurrence of breast cancer at different ages, and the consumption of different types of alcohol.

For consumption at different ages, detailed data are given in the paper for consumption during a recent age interval (but still preceding that in which diagnosis occurred) compared with consumption before age 30. The full results have been condensed in **Ex. 15.2** to show only the overall relative risk per 13 g/day alcohol consumption, derived from the multivariate model. The analysis has to be restricted to subjects over age 40, as obviously this distinction cannot be made for younger subjects. There was a significant positive association with consumption during the recent time period ($RR = 1.21$), but the association with consumption before age 30 was weak and not significant ($RR = 1.09$). The data were also subdivided by age of diagnosis of breast cancer, into pre-menopausal and post-menopausal women, and the results then become more complex; the situation just described applied to post-menopausal women, but for pre-menopausal women the association with alcohol intake before age 30 was stronger than that for recent consumption, which is non-significant. Of course, these two time periods will overlap for many of these younger women, and so the interpretation is not as clear as it is for post-menopausal women.

The other comparison made, for women aged over 40, was to assess the joint effect of consumption before age 30 and in a recent time period. The results are given in the paper for 16 subgroups representing four categories of consumption in each time period, and the summary effects are shown

---

ASSOCIATIONS IN SUBGROUPS

*Relative risk per 13 g/day alcohol intake, from multivariate model*

| | RR | 95% confidence limits |
|---|---|---|
| *All subjects* | | |
| all subjects, lifetime average consumption (Table 4) | 1.31 | 1.20–1.43 |
| all subjects, recent time interval (Table 1) | 1.24 | 1.15–1.33 |
| *Subjects over age 40* | | |
| recent time interval (all other results Table 2) | 1.21 | 1.09–1.34 |
| consumption before age 30 | 1.09 | 0.95–1.24 |
| *Subjects over age 40, post-menopausal* | | |
| recent time interval | 1.26 | 1.12–1.42 |
| consumption before age 30 | 1.03 | 0.88–1.20 |
| *Subjects over age 40, pre-menopausal* | | |
| recent time interval | 1.05 | 0.85–1.31 |
| consumption before age 30 | 1.34 | 1.02–1.75 |

**Ex. 15.2.** Relative risks per 13 g/day alcohol consumption, from logistic regression model, in various subgroups. Data from Longnecker *et al*. [1]

in **Ex. 15.3**. These results are 'mutually adjusted'; that is the relative risk for alcohol consumption before age 30 is adjusted for alcohol consumption in the recent time period, and vice versa. The results show that there is no association with consumption before age 30 in women with high alcohol consumption in a recent time period, and vice versa. (Ex. 15.3, subtable A, relative risk 1.00; subtable B, relative risk 1.01). However, in women with no recent consumption, alcohol consumption before age 30 has a strong effect ($RR = 1.72$); similarly in women with no consumption before age 30, recent alcohol consumption has a strong effect ($RR = 1.90$). The authors suggest that this is consistent with a cumulative effect. These data do not support the prior hypothesis of a specific effect of alcohol consumption in early life.

With regard to the age of the women at diagnosis, comparing pre-menopausal with post-menopausal breast cancer showed that results were generally similar for these two groups. Although the association was stronger in post-menopausal than in pre-menopausal women, a statistical test of this interaction showed that the difference in effect was not significant.

Data are presented for daily intake of alcohol from three groups of drinks: beer, wine, and liquor. Using data on alcohol consumption in the most recent

EFFECTS OF ALCOHOL CONSUMPTION AT DIFFERENT AGES

A. RR for 13 g/day consumption before age 30, in categories by recent consumption

| Recent consumption g/day | RR for consumption before age 30 | 95% confidence limits |
|---|---|---|
| 0 | 1.72 | 1.20–2.46 |
| >0–5 | 1.12 | 0.92–1.37 |
| 6–18 | 0.96 | 0.76–1.23 |
| >=19 | 1.00 | 0.79–1.26 |

B. RR for 13 g/day recent consumption, in categories of consumption before age 30

| Consumption before age 30 g/day | RR for recent consumption | 95% confidence limits |
|---|---|---|
| 0 | 1.90 | 1.46–2.46 |
| >0–5 | 1.19 | 1.05–1.35 |
| 6–18 | 1.11 | 0.90–1.37 |
| >=19 | 1.01 | 0.78–1.34 |

**Ex. 15.3.** Relative risks per 13 g/day alcohol consumption, from logistic regression model, by age at consumption, stratified for consumption at other ages. Data from Table 3 of Longnecker et al. [1]

age interval, the multivariate model was fitted with a continuous variable for each measure of alcohol consumption. As these factors are fitted simultaneously, the resulting relative risk is the estimate of the change in risk with a unit change in alcohol consumption, here categorized as 13 g/day, adjusting for the other sources of alcohol. The relative risk estimates for beer, liquor, and wine were 1.25, 1.18, and 0.93, respectively; the coefficients for beer and liquor are statistically significant, but that for wine is not significant. Thus the results show no association with wine, but positive associations with beer and liquor. We need to assess this result with regard to possible observational bias and confounding. The weaker association with the consumption of wine could arise if the degree of non-differential classification for this exposure were greater than that for the other types of alcohol, or if there were other confounding effects related to this exposure. If there is under-reporting of heavy consumption, this reduces the range of reported consumption, which thus reduces the ability to detect a real association; such an effect might have a greater influence where the range may be relatively small, as in wine consumption.

## Conclusions with regard to internal validity

The internal validity of the result of this study is high. It is a large study. It has been carefully conducted with standardized and, to a large extent, interviewer-blind data collection, although of course the subjects providing the data are well aware of whether or not they have had breast cancer. The possibility of observation bias remains, but the regularity of the dose–response relationships, the good result from an examination of re-test reliability of the questionnaire, and previous information suggesting that interview data collected in this way are reasonably reliable and unlikely to be influenced by bias, together make observation bias a less likely explanation of the results. Non-differential error will make the results underestimate the true association. Confounding by the accepted risk factors for breast cancer has been dealt with by collecting data on these items and controlling them in a multivariate analysis; the fact that this gave very little change in the risk ratios suggest that confounding by these factors is minor, and also suggests that further control, for example by having more comprehensive data on such factors, would be unlikely to greatly modify the result. However, the influence of unrecognized confounders cannot be dismissed. Diet has not been assessed and could be a confounder. Chance variation can be much more confidently excluded, as the study is large, and the tests show that the probability of such results occurring by chance is extremely small. The time relationships are consistent with causality, the relationship is reasonably strong, and there is a very clear and regular dose–response relationship. The results suggest generally similar affects for pre-menopausal and post-menopausal women, and suggest that the relationship with alcohol consumption is confined to alcohol taken in the form of beer or liquor, rather than wine. A causal explanation of the association seems more likely than any of the alternative non-causal explanations, and it is reasonable to proceed on this basis. The most plausible non-causal explanation would be confounding by other dietary factors, or other unrecognized factors.

## D. External validity: generalization of the results

### 14. Can the study results to applied to the eligible population?

The relationship of participants to eligible subjects brings us to the question of response rates and missing data. **Ex. 15.4** shows the typical complexity of a large population-based case–control study. The 6862 cases participating fully in the trial are derived from an eligible population of 8579. Of these, 14.9 per cent were not approached for interview for the reasons shown, 5.6 per cent of those approached refused the interview, and a further 3.3 per cent had missing data on some of the key variables. Therefore the voluntary response rate is extremely high at 91 per cent, and the participation rate (the participant group divided by the eligible population) is also substantial at 78 per cent.

For the control group, the 9163 controls are derived from 11 238 eligible control subjects. The proportion not approached (2.5 per cent) is much lower than that of the cases, because fewer died before interview and there was no requirement for a doctor to give permission. On the other hand, the 14 per cent refusal rate for interviews is much higher than that of the cases, although it is still very reasonable; a similar proportion of the interviews (2.8 per cent) were incomplete. The voluntary response rate for controls was 83.6 per cent, which is very high for a study of this nature in the USA, and the participation rate at 81.5 per cent is also high and very similar to that of the case series.

These results are impressive. The cases will tend to exclude women with very advanced disease who died before interview, and those whose doctor refused permission may also have had more advanced disease. This is relevant if the association between alcohol and breast cancer also relates to the extent of disease at diagnosis, for example by affecting the growth speed of the tumour or the speed of diagnosis. Apart from that, the exclusion and voluntary refusals are minor. We might well expect that they could be related to alcohol consumption, and that the higher refusal rate amongst those approached for interview in the control group compared with the cases could lead to the exclusion of more controls with particularly high alcohol intakes. If this bias did occur, it would tend to exaggerate the observed relative risks; the recorded level of alcohol

PROGRESS OF A CASE-CONTROL STUDY

| | Cases | | | Controls | | |
|---|---|---|---|---|---|---|
| | In study | Excluded | | In study | Excluded | |
| *Source population (SP)* | 11879 | % of source | | 16217 | % of source | |
| no phone number | | 2641 | 22.2 | | 4442 | 27.4 |
| previous breast cancer | | 273 | 2.3 | | 296 | 1.8 |
| no driver's licence | | 297 | 2.5 | | 47 | 0.3 |
| inadequate English | | 51 | 0.4 | | 87 | 0.5 |
| missing data | | 38 | 0.3 | | 107 | 0.7 |
| Total excluded | | 3300 | 27.8 | | 4979 | 30.7 |
| *Eligible population (EP)* | 8579 | % of eligible | | 11238 | % of eligible | |
| died before interview | | 463 | 5.4 | | 126 | 1.1 |
| doctor refused permission | | 761 | 8.9 | | 0 | 0.0 |
| not located | | 55 | 0.6 | | 153 | 1.4 |
| Total not approached | | 1279 | 14.9 | | 279 | 2.5 |
| *Approached for interview (AI)* | 7300 | % | | 10959 | % | |
| refused interview | | 412 | 5.6 | | 1535 | 14.0 |
| *Participants in study (PS)* | 6888 | % | | 9424 | % | |
| missing data | | 226 | 3.3 | | 261 | 2.8 |
| *Participants in analysis (PA)* | 6662 | | | 9163 | | |
| Voluntary response rate (overall) | | =PS/AI | 94.4% | | 86.0% | |
| Voluntary response rate (full data) | | =PA/AI | 91.3% | | 83.6% | |
| Participation rate | | =PA/EP | 77.7% | | 81.5% | |
| Eligible / source population | | =EP/SP | 72.2% | | 69.3% | |
| Participants / source population | | =PA/SP | 56.1% | | 56.5% | |

**Ex. 15.4.** Derivation of the case and control groups contributing to the analysis of alcohol consumption and breast cancer in Longnecker *et al.* [1]

consumption in participating controls would underestimate the consumption in all eligible controls, with this bias occurring to a lesser extent among the cases.

## 15. Can the study results be applied to the source population?

The definition of the source population is, for the cases, women diagnosed with breast cancer who were resident in the four geographical areas in 1988–1991, and for the controls, women in the general population for the four areas. The eligibility criteria that restrict the study and were applied to both cases and controls were that the women had to have a listed telephone number (which excluded 22 per cent of cases and 27 per cent of controls) and possess a drivers' licence (which excluded 3 per cent of cases and 1 per cent of controls) (Ex. 15.4). There is no discussion of the effects of these exclusions. There should be little effect on internal validity, as the restrictions apply to both cases and controls, and an internal bias will only occur if the selection criteria had differential effects for cases compared with controls. The restriction by the telephone criterion may mean that women in unfavourable socio-economic circumstances may be underrepresented; this restriction might exclude some women who have alcohol-related problems. Some women with particular occupational roles might be excluded, given that many telephone numbers in the USA are unlisted. However, it seems unlikely that these exclusions would greatly affect the relationship between alcohol consumption and breast cancer occurrence examined in this study.

## 16. Can the study results be applied to other relevant populations?

This study shows an association in recently diagnosed women in the USA, who were almost all white. Breast cancer is a disease that varies considerably in frequency, being more common in populations of European origin than in, for example, Asian or African populations. Alcohol consumption in women is a culturally specific exposure, and its associations with other social, economic, and cultural factors vary considerably in different societies. This means that the confounding relationships could be different in different societies. On the other hand, despite the considerable range of incidence rates of breast cancer, other breast cancer risk factors such as reproductive factors have reasonably consistent associations with the disease in a wide range of cultures. A fundamental biological association between alcohol consumption and breast cancer would be expected to be universal. Therefore, in general, the reasonably high internal validity suggests a biological causal relationship between alcohol consumption and breast cancer, which can be applied widely. The details of the relationship, such as the specificity to consumption of beer or liquor rather than wine, might suggest possible differences in confounding relationships, in that the social factors linked to these different drinks may vary. It would be reasonable to consider these results as applicable to generally similar societies, i.e. affluent Western societies with women of predominantly European origin, but there would be more caution in applying the results to other social, ethnic, or racial groups.

## E. Comparison of the results with other evidence

### 17. Are the results consistent with other evidence, particularly evidence from studies of similar or more powerful study design?

When published, this study, primarily because of its size, was one of the best individual case–control studies of this topic. Other case–control and cohort studies are reviewed in the discussion. Many studies have found a positive association between alcohol consumption and breast cancer; the inconsistencies are in terms of whether drinking at different ages has different affects, and in terms of specific relationships to the type of alcohol. The further studies published after this one are briefly discussed later in this chapter.

## 18. Does the total evidence suggest any specificity?

The main issues with regard to specificity on the basis of the total evidence are the two which have been discussed, age specificity in the exposure, and specificity to different types of alcohol. There are no consistent results from the total range of human-based evidence available for either of these aspects, and therefore no firm conclusion can be reached.

## 19. Are the results plausible in terms of a biological mechanism?

The possible biological mechanisms of this association are discussed in some detail in this paper. Several mechanisms by which alcohol intake could increase breast cancer risk have been suggested, although none of these is established. Some animal experiments have shown that alcohol intake increases the risk of breast tumours and the proliferation rate of breast tissue cells, although the animal results are also inconsistent. Alcohol is not generally accepted as a simple carcinogen, i.e. an initiator of the cancer transformation process in cells. However, it is recognized as a promoter, i.e. a chemical which promotes the development of cells which have already gone through the first cancer transformation step, by acting on other aspects of cancer cell changes, or through hormonal, immunological, or other mechanisms. Therefore we can conclude that the association is plausible, although the mechanism is unclear. The authors quote studies showing that alcohol appears to increase serum oestradiol levels, which is relevant as there is other work linking high oestradiol levels to breast cancer risk.

## 20. If a major effect is shown, is it coherent with the distribution of the exposure and the outcome?

The overall association is not strong enough to make an argument of coherence tenable. Breast cancer is a common disease, and several other factors have associations as strong as or stronger than that produced here. Therefore, in general, we would not anticipate a clear relationship between alcohol consumption and breast cancer incidence, for example on a geographical or secular trend basis. Having said that, the high incidence rate in Western countries, and perhaps the increasing trend in breast cancer incidence over recent decades, is consistent with differences in alcohol consumption. A positive association between breast cancer mortality and estimated alcohol intake per capita, comparing countries, has been shown [5], although the association with fat intake was greater. The limitation is that this type of evidence is open to so many other interpretations that it adds little to the argument for causality; the current study uses a much more powerful method of inquiry.

## Conclusions

In conclusion, this large case–control study has shown a regular positive association between recorded alcohol intake and breast cancer risk (**Ex. 15.5**). The most convincing aspect of this is the clear and regular dose–response relationship. The least convincing aspect is the complex relationship with consumption at different ages, with curious results when age at diagnosis is also taken into consideration, which do not lead to a clear conclusion. The overall association is unlikely to be due to observation bias. Confounding by most well-established risk factors for breast cancer has been dealt with. Confounding by diet has not been addressed, and the disease is sufficiently complex that the possibility of unrecognized confounding factors remains. The associations seen are highly statistically significant. The results are generally consistent with the results of other observational studies, most of which, however, would be open to the same limitations. A reasonable conclusion is that a causal explanation is the most likely explanation of the results seen, but that confounding cannot be excluded. The aspect of the results suggesting that the association is specific to beer or liquor consumption, rather than wine consumption, is not consistent with the totality of other evidence, and can be regarded only as tentative.

## Subsequent development

This study was a substantial contribution to knowledge about alcohol consumption and breast cancer, and its most important result was to show that risk increased even at moderate levels of consumption, of even one standard drink per day. The other major finding was that consumption before the age of 30 was less important than average lifetime consumption or alcohol consumption in recent years. The association with even low levels of consumption has been confirmed, particularly in a large pooled analysis of 53 epidemiological studies, including over 58 000 women with breast cancer, done by the same group who explored other risk factors for breast cancer, such as oral contraceptive use and a previous abortion, as discussed earlier in this book [6]. This meta-analysis showed that the risk of breast cancer increased by 7 per cent for each extra unit of alcohol (10 g) consumed per day, and estimated

## ASSESSMENT OF A LARGE CASE–CONTROL STUDY

A. *Description of the evidence*

| | | |
|---|---|---|
| 1 | Exposure | Alcohol consumption at different ages, dosages, and types |
| 2 | Outcome | Breast cancer incidence |
| 3 | Design | Retrospective case–control study, population based; telephone interviews |
| 4 | Study population | Breast cancer cases in 4 states in USA, 1988-91; controls from community sources |
| 5 | Main result | Increased risk with increasing alcohol consumption, even at moderate levels; consumption before age 30 not specifically hazardous |

B. *Non-causal explanations*

| | | |
|---|---|---|
| 6 | Observation bias | Systematic methods and single blind design may protect; evidence of acceptably high re-test consistency; cannot exclude some bias |
| 7 | Confounding | Controlled for most known confounders by multivariate methods. Confounding by diet still possible |
| 8 | Chance | Large study gives precise estimates; chance can be confidently excluded |

C. *Features consistent with causation*

| | | |
|---|---|---|
| 9 | Time relationship | Positive association seen with lifetime, recent and before age 30 consumption, varying in different age groups of cases; consistent with a cumulative effect rather than specific to one age range at consumption |
| 10 | Strength | Overall effect not very strong: relative risk up to 2 at maximum consumption |
| 11 | Dose response | Clearly seen over finely divided range; consistent with linear increase, no evidence of threshold effect |
| 12 | Consistency | Not consistent between pre- and post-menopausal women; generally positive but differences in detail |
| 13 | Specificity | Specific to beer or liquor consumption; no effect seen with wine consumption |

D. *External validity*

| | | |
|---|---|---|
| 14 | Eligible population | High participation rates; little difficulty in generalizing to eligible population |
| 15 | Source population | Eligible subjects had to have a listed phone and a drivers' licence; may exclude some social groups |
| 16 | Target populations | Applicable to women in most developed countries; predominantly white ethnic groups |

E. *Comparison with other evidence*

| | | |
|---|---|---|
| 17 | Consistency | Consistent with earlier studies; adds precision in dose response |
| 18 | Specificity | Specificity to beer or liquor not supported by other studies. Relationships in different age groups still unclear for all evidence |
| 19 | Plausibility | Plausible, although mechanism of action unknown |
| 20 | Coherence | Relationship too weak, and may be other aetiological factors for breast cancer, to expect clear coherence |

**Ex. 15.5.** Summary of assessment of the case–control study of breast cancer and alcohol consumption: Longnecker *et al.* [1]

that about 4 per cent of breast cancers in developed countries were attributable to alcohol use. Of course, the individual studies have given varied results; for example, the well-known Framingham cohort study did not show any relationship of alcohol to breast cancer, and reasons for this have been discussed [7]. The finding that risk is increased more by recent alcohol intake than by consumption in early life has also been shown in some other cohort and case–control studies [8,9], but there is less consistency on this [10]. The issue of whether risk of breast cancer varies by the type of alcohol consumed has not been confirmed, with some other studies showing no such variation [10,11]. The association with alcohol use may also vary with the type of breast cancer, being greater with oestrogen-receptor-positive tumours [12]. Considerable work has been done on the possible mechanisms for the association of breast cancer with alcohol, which may be closely related to aspects of obesity and to folate consumption and metabolism [13,14]. Alcohol intake is associated with several cancers in addition to breast cancer; again, the mechanism of its carcinogenic effect is not yet known, and the possibilities include toxic effects of the main metabolite acetaldehyde, increased oestrogen concentration, the production of reactive oxygen and nitrogen compounds, a solvent action in combination with tobacco carcinogens, and effects on folate metabolism [15].

## References

1. Longnecker MP, Newcomb PA, Mittendorf R, Greenberg ER, Clapp RW, Bogdan GF *et al.* Risk of breast cancer in relation to lifetime alcohol consumption. *J Natl Cancer Inst* 1995; **87**: 923–929.
2. Longnecker MP. Alcohol consumption in relation to risk of breast cancer: meta-analysis and review. *Cancer Causes Control* 1994; **5**: 73–82.
3. Hunter DJ, Spiegelman D, Adami H-O, *et al.* Cohort studies of fat intake and the risk of breast cancer: a pooled analysis. *N Engl J Med* 1996; **334**: 356–361.
4. Holmes MD, Willett WC. Does diet affect breast cancer risk? *Breast Cancer Res* 2004; **6**: 170–178.
5. Schatzkin A, Piantadosi S, Miccozzi M, Bartee D. Alcohol consumption and breast cancer: a cross-national correlation study. *Int J Epidemiol* 1989; **18**: 28–31.
6. Hamajima N, Hirose K, Tajima K, *et al.* Alcohol, tobacco and breast cancer: collaborative reanalysis of individual data from 53 epidemiological studies, including 58,515 women with breast cancer and 95,067 women without the disease. *Br J Cancer* 2002; **87**: 1234–1245.
7. Longnecker MP. Invited commentary: the Framingham results on alcohol and breast cancer. *Am J Epidemiol* 1999; **149**: 102–104.
8. Horn-Ross PL, Canchola AJ, West DW, *et al.* Patterns of alcohol consumption and breast cancer risk in the California Teachers Study cohort. *Cancer Epidemiol Biomarkers Prev* 2004; **13**: 405–411.

9. McDonald JA, Mandel MG, Marchbanks PA, *et al.* Alcohol exposure and breast cancer: results of the women's contraceptive and reproductive experiences study. *Cancer Epidemiol Biomarkers Prev* 2004; **13**: 2106–2116.

10. Singletary KW, Gapstur SM. Alcohol and breast cancer: review of epidemiologic and experimental evidence and potential mechanisms. *JAMA* 2001; **286**: 2143–2151.

11. Petri AL, Tjonneland A, Gamborg M, *et al.* Alcohol intake, type of beverage, and risk of breast cancer in pre- and postmenopausal women. *Alcohol Clin Exp Res* 2004; **28**: 1084–1090.

12. Suzuki R, Ye W, Rylander-Rudqvist T, Saji S, Colditz GA, Wolk A. Alcohol and post-menopausal breast cancer risk defined by estrogen and progesterone receptor status: a prospective cohort study. *J Natl Cancer Inst* 2005; **97**: 1601–1608.

13. Dumitrescu RG, Shields PG. The etiology of alcohol-induced breast cancer. *Alcohol* 2005; **35**: 213–225.

14. Le Marchand L, Haiman CA, Wilkens LR, Kolonel LN, Henderson BE. MTHFR polymorphisms, diet, HRT, and breast cancer risk: the multiethnic cohort study. *Cancer Epidemiol Biomarkers Prev* 2004; **13**: 2071–2077.

15. Boffetta P, Hashibe M. Alcohol and cancer. *Lancet Oncol* 2006; **7**: 149–156.

# Answers to self-test questions

## Chapter 1

### Q1.1

A factor is a cause of an event if its operation increases the frequency of the event.

### Q1.2

(a) Sufficient causation for this person (with common-sense assumptions about the general circumstances).

(b) Necessary causation (but note that clinical polio is defined as involving infection with the virus).

(c) Common causation, i.e. neither necessary (the lung cancer could be due to other factors) nor sufficient (lung cancer does not always occur even after heavy smoking).

(d) Sufficient and necessary causation. Most examples of sufficient and necessary causation are situations where there is enough knowledge to relate a specific genetic or biochemical abnormality to a clearly defined disease state.

(e) Common causation (if the evidence supports that interpretation), neither necessary nor sufficient.

### Q1.3

(a) The prevalence of wearing glasses is 8 in 40, or 20 per cent.

(b) The incidence rate of road accidents was 1 per 1000 per year.

(c) The in-hospital mortality rate is 14 per cent (this is a cumulative incidence rate of death, but it would be better if the time period was known).

(d) The prevalence of breast malignancy is 25 per cent.

## Q1.4

(a) The initial prevalence of hypertension is 16 per cent; the final prevalence is 28 per cent.

(b) The cumulative incidence of hypertension over 3 years is 120/840 = 14.3 per cent (as the number at risk at the beginning of the observation time is 840).

(c) In the 3 years recorded, the incidence is 120 new cases and the average population at risk is 780 (840 at risk at the start, 720 at risk after 3 years), so that the incidence rate is 120/780 over 3 years = 5.1 per cent per year.

## Q1.5

(a) Population at risk at 1 January 2001 = 1000 − 180 = 820.

(b) Prevalence rate at 1 January 2002 = 200/1000 = 20 per cent.

(c) Number of new cases over 2 years = 250 − 180 = 70. Initial population at risk = 820. Cumulative incidence over 2 years = 70/820 = 8.5 per cent.

(d) Number of new cases in 2002 = 250 − 200 = 50.
Population at risk at start of 2002 = 800; at end of 2002 = 750. Therefore average population at risk in 2002 = 775; hence average incidence rate in 2002 = 50/775 = 6.5 per cent per year.

# Chapter 2

## Q2.1

(a) Cohort study, as the subjects are selected on their exposure, air travel; cross-sectional.

(b) Case–control study, retrospective. The subjects are selected on their outcome, which is hypertension.

(c) Cohort study, retrospective. The comparison is based on the exposure, which is occupation.

(d) Case–control study, retrospective. The comparison is based on the outcome, which is infarction.

(e) Cohort study, prospective. The comparison is based on the exposure, which is smoking.

(f) Case–control study nested in a cohort study.

(g) Non-randomized intervention study (clinical trial): equally can be regarded as a cohort study.

## Q2.2

(a) Perhaps, but as the time direction is unspecified, diabetes may lead to unemployment, or both may be consequences of other causal factors.

(b) Perhaps, but maybe those who smoke at age 85 are less likely to survive to age 95.

(c) Perhaps, but in this retrospective case–control study the accuracy of the information on stressful events is questionable. A prospective study, where data on stressful events were collected before the breast cancer diagnosis would be stronger.

(d) Perhaps, but this cross-sectional study will exclude any workers who developed repetitive strain injury and then stopped work. A prospective study of workers from their first employment would be better.

## Q2.3

A cohort study addresses the question of the effects of a particular exposure, and will allow multiple endpoints to be assessed. The major disadvantages for an outcome such as cancer occurrence will be the large size of study (both exposed and unexposed comparison groups) which will be needed, and the long time period of follow-up necessary. The potential of the outcome ascertainment being biased by knowledge of the exposure is also a potential problem.

## Q2.4

A case–control study can assess a large number of potential exposure factors, and is feasible even with a fairly small number of cases of the newly recognized disease. Questions can be asked about exposures at various times in the past, avoiding the time delay of prospective studies. The main difficulties are that the retrospective assessment of exposures will be open to inaccuracy, and perhaps bias. Defining an appropriate control group may be difficult.

## Q2.5

Randomized trials are a direct method of testing a causal hypothesis by observing whether subjects offered the intervention under test have a different frequency of outcome to an appropriate comparison group. Randomization on an adequately large sample should mean that the two groups being compared are similar in all relevant factors, so that, without the intervention, they would have the same frequency of outcome. Randomization demands a precise protocol and concurrent controls, so that methods to avoid bias in the outcome assessment, such as double-blind techniques, can be used.

## Chapter 3

### Q3.1

(a) The mortality rates are 7.3 per cent in the treated group and 26.9 per cent in the controls. These are cumulative mortality rates over the follow-up period (which was 6 months).

(b) The relative risk of death is 0.27, or the relative risk of survival is 3.7.

(c) The odds ratio for death is 0.21, or the odds ratio of survival is 4.7. It is larger than the relative risk (greater difference from 1) as the risk of death is high.

(c) The attributable risk is −19.6 per cent.

(d) The attributable benefit is 19.6 per cent (i.e. 19.6 per cent of treated subjects benefit from the treatment in regard to this outcome).

(e) The number needed to treat for one death prevented is 100/19.6 = 5. There were 10 less deaths than expected in the 55 subjects treated.

### Q3.2

(a) The mortality rates are 3.84 deaths per 1000 man-years in the high fat group, and 2.91 per 1000 man-years in the lower fat group

(b) The relative risk (high fat compared with lower fat) is 1.32.

(c) The attributable risk of the high fat diet in this population is 0.93 deaths per 1000 man-years, if causality is accepted.

(d) The preventable proportion in the high fat diet group is 0.93/3.84 = 24.2 per cent, again if causality is accepted.

(e) The preventable proportion in this whole population, in which the death rate is 3.25 per 1000 man-years, is (3.25 − 2.91)/3.25 = 10.5 per cent, again if causality is accepted, and if the study is representative in terms of the exposure distribution.

### Q3.3

(a) Assuming an additive model, the expected incidence rate for joint exposure is 50 + 50 + 350 = 450 per 10 000 person-years

(b) Assuming a multiplicative model, the relative risk for smoking is 8, and for air pollution is 2; therefore the joint relative risk is 8 × 2 = 16, and the expected incidence rate for joint exposure is 50 × 16 = 800 per 10 000 person-years.

## Q3.4

(a) The relative risk cannot be directly assessed. The best estimate will be the odds ratio; it will be somewhat different from the relative risk as this disease is quite common

(b) The odds ratio is $(180 \times 680)/(320 \times 120) = 3.19$, showing an increased risk in those with a prior knee injury.

(c) The attributable proportion in the exposed group $= (3.19 - 1)/3.19 = 68.7$ per cent, if the association is causal.

## Q3.5

This describes incidence-based sampling, so that now the cross-products ratio of 3.19 is a valid estimate of relative risk. The odds ratio is not directly obtained.

## Q3.6

(a) Assuming causality, and using the relative risk of 5.1, the preventable proportion is $(5.1 - 1.0)/5.1 = 80$ per cent. (Using 4.8 yields 79 per cent; the difference is a rounding error.)

(b) This is another application of the number needed to treat; as the risk difference is 3.8 per 100 000 population, the number affected is about 26 000 to reduce firearm-based murders by one per year

(c) Here we use the total results; the preventable proportion is calculated as either $(1.6 - 1)/1.6 = 38$ per cent or $(11.3 - 6.9)/11.3 = 39$ per cent. This assumes that the results show causality, and that a change in the laws would produce the same effect as is seen in these observational data based on past experience.

# Chapter 4

## Q4.1

The participants are the children whose data are analysed even though their parents or other informants provide the data. The eligible population comprises all children with leukaemia seen in the particular hospital, in some specified time period, excluding those in a terminal stage. The age range and the definition of 'terminal stage' need to be clarified. The source population is all children seen in that hospital. The target population is probably all children with leukaemia in the country concerned, or internationally, but may be restricted to certain types of leukaemia or in other ways.

## Q4.2

The internal validity concept addresses whether this association is due to a causal relationship between measles and leukaemia in the children participating in this study, or is produced by observation bias, confounding, or chance. The issue of external validity is whether the association, if internally valid, can be applied to 'measles' and 'childhood leukaemia' on a wider basis, for example in all children, in those in certain age groups, in those with different types of measles or leukaemia, or in different geographical areas and times.

## Q4.3

Selection bias can affect the external validity if the participants are not representative of a wider population, it can affect the internal validity if selection effects are different in the groups being compared, or it may modify the hypothesis being tested.

## Q4.4

The source population is 1000, and the eligible population is 900. Of these, a total of 160 are not approached for administrative reasons, and so 740 are approached, of whom 500 agree to be interviewed, but only 450 give the information that is used in the analysis.

The participation rate (full participants divided by eligible subjects) is 450 out of 900, 50 per cent; the voluntary response rate for full participation is 450 out of 740, 61 per cent, and for any co-operation is 500 out of 740, 68 per cent. Thus the full participants represent 50 per cent of the eligible subjects and 45 per cent of the source population. The study results depend on the full participants, and the 50 per cent figure is the best indicator of their relationship to the ideal, which would be to have information on all eligible subjects.

## Q4.5

Fifty per cent of those randomized to the intervention accepted the intervention, and of those 50 per cent quit smoking (total 25 per cent quit); 50 per cent did not accept, and of those 10 per cent quit (total 5 per cent). Therefore the success rate in the whole group randomized to intervention is 30 per cent. This can be compared with the success rate in the whole group randomized to no intervention (20 per cent), giving a relative risk of cessation of 1.5 (30/20), an odds ratio of 1.7, or a difference in rate of quitting of 10 per cent. All these are valid results. This comparison assesses the effect of *offering* the programme, and as it is based on the randomization, should have protection against confounding. Any comparison based on the 50 per cent success rate in those who accept the programme is no longer a randomized comparison, and must be interpreted as very likely to be influenced by confounding factors which relate to acceptance of the programme.

## Q4.6

The exposed group should truly be exposed, they should be studied from the beginning of exposure or from some defined period after it, they should be representative of a defined eligible population of exposed subjects, and they should be chosen so that the further investigations and follow-up can be carried out in a similar manner as in the comparison group.

## Q4.7

The controls will be chosen either to be representative of unaffected subjects, or to be representative of the entire study base; in this case, the former is more likely. They should be chosen so that the information can be gained in the same way as in the cases, i.e. by telephone interviews. They should be representative of the same eligible population which provides the cases. Therefore it would be wise to select controls who are also patients in the same general practices.

## Q4.8

In a single-blind trial, participating subjects are unaware of which intervention they are receiving; in a double-blind trial, neither the subjects nor those making the observations of outcome are aware of the intervention being received. This is frequently accomplished in drug trials by using an identical placebo to the active drug.

## Q4.9

An internal control group would consist (for example) of other employees who were not exposed to that particular chemical; an external comparison group might consist of members of a different workforce or industry, or the general population of the geographical area or country. An internal control group will in general give better comparability, if an adequately large group can be found, and if there is little danger of contamination (in both chemical and epidemiological terms) by that control group also being exposed to the chemicals under study.

# Chapter 5

## Q5.1

Observation bias; because confounding and chance variation can only be assessed by using the data, which if biased will be misleading.

## Q5.2

Bias refers to inaccuracy that is different in the different groups of subjects being compared; error refers to inaccuracy that is similar in the different groups.

## Q5.3

Non-differential error will nearly always make the observed association closer to the null value than is the true association.

## Q5.4

Observation bias, having different effects on the different groups being compared, can affect the results of a study in either direction, increasing or decreasing the measure of association compared with the true value.

## Q5.5

In a single-blind assessment, the observer is unaware of the exposure or disease status of the subject; in a double-blind comparison, the subject is also usually unaware of their exposure or treatment classification; in a triple-blind design, the analysis is done without knowledge of the allocation of subjects.

## Q5.6

Having a clear definition of the factors being assessed, and appropriate choices of instruments, standardization of methods, and good quality control, applied in identical fashions to all groups of subjects being assessed.

## Q5.7

(a) The proportion showing agreement $= 0.6 + 0.2 = 0.8 = 80$ per cent.

(b) The expected agreement by chance $= 0.7 \times 0.7 + 0.3 \times 0.3 = 0.58 = 58$ per cent.

(c) Kappa $= (0.80 - 0.58)/(1 - 0.58) = 0.52 = 52$ per cent.

## Q5.8

If kappa = 0.52 and observed odds ratio = 1.8, the estimated true odds ratio = (0.52 + 1.8 − 1)/0.52 = 2.5.

## Q5.9

A kappa value of 0.9 shows very good agreement, 0.7 reasonable agreement, 0.5 moderate agreement, and 0.2 poor agreement, but this categorization is very approximate. Kappa values may be misleading, particularly when the prevalence of the factor assessed is very low or very high.

## Q5.10

Sensitivity = 50/60 = 83 per cent.

Specificity = 890/940 = 95 per cent.

Predictive value positive = 50/100 = 50 per cent.

## Q5.11

As the validity coefficient is 0.9, the true odds ratio is exp $(\ln 1.2/0.9^2) = 1.25$.

## Q5.12

The observed odds ratio is $(0.5 \times 0.75)/(0.5 \times 0.25) = 3.0$.

Using the formula shown in Ex. 5.9, the estimated 'true' proportion exposed is 60 per cent for the cases and 27 per cent for the controls; the true odds ratio is $(0.6 \times 0.73)/(0.4 \times 0.27) = 4.1$.

# Chapter 6

## Q6.1

Because D is associated with X, the results will show a negative association, i.e. an apparent protective effect, of high intakes of D on cancer incidence rates.

## Q6.2

As D itself has no effect, the randomized trial will show no effect on cancer incidence.

## Q6.3

It is quite likely that the teachers who volunteer will be the more enthusiastic teachers and they will put extra effort into the programme because it is innovative.

For that reason, children in the new curriculum will show better results. Any true effect of the new curriculum, positive or negative, will be supplemented (confounded) by this effect due to selection of teachers.

## Q6.4

In assessing confounding, whether the difference in a characteristic between two groups being compared is statistically significant is not relevant; the size of the confounding effect produced depends on the size of the difference between the two groups, and also on the strength of the association between that factor and the outcome. Assessing the change in relative risk with or without control for the confounding factor is the appropriate way to assess if there is substantial confounding.

## Q6.5

The ratio of success rates, comparing hospital B with hospital A, is 1.5 for early disease and 1.6 for late disease. However, the overall success rate is 37.5 per cent in hospital A, and 46.7 per cent in hospital B, giving a crude ratio of only 1.24. This is lower than the true effect, because hospital B, although it has superior results, has a higher proportion of patients with late disease.

## Q6.6

The Mantel–Haenszel relative risk is 1.53, which is intermediate between the relative risks for each category of patients. See Ex. 6.17 (p. 185).

## Q6.7

This rate, which we could call the stage-standardized rate, is 28.8 per cent for hospital A and 45.0 per cent for hospital B. The stage-standardized risk ratio is the ratio of these two results, which is 1.56. It differs from the Mantel–Haenszel estimate because although both are weighted averages, the weighting factors are different.

## Q6.8

The crude odds ratio is 2.22; the sex-specific odds ratios are 1.5 in men and 0.80 in women. The fact that the overall odds ratio is higher than either of the sex-specific odds ratios demonstrates confounding; here because exposure to injury is more common in men (in the controls) and arthritis is more common in men (in this study, in the unexposed). The Mantel–Haenszel odds ratio is 1.44, being predominantly influenced by the results for men, as these are based on larger numbers. However, the effects appear to be different in the two genders, and so there is effect modification and the summary estimate is less useful; it is better to report the results for men and women separately.

## Q6.9

The matched odds ratio is 200/50 = 4. The (incorrect) unmatched odds ratio is 3.2. See Ex. 6.26, p. 199.

## Q6.10

The odds ratio for ever use of oral contraceptives on the crude analysis is $\exp(0.45) = 1.57$. However, controlling for weight changes this to an odds ratio of 0.92. Thus the positive association disappears. This would occur either if oral contraceptive use is more common in women of greater weight and greater weight is positively associated with cardiovascular risk; or if oral contraception was less common in heavier women and such women had a lower risk of cardiovascular events. Of course, the odds ratios and the change in them may also be due to chance variation, which would need to be assessed.

# Chapter 7

## Q7.1

First you should consider whether the studies have been appropriately performed and whether observation bias and confounding have been dealt with. Assuming that they have, the first study shows a relative risk of 2.2, and the probability of this or a larger difference occurring by chance is less than 0.01, from the chi-square statistic (the Excel routine gives the $P$-value as 0.002). Therefore, for practical purposes, we can exclude chance variation as a possible explanation, and so if the other issues have been dealt with, we can conclude that the treatment increases recovery. The second study shows a greater benefit with a relative risk of 4.6, but the chi-square statistic gives a probability value of 0.18; that is, about 18 per cent of trials similar to this study would produce a relative risk of 4.6 or greater, or an equivalently large effect in the opposite direction, if there were no true effect. The implication is that this study must be small, and we cannot be confident about the result. These results of the second trial could occur if the treatment were effective, had no effect, or even was detrimental.

## Q7.2

Calculation by the methods shown in Ex. 7.4 gives $a = 16$, $E = 5.09$, $V = 4.60$, and $\chi^2 = 25.8$, giving a $P$-value of less than 0.000 001 (Appendix Table 15 or 16). The relative risk is 4.0, with 95 per cent limits of 2.25 to 7.12, using the formula for the standard deviation of ln $RR$ in Appendix Table 2, part 4A.

## Q7.3

The odds ratio is 3.45; for the Mantel–Haenszel calculation $a = 34$, $E = 17.2$, $V = 11.42$, and the $\chi^2$ statistic is 24.7. This corresponds to a $P$-value of less than 0.001. The 95 per cent limits are 2.08 to 5.72, using the formula for the standard deviation of ln $RR$ in Appendix Table 1, part 4A. A positive association is seen, and is very unlikely to be due to chance variation. The other non-causal explanations (observation bias and confounding) need to be assessed.

## Q7.4

The best estimate of the true relative risk is 2.25. There is a range of true relative risks compatible with this result; 95 per cent of this range is from 0.88 to 5.75 and thus there is a 5 per cent probability that the true $RR$ is below 0.88 or above 5.75. As this range includes the null hypothesis value of 1.0, the result is not 'statistically significant' at the 5 per cent two-sided level.

## Q7.5

Assuming equal-sized groups, $P_1 = 0.1$ and $P_2 = 0.2$. The $K$ constant for 90 per cent power, using a one-sided test at 0.05 level, is 8.6. This yields $n = 215$ which is the minimum number required in each of two equal groups.

## Q7.6

A smaller number would be possible if the background rate of cessation were higher and the effect the same on a ratio basis, i.e. a doubling of cessation rate, or if a larger absolute difference would be accepted as the quantity measurable, for example a difference between 10 per cent and 30 per cent. This might be achievable by studying a different group, or using a longer follow-up time (or in this situation perhaps a shorter follow-up time, if the effect decreases over time, but the relevance of the outcome variable must not be compromised). If the power criterion is weakened, accepting a study with, say, only 80 per cent chance of detecting a true result, the numbers required are smaller, but the risk of missing a true effect is larger. A one-sided test has already been chosen. Thus if $P_1 = 0.2$ and $P_2 = 0.4$, and power = 80 per cent, $n = 62$.

## Q7.7

From the formula on Ex. 7.16, $P_2 = 0.1$ and $OR = 2$, and hence $P_1 = 0.18$; $K = 7.9$ and hence hence $n = 282$. This is the minimum number of cases and controls assuming equal-sized groups.

## Q7.8

If four controls per case are used, with other parameters being the same, a study with 179 cases and four times this number of controls will provide equivalent power (Ex. 7.16).

## Q7.9

The odds ratio is 4 and the chi-square statistic is 90, giving $P < 0.000\,001$. For 99 per cent limits, we use $Z = 2.58$ in the approximate calculation shown in Ex. 7.7, giving limits of 2.74 and 5.83.

## Q7.10

The odds ratios are 4.0 for men and 13.5 for women. The heterogeneity chi-square is 5.81 (using Appendix Table 1, part 5E) on 1 d.f., which is significant. Therefore the summary odds ratio is less useful; the results are best given as odds ratios of 4.0 (95 per cent limits 2.1 to 7.5) for men and 13.5 (95 per cent limits 6.3 to 29.0) for women.

## Q7.11

The curves show better survival for group B, especially in the first 12 months. The survival at 18 months is 75.0 per cent in group B compared with 28.6 per cent in group A. This is consistent with the significant difference shown by the log-rank statistic, but this comparison at only one time point is a less useful than the overall difference shown by the log-rank analysis. However, as an artificial example, the trial is much too small, and the confidence limits are very wide: 0 to 60 per cent in group A, and 45 to 100 per cent in group B.

# Chapter 8

## Q8.1

Publication bias exists if the results of a study influence whether it is published or presented, or whether it is easily retrieved. The most likely effect is that small studies which show strong, significant, or unusual results are more likely to be published than small studies which show null results, or results in the expected direction. Publication bias can also mean that research in different countries, reported in different languages and from different disciplines, may differ in accessibility.

## Q8.2

The prime argument for including all studies is to avoid publication bias. The main argument against is that some studies may have clear methodological weaknesses, and including them may bias the overall result. Some reviews use explicit quality criteria to select studies for inclusion, or else use quality criteria to rank studies and assess the influence on the overall result of including studies cumulatively in regard to the quality score.

## Q8.3

Using the Peto method gives an odds ratio of 2.78, with a normal deviate of 3.66 ($P < 0.001$); the 95 per cent confidence limits for the odds ratio are 1.61 to 4.80. Using the Mantel–Haenszel method, the odds ratio is 2.79, with the same statistical test. The heterogeneity statistic is small ($\chi^2$ is 0.11 by the Peto method, and 0.04 by the Mantel–Haenszel method).

## Q8.4

Using the method shown in Ex. 8.5, the summary odds ratio is 3.21, with 95 per cent limits of 2.81 to 3.65. The heterogeneity statistic is 3.66, on three degrees of freedom, giving $P = 0.3$ (Appendix Table 16), which is non-significant. The analysis is heavily weighted by the third study; its narrow confidence limits show that it must be much larger than the rest.

# Appendix

# Methods of statistical analysis: formulae and worked examples

This appendix presents tables showing the calculations of measures of association and of statistical tests, for the main study designs discussed showing for each the formulae and worked examples. There are also reference tables for statistical issues.

## Introduction

## Introduction

These tables will enable the reader to analyse most studies where the factors involved are discrete rather than continuous variables. Of course, major analyses should not be done without consideration of alternative methods and discussion with colleagues, including those more skilled in statistical and epidemiological methods.

The formulae are primarily those derived from the work of Mantel and Haenszel. These involve approximations which are appropriate if the numbers of observations available are adequate: in a 2 × 2 table each expected value should be greater than 5. For the formulae used to produce summary risk estimates and test statistics after confounder control by stratification, it is the total number of observations which is relevant; the formulae can be applied even if some strata have few observations. The statistics used to test whether an odds ratio or attributable risk estimate is constant over several strata *do* depend upon having reasonable numbers of observations within each stratum.

The one exception in this Appendix to the limitation of small numbers is the 'exact' test for a 2 × 2 table presented in Table 4. This can be applied to simple tables with small numbers. For all the other designs considered, more precise formulae ('exact' tests) are also available, but these will usually give similar results except where the numbers of observations are small.

The sources of the formulae are given with each table. There are many texts which review these and related methods in detail, and discuss the situations in which more complex formulae may be appropriate, and provide information on them.

## Table.1. Case–control studies. Unmatched: formulae

1. *Format of table*

|            | Cases (affected) | Controls (unaffected) | Total |
|------------|------------------|------------------------|-------|
| Exposed    | $a$              | $b$                    | $N_1$ |
| Unexposed  | $c$              | $d$                    | $N_0$ |
| Total      | $M_1$            | $M_0$                  | $T$   |

2. *Risks*

Odds ratio, $OR = \dfrac{a}{b} \bigg/ \dfrac{c}{d} = \dfrac{ad}{bc}.$

3. *Statistical tests*

Observed exposed cases $= a$

Expected value of $a$ $\quad = E = N_1 M_1/T$

Variance of $a$ $\quad\quad\quad = V = N_1 N_0 M_1 M_0/T^2(T–1)$

3A Chi–squared statistic, $\chi^2$, with 1 degree of freedom

$$= \frac{(a-E)^2}{V} = \frac{\left(a - N_1 M_1/T\right)^2}{\dfrac{N_1 N_0 M_1 M_0}{\left\{T^2(T-1)\right\}}}$$

3B $\chi$ statistic, or normal deviate $= \chi = \sqrt{\chi^2}$ .

3C Continuity correction: reduce absolute value of numerator by $\frac{1}{2}$ before squaring; i.e. replace numerator by $(|a - E| - \frac{1}{2})^2$, where $|a - E|$ means the absolute value of $(a - E)$, irrespective of being positive or negative.

4. *Confidence limits (C.L.)*

$y\%$ limits for logarithm of odds ratio $= \ln\ OR \pm Zy(\text{dev}\ln OR)$, where $Zy$ = appropriate normal deviate (see Table 15) and dev ln $OR$ = standard deviation of in $OR$

4A dev ln $OR = \sqrt{\dfrac{1}{a} + \dfrac{1}{b} + \dfrac{1}{c} + \dfrac{1}{d}}.$

## Table.1. Case–control studies. Unmatched: worked example

Data from the case–control study shown in Ex.6.24 and in Ex.7.9: association between cervical carcinoma and smoking.

1. Crude table:

|             | Cases | Controls | Total |
|-------------|-------|----------|-------|
| Smokers     | 130   | 45       | 175   |
| Non-smokers | 87    | 198      | 285   |
| Total       | 217   | 243      | 460   |

2. Odds ratio $= (130 \times 198)/(45 \times 87) = 6.57$

3A,B Statistical test:

$$a = 130 \quad E = 175 \times 217/460 = 82.55$$
$$V = (175 \times 285 \times 243 \times 217)/(460 \times 460 \times 459) = 27.08$$
$$\chi^2 = (130 - 82.55)^2/27.08 = 83.14 \quad \chi = \sqrt{83.14} = 9.12$$
$$\text{d.f.} = 1 \quad P < 0.000001 \text{ (Appendix Table 15 or 16)}$$

3C With continuity correction $\chi^2 = 81.4$

4A dev ln $OR = \sqrt{(1/130 + 1/45 + 1/87 + 1/198)}$
$$= 0.216$$
and 95% c.l. $= \exp[\ln 6.57 \pm (1.96 \times 0.216)]$
$$= 4.3, 10.0$$

## Table 1. formulae, continued

5. *Stratified analysis over I subtables of above format, values $a_i$ etc.*

5A  Summary odds ratio $= OR_s = \dfrac{\sum\limits_i a_i d_i/T_i}{\sum\limits_i b_i c_i/T_i}$

5B  Summary $\chi^2$ statistic, 1 d.f. $= \dfrac{\left(\sum\limits_i a_i - \sum\limits_i E_i\right)^2}{\sum\limits_i V_i}$

Each term analogous to 3 above.

5C  Continuity correction: reduce absolute value of numerator by $\frac{1}{2}$ before squaring.

5D  A formula for the variance of the logarithm of the summary odds ratio is given by Robins *et al.*[1]

For each stratum, these quantities are calculated. The subscripts have been omitted.

$$F = ad(a+d)/T^2 \qquad G = \left[ad(b+c)+bc(a+d)\right]/T^2 \qquad H = bc(b+c)/T^2$$
$$R = ad/T \qquad S = bc/T$$

Then the variance of ln Mantel-Haenszel summary odds ratio is:

$$\text{variance} = \frac{\sum F}{2\left(\sum R\right)^2} + \frac{\sum G}{2\sum R \sum S} + \frac{\sum H}{2\left(\sum S\right)^2}$$

and $y\%$ confidence limits for $\ln OR_s$

$$= \ln OR_s \pm Z_y \sqrt{\text{variance}}$$

5E  Test of homogeneity $= \sum\limits_i \dfrac{\left(\ln OR_i - \ln OR_s\right)^2}{\text{var} \ln OR_i}$ where variance of

$\ln OR_i$ = square of standard deviations given in 4A above. Gives a $\chi^2$ on $I - 1$ degrees of freedom.

| Sources: | 3A, 5A, 5B | Mantel and Haenszel [2] |
|---|---|---|
| | 4A | Wolff [3] |
| | 5D | Robins *et al.* [1] |
| | 5E | Rothman and Greenland [4] |

## Table 1. worked example, continued

5. Stratified analysis:
   Data are shown in Ex.7.9. Totals in the three subtables are 113, 211, 136
   (p. 244).

5A Summary $OR = \dfrac{(41 \times 53/113) + (66 \times 83/211) + (23 \times 62/136)}{(6 \times 13/113) + (25 \times 37/211) + (14 \times 37/136)}$

$= 6.27$

5B Summary $\chi^2$: calculate for each subtable $a_i$, $E_i$, $V_i$; and sum each of these.

|          |   | $a_i$ | $E_i$ | $V_i$ |
|----------|---|-------|-------|-------|
| Subtable | 1 | 41    | 22.46 | 6.91  |
|          | 2 | 66    | 44.42 | 12.99 |
|          | 3 | 23    | 16.32 | 6.69  |
| Sum      |   | 130   | 83.20 | 26.59 |

$$\chi^2 = (130 - 83.2)^2 / 26.59 = 82.4 \quad \chi = \sqrt{82.4} = 9.08$$

5C. $\chi^2$ with continuity correction $= 80.6$
   d.f. $= 1$ $P < 0.000001$ (Appendix Table 15)

5D Using Robins formula, var ln $OR_{MII} = 0.0456$,
   and 95% confidence limits of $OR_{MH} = 4.12, 9.53$.

5E Test of homogeneity: calculate for each table $OR_i$,

and use formula 4A to obtain dev ln $OR_i$

|          |   | $OR_i$ | dev ln $OR_i$ (formula 4A) |
|----------|---|--------|----------------------------|
| Subtable | 1 | 27.86  | 0.536                      |
|          | 2 | 5.92   | 0.307                      |
|          | 3 | 2.75   | 0.398                      |

Hence test of homogeneity $=$ sum of $\{(\ln OR_i - \ln OR_s)^2 / \text{var} \ln OR_i\}$
where var ln $OR_i =$ dev ln $OR_i^2$ and $OR_s = 6.27$
or, equivalently, test $=$ sum of $\{(\ln OR_i / \ln OR_s) / \text{dev} \ln OR_i\}^2$

$$\chi^2 = (7.74 + 0.04 + 4.29) = 12.1$$

$$P = 0.002$$

d.f. $= 2$, $P$-values from Appendix Table 16. The odds ratios vary significantly.

## Table 2. Cohort studies, count data: formulae

1. *Format of table*

|  | Affected | Unaffected | Total | Risk |
|---|---|---|---|---|
| Exposed | $a$ | $b$ | $N_1$ | $a/N_1 = r_e$ |
| Unexposed | $c$ | $d$ | $N_0$ | $c/N_0 = r_0$ |
| Total | $M_1$ | $M_0$ | T |  |

2. *Risks*

Relative risk $= r_e/r_0$  Odds ratio $= \dfrac{ad}{bc}$  Attributable risk $= r_e - r_0$

3. *Statistical tests*

Observed exposed cases $= a$

Expected value of $a = E = N_1 M_1 / T$

Variance of $a = V = N_1 N_0 M_1 M_0 / T^2 (T-1)$

3A  Chi–squared statistic, $\chi^2$, with 1 degree of freedom $= (a-E)^2 / V$

$$= \frac{\left(a - N_1 M_1 / T\right)^2}{\dfrac{\left(N_1 N_0 M_1 M_0\right)}{\left\{T^2 (T-1)\right\}}}$$

3B  $\chi$ statistic, or normal deviate $= \chi = \sqrt{\chi^2}$ .

3C  Continuity correction: reduce absolute value of numerator by $\frac{1}{2}$ before squaring, i.e. replace numerator by $(|a - E| - \frac{1}{2})^2$, $|a - E|$ means the absolute value of $(a-E)$, irrespective of being positive or negative.

4. *Confidence limits (C.L.)*

   (i) for logarithm of *RR*

      $= \ln RR + Zy$ dev $\ln RR$

  (ii) for logarithm of *OR*; analogous to *RR*, hence

      $= \ln OR \pm Zy$ dev $\ln RR$

 (iii) for attributable risk

      $= AR \pm Zy$ dev $AR$

where $Zy =$ appropriate normal deviate (see Table 15) and dev $=$ standard deviation

TABLE 2. COHORT STUDIES, COUNT DATA | 513

## Table 2. Cohort studies, count data: worked example

Data from a prospective cohort study; association between maternal epilepsy in pregnancy and malformation in infants; Shapiro *et al.* [5] (Ex. 3.2 showed another study in the same format).

1. Crude table:

| | Malformed | Not malformed | Total | Prevalence of malformation (%) |
|---|---|---|---|---|
| Exposed— epilepsy | 32 | 273 | 305 | 10.49 |
| Unexposed— no epilepsy | 3216 | 46761 | 49977 | 6.43 |
| Total | 3248 | 47034 | 50282 | |

2. Relative risk = 1.63     Odds ratio = 1.70     Attributable risk = 4.06%

3A Statistical test:

$a = 32$   $E = 305 \times 3248/50282 = 19.70$

$V = (305 \times 49977 \times 47034 \times 3248)/(50282 \times 50282 \times 50281)$

$= 18.32$

3B $\chi^2 = (a - E^2)/V = 8.26$   $\chi = \sqrt{\chi^2} = 2.87$

d.f. = 1       $P < 0.01$ (Appendix Table 15 or 16)

3C With continuity correction $\chi^2 = 7.60$.

### Table 2. formulae, continued

4A   Formulae for standard deviation

$$\text{(i)} \quad \text{dev ln } OR = \sqrt{\frac{b}{aN_1} + \frac{d}{cN_0}}$$

$$\text{(ii)} \quad \text{dev ln } OR = \sqrt{\frac{1}{a} + \frac{1}{b} + \frac{1}{c} + \frac{1}{d}}$$

$$\text{(iii)} \quad \text{dev } AR = \sqrt{\frac{ab}{N_1^3} + \frac{cd}{N_0^3}}$$

5.   *Stratified analysis*

5A   Risks

(i) Summary $RR_s$     (ii) Summary $OR_s$     (iii) Summary $AR_s$

$$\frac{\sum_i a_i N_{0i}/T_i}{\sum_i c_i N_{1i}/T_i} \qquad \frac{\sum_i a_i d_i/T_i}{\sum_i b_i c_i/T_i} \qquad \frac{\sum_i w_i AR_i}{\sum_i w_i}$$

$$\text{where } w_i = 1/\left(\text{dev } AR_i\right)^2$$

5B   Summary $\chi^2$ statistic on 1 d.f. $= \dfrac{\left(\sum_i a_i - \sum_i E_i\right)^2}{\sum_i V_i}$

Each term analogous to 3 above.

5C   Continuity correction: reduce absolute value of numerator by $\frac{1}{2}$ before squaring.

TABLE 2. COHORT STUDIES, COUNT DATA | 515

## Table 2. worked example, continued

4A  Confidence limits:

for $RR$, dev $\ln RR = 0.168$; limits $= \exp(\ln RR \pm 1.96 \times \text{dev} \ln RR)$
$$= 1.17, 2.27$$

for $OR$, dev $\ln OR = 0.188$; limits $= \exp(\ln OR \pm 1.96 \times \text{dev} \ln OR)$
$$= 1.18, 2.46$$

for $AR$, dev $AR = 1.758\%$; limits $= AR \pm 1.96 \times \text{dev} AR$
$$= 0.61, 7.51\%$$

5.  Stratified analysis:
Analogous to Table 1. If the above data were one stratum of a stratified table, the weight $w_i$ for use in formula 5A(iii) would be $1/(\text{dev} AR_i)^2 = 1/(0.0176)^2$.

## Table 2. formulae, continued

5D  Tests of homogeneity; $\chi^2$ on $I$–1 degrees of freedom; variances are squares of standard deviations given in 4.

| Relative risk | Attributable risk |
|---|---|
| $$\sum_i \frac{\left(\ln RR_i - \ln RR_s\right)^2}{\mathrm{var}\ln RR_i}$$ | $$\sum_i \frac{\left(AR_i - AR_s\right)^2}{\mathrm{var}\ AR_i}$$ |

Sources:  3A, 5A, 5B  Mantel and Haenszel [2]

4A  Rothman and Greenland [4], Wolff [3]

5D  Rothman and Greenland [4]

## Table 3. Cohort studies, person-time data: formulae

1. *Format of table*

|  | Affected | Person-time | Risk |
|---|---|---|---|
| Exposed | $a$ | $N_1$ | $a/N_1 = r_e$ |
| Unexposed | $c$ | $N_0$ | $c/N_0 = r_0$ |
| Total | $M_1$ | $T$ |  |

2. *Risks*

   Relative risk $= r_e/r_0$     Attributable risk $= r_e - r_0$

3. *Statistical tests*

   Observed exposed cases $= a$

   $\qquad$ Expected value of $a = E = N_1 M_1 / T$
   $\qquad\qquad$ Variance of $a = V = N_1 N_0 M_1 / T^2$

3A   Chi-squared statistic, $\chi^2$ with 1 degree of freedom $= (a - E)^2 / V$

$$= \frac{\left(a - N_1 M_1 / T\right)^2}{\left(N_1 N_0 M_1\right)/T^2}$$

3B   $\chi$ statistic, or normal deviate $= \chi = \sqrt{\chi^2}$

3C   Continuity correction: reduce absolute value of numerator by $\frac{1}{2}$ before squaring; i.e. replace numerator by $(|a - E| - \frac{1}{2})^2$, $|a - E|$ means the absolute value of $(a{-}E)$, irrespective of being positive or negative.

4. *Confidence limits (C.L.)*

   (i) for logarithm of $RR$     (ii) for attributable risk
   $\quad = \ln RR \pm Zy$ dev $\ln RR$ $\qquad = AR \pm Zy$ dev $AR$
   where $Zy =$ appropriate normal deviate (Table 15) and dev $=$ standard deviation

4A   Formulae for standard deviation

$$\text{dev } \ln RR = \sqrt{\frac{1}{a} + \frac{1}{c}} \qquad \text{dev } AR = \sqrt{\frac{a}{N_1^2} + \frac{c}{N_0^2}}$$

TABLE 3. COHORT STUDIES, PERSON-TIME DATA | 519

## Table 3. Cohort studies, person-time data: worked example

Data from the prospective cohort study shown in Ex.6.7; association between exercise and coronary heart disease mortality.

1. Crude table:

|  | Deaths | Man-years | Rate/10 000 |
|---|---|---|---|
| Light or moderate exercise | 532 | 65 000 | 81.85 |
| Heavy exercise | 66 | 27 700 | 23.83 |
| Total | 598 | 92 700 |  |

2. Relative risk $= 81.85/23.83 = 3.43$
   Attributable risk $= 81.85 - 23.83 = 58.02/10\ 000$ man-years

3A Statistical test:

$$a = 532 \quad E = 65\ 000 \times 598/92\ 700 = 419.31$$
$$V = 65\ 000 \times 27\ 700 \times 598/92\ 700^2 = 125.30$$

3B $\chi^2 = (a - E)^2/V = 101.35$ $\quad \chi = \sqrt{101.35} = 10.07$
   d.f. $= 1$ $\quad P < 0.000001$ (Appendix Table 15 or 16)

3C With continuity correction $\chi^2 = 100.45$.

4A dev $\ln RR = 0.131$ $\quad$ 95% limits $= \exp\{\ln 3.43 \pm (1.96 \times 0.131)\}$
   $= 2.66, 4.44$
   dev $AR = 4.60/10\ 000$ $\quad$ 95% limits $= 58.0 \pm (1.96 \times 4.60)$
   $= 49.0, 67.0$

## Table 3. formulae, continued

5. *Stratified analysis over 1 subtables of above format, values, $a_i$ etc.*

5A

Summary relative risk, $RR_s$

$$= \frac{\sum_i a_i N_{0i}/T_i}{\sum_i c_i N_{1i}/T_i}$$

Summary attributable risk, $AR_s$

$$= \frac{\sum_i w_i AR_i}{\sum_i w_i}$$

$$w_i = 1/\left(\mathrm{dev}\, AR_i\right)^2$$

5B   Summary $\chi^2$ statistic $= \dfrac{\left(\sum_i a_i - \sum_i E_i\right)^2}{\sum_i V_i}$

Each term analogous to 3 above.

5C   Continuity correction: reduce absolute value of numerator by $\frac{1}{2}$ before squaring.

5D   Tests of homogeneity; $\chi^2$ on $I-1$ degrees of freedom; variances are squares of standard deviations given in 4.

Relative risk

$$= \sum_i \frac{\left(\ln RR_i - \ln RR_s\right)^2}{\mathrm{var}\ln RR_i}$$

Attributable risk

$$= \sum_i \frac{\left(AR_i - AR_s\right)^2}{\mathrm{var}\, AR_i}$$

Odds ratio: analogous to relative risk

Sources: 3A   Mantel and Haenszel [2]

5D   Rothman and Greenland [4]

TABLE 3. COHORT STUDIES, PERSON-TIME DATA | 521

# Table 3. Cohort studies, person-time data: worked example

5.  Stratified analysis. Analogous to Appendix Table 1

## Table 4. Cohort (count data) or case–control, with small numbers; exact test for a fourfold table: formulae

1. *Format of table*

|  | Affected | Unaffected | Total |
|---|---|---|---|
| Exposed | $a$ | $b$ | $N_1$ |
| Unexposed | $c$ | $d$ | $N_0$ |
| Total | $M_1$ | $M_0$ | $T$ |

2. *Risks*

   As in Table 2; the small numbers make no difference.

3. *Statistical test*

   Probability of a particular table occurring $= \dfrac{N_1! N_0! M_1! M_0!}{T! a! b! c! d!}$.

   To calculate one-sided probability of $a$ or a more extreme value: if $a$ is greater than expected, i.e. $a > N_1 M_1 / T$, calculate quantity above for each value of $a$ from observed value to the maximum, given when $a = N_1$ or $a = M_1$; sum these values. If $a$ is less than expected, calculate for values of $a$ down to zero. For two-sided tests, the one-sided value is usually doubled.

   ! represents a factorial; e.g. 5! is $5 \times 4 \times 3 \times 2 \times 1$.

Sources: This test was developed independently in the 1930s by R.A. Fisher, J.O. Irwin, and F. Yates.

Exact confidence limits and stratified analysis will not be presented: see, for example, Breslow and Day [6] or Armitage et al. [7].

TABLE 4. COHORT (COUNT DATA) OR CASE-CONTROL, EXACT TEST | 523

## Table 4. Cohort (count data) or case–control, with small numbers; exact test for a fourfold table: worked example

Saral *et al.* [8] performed a double-blind randomized trial of the drug acyclovir, compared with placebo, as prophylaxis against herpes simplex infection in 20 bone marrow transplant recipients who were seropositive for herpes simplex before randomization; the outcome was development of active herpes simplex infection.

1.  Table of results:

|  | Infection | No infection | Total |
|---|---|---|---|
| Acyclovir | 0 | 10 | 10 |
| Placebo | 7 | 3 | 10 |
| Total | 7 | 13 | 20 |

2.  Risk: the relative risk and odds ratio are both zero.

3.  Statistical test:
    probability of this set of data, given the null hypothesis

$$P = \frac{10!10!13!7!}{20!0!10!7!3!}$$

$$= \frac{10!13!}{20!3!} \quad (0!=1)$$

$$= \frac{10 \times 9 \times 8 \times 7 \times 6 \times 5 \times 4}{20 \times 19 \times 18 \times 17 \times 16 \times 15 \times 14}$$

$$= 0.0015$$

This is the one sided $P$-value; the two sided value of $P = 0.003$. As the result obtained was an extreme one, only one calculation is necessary. Otherwise, further calculations are needed. For example, suppose there had been two infections in the acyclovir group compared with seven in the placebo. To assess significance, we add the probability of the observed table to the probability of more extreme results with the same marginal totals: the observed table is:

|  | Infection | No infection | Total |  |
|---|---|---|---|---|
| Aciclovir | 2 | 8 | 10 | $P = \dfrac{10!10!11!9!}{20!2!8!7!3!}$ |
| Placebo | 7 | 3 | 10 | |
| Total | 9 | 11 | 20 | $= 0.032$ |

TABLE 4. COHORT (COUNT DATA) OR CASE-CONTROL, EXACT TEST | 525

## Table 4. worked example, continued

More extreme results, given that $a$ is less than its expected value, are $a = 1$ and $a = 0$ with the same marginal totals:

|           | Infection | No infection | Total |              |
|-----------|-----------|--------------|-------|--------------|
| Acyclovir | 1         | 9            | 10    | $P = 0.0027$ |
| Placebo   | 8         | 2            | 10    |              |
| Total     | 9         | 11           | 20    |              |

|           | Infection | No infection | Total |                |
|-----------|-----------|--------------|-------|----------------|
| Acyclovir | 0         | 10           | 10    | $P = 0.00006$  |
| Placebo   | 9         | 1            | 10    |                |
| Total     | 9         | 11           | 20    |                |

giving the final $P$-value (one-sided) of $0.032 + 0.0027 + 0.00006 = 0.035$ or (two-sided) $= 0.07$

## Table 5. Case–control, 1:1 matching: formulae

1.  *Format of table: numbers of pairs*

|        |           | Controls |           |
| ------ | --------- | :------: | :-------: |
|        |           | Exposed  | Unexposed |
| Cases  | Exposed   | $u$      | $s$       |
|        | Unexposed | $t$      | $v$       |

2.  *Risks*

Odds ratio $= s/t$

3A  *Statistical tests*

$$\chi^3 \text{ statistic on 1 d.f. } = \frac{(s-t)^2}{s+t}$$

3B  $\chi$ statistic, or normal deviate $= \sqrt{\chi^2}$ .

3C  Continuity correction: reduce absolute value of numerator by 1 before squaring; it becomes $(|s-t| - 1)^2$.

4.  *Confidence limits*

The derivation of confidence limits is complex. Approximate test-based limits can be based on the statistic by the methods shown in Ex.7.7.

Sources:  McNemar [9]. Stratified analysis of matched data is not frequently performed; matched multivariate models are more useful.

TABLE 5. CASE–CONTROL, 1:1 MATCHING | 527

## Table 5. Case–control, 1:1 matching: worked example

Data from the case–control study shown in Ex. 6.24 and Ex.7.9, association between nasal cancer and smoking.

1. Table:

|       |             | Controls |             |
|-------|-------------|----------|-------------|
|       |             | Smokers  | Non-smokers |
| Cases | Smokers     | 31       | 30          |
|       | Non-smokers | 7        | 52          |

2. Odds ratio = 30/7 = 4.29

3A, B $\chi^2$ statistic $=(30-7)^2/(30+7)=14.30$     $\chi = \sqrt{14.30} = 3.78$

3C  With continuity correction, $\chi^2 = 13.1$.

4. 95% confidence limits for $OR$, test-based $= \exp\left\{\ln 4.29 \left(1 \pm 1.95/3.78\right)\right\}$
$$= 2.0, \ 9.1$$

## Table 6. Case–control studies, fixed 1:$m$ matching: formulae

1. *Format of table: numbers of pairs*

| Cases | No. of controls exposed (maximum = $M$) | | | | | |
|---|---|---|---|---|---|---|
| | 0 | 1 | 2 | ... | $m$ | ... |
| Exposed | $a_0$ | $a_1$ | $a_2$ | ... | $a_m$ | ... |
| Unexposed | $c_0$ | $c_1$ | $c_2$ | ... | $c_m$ | ... |

The pairs of sets $(a_{m-1}, c_m)$ form the basis for the calculations. The values $a_m$ (sets where all are exposed) and $c_0$ (sets where none is exposed) do not contribute.

2. *Risks*

$$\text{Odds ratio} = \frac{\sum_{m=1}^{M}(M+1-m)a_{m-1}}{\sum_{m=1}^{M}mc_m}$$

$$= \frac{Ma_0+(M-1)a_1+(M-2)a_2+\cdots+a_{M-1}}{c_1+2c_2+3c_3+\cdots+Mc_M}$$

3. *Statistical tests*

$$\chi^2 \text{ statistic on 1 d.f.} = \frac{\left\{\sum_{m=1}^{M}(M+1-m)a_{m-1}-\sum_{m=1}^{M}mc_m\right\}^2}{\sum_{m=1}^{M}(a_{m-1}+c_m)m(M+1-m)}$$

For the continuity correction, reduce the absolute value of the numerator by $\frac{1}{2}(M+1)$ before squaring.

4. *Confidence limits*
   The derivation of confidence limits is complex. Approximate test-based limits can be based on the $\chi$ statistic by the methods shown in Ex. 7.7.

   Sources:  2,3 Based on Mantel and Haenszel [2]
   
   For more complex matched designs, see Breslow and Day [6], pp.169–187.

TABLE 6. CASE–CONTROL STUDIED, FIXED 1:M MATCHING | 529

## Table 6. Case–control studied, fixed 1:*m* matching: worked example

Data from Collette *et al.* [10]; a 1:3 matched case–control study assessing the value of screening for breast cancer by physical examination and xeromam-mography. The cases were women from the defined population who had died from breast cancer; the controls were age-matched women randomly selected from this population.

1. *Table:*

|  | | No. of matched controls screened (*m*) | | | |
|---|---|---|---|---|---|
|  | | 0 | 1 | 2 | 3 |
| Cases: | screened | 1 | 4 | 3 | 1 |
|  | unscreened | 11 | 10 | 12 | 4 |

Here $M = 3$; summations are from $m = 1$ to $m = 3$.

2. Odds ratio $= \dfrac{(3\times1)+(2\times4)+(1\times3)}{(1\times10)+(2\times12)+(3\times4)}$

$= 14/46 = 0.30$

3. $\chi^2$ statistic $= \dfrac{(14-46)^2}{(11\times1\times3)+(16\times2\times2)+(7\times3\times1)}$

$= 1024/118$

$= 8.68 \qquad \chi = 2.95$

With continuity correction, $\chi^2 = 7.63$

4. 95% confidence limits for *OR* (test-based) $= \exp[\ln 0.30 \, (1 \pm 1.96/2.95)]$

$= 0.13, 0.67$

## Table 7. Cohort (count data) or case–control studies: test for trend: formulae

1. *Format of table*

| Exposure level | | Cases (affected) | Controls (unaffected) | Total | Score |
|---|---|---|---|---|---|
| | 0 (referent) | $c$ | $d$ | $N_0$ | $x_0$ |
| | 1 | $a_1$ | $b_1$ | $N_1$ | $x_1$ |
| | 2 | $a_2$ | $b_2$ | $N_2$ | $x_2$ |
| | 3...k | $a_k$ | $b_k$ | $N_k$ | $x_k$ |
| Total | | $M_1$ | $M_0$ | $T$ | |

2. *Risks*

Odds ratio for exposure level $k = \dfrac{a_k d}{b_k c} = \dfrac{a_k}{b_k} \Big/ \dfrac{c}{d}$

3. *Statistical tests*

3A For each level $k$ against the referent level: tests and confidence limits as in Appendix Table 1.

Heterogeneity $\chi^2$ for the table above, on $k-1$ degrees of freedom

$$= (T-1)\left(\frac{1}{M_1} + \frac{1}{M_0}\right) \sum_k \frac{(a_k - E_k)^2}{N_k}$$

where $E_k$ = expected value of $a_k = N_k M_1 / T$.

This test assesses whether the odd ratios, or more directly the proportions of cases, in the various exposure levels are consistent with the overall value—it does not take into account the order of the levels of exposure.

3B Test for trend from regression of the values $a_k - E_k$ on the score $x_k$; $\chi^2$ on 1 d.f.

$$= \frac{T^2(T-1)\left\{\sum_k x_k (a_k - E_k)\right\}^2}{M_1 M_0 \left\{T \sum_k x_k^2 N_k - \left(\sum_k x_n N_k\right)^2\right\}}.$$

For a continuity correction, if $x_k$ scores are one unit apart, replace

$\left\{\sum_k x_k (a_k - E_k)\right\}^2$ by $\left\{\left|\sum_k x_k (a_k - E_k)\right| - \dfrac{1}{2}\right\}^2$.

TABLE 7. COHORT OR CASE–CONTROL, TEST FOR TREND | 531

## Table 7. Cohort (count data) or case–control studies: test for trend: worked example

These are data from a case–control study relating the occurrence of twin births to maternal parity (the number of previous births the mother has had). The cases were births, the controls a sample of single births. From Elwood [11]

1.  Table and elements of calculations:

| Category | Cases (twins) | Controls (single births) | Total | Score | Odds ratio | E | $a - E$ |
|---|---|---|---|---|---|---|---|
| Parity 0 | 716 | 1833 | 2549 | 0 | 1.0(R) | 848.07 | −132.07 |
| 1 | 582 | 1269 | 1851 | 1 | 1.17 | 615.84 | −33.84 |
| 2 | 454 | 853 | 1307 | 2 | 1.36 | 434.85 | −19.15 |
| 3+ | 720 | 1003 | 1723 | 3 | 1.84 | 573.25 | 146.75 |
| Total | 2472 | 4958 | 7430 | | | | |

2.  Risks:

Given above: e.g. for parity 2 odds ratio $= (454 \times 1833)/(853 \times 716)$
$$= 1.36$$

3A  Global or heterogeneity $\chi^2$. For each level $E_k = N_k M_1 / T$
e.g. for parity 2, $E_2 = 1307 \times 2472 / 7430 = 434.85$

$$\chi^2 = 7430\left(\frac{1}{2472} + \frac{1}{4958}\right)\left(\frac{(716 - 848.07)^2}{2549} + \text{etc. for each level}\right)$$

$= 91.16$ d.f. $= 3$   $P < 0.001$ (Appendix Table 16).

3B  Test for trend:

$$\chi^2 = \frac{7430^2 \times 7429\left(-33.84 + 2 \times 19.15 + 3 \times 146.7\right)^2}{2472 \times 4958\left\{7430\left(1851 + 4 \times 1307 + 9 \times 1723\right) - \left(1851 + 2 \times 1307 + 3 \times 1723\right)^2\right\}}$$

$$= \frac{7430^2 \times 7429 \times 444.71^2}{2472 \times 4958\left(7430 \times 22\ 586 - 9634^2\right)}$$

$= 88.24$   With continuity correction, $\chi^2 = 88.04$
d.f. $= 1$   $P < 0.000001$ (Appendix Table 15).

**Table 7. formulae, continued**

3C An approximate test of departure from the linear trend is given by the difference between the heterogeneity and the trend $\chi^2$ statistics, on $k - 2$ degrees of freedom: this tests the adequacy of the linear trend in describing the data.

4. *Stratified analysis*

The trend statistic above can be generalized to a stratified analysis over $I$ subtables of the format above, but the formula is tedious for hand calculation; see Breslow and Day [6] pp.148–150.

The stratified $\chi^2$ statistic on 1 d.f. is

$$= \frac{\left\{ \sum_k x_k \left( \sum_i a_{ki} - \sum_i E_{ki} \right) \right\}^2}{\sum_i \dfrac{M_{0i}}{T_i - 1} \left\{ \sum_k x_k^2 E_{ki} - \dfrac{1}{M_{1i}} \left( \sum_k x_k E_{ki} \right)^2 \right\}}.$$

where $E_{ki} = N_{ki} M_{1i} / T_i$.

Sources: 3A: Armitage [12], Armitage *et al.* [7]
  3B  Mantel [13]

TABLE 7. COHORT OR CASE–CONTROL, TEST FOR TREND | 533

## Table 7. worked example, continued

3C  Test for departure from linear trend:

$\chi^2 = 91.2 - 88.2 = 3.0$   d.f. = 2    $P > 0.2$   (Table 16).

## Table 8. Formulae for sample size determination: formulae

1. *Unmatched studies, equal groups*

basic formula

$$n = \frac{(p_1 q_1 + p_2 q_2) \cdot K}{(p_1 - p_2)^2}$$

approximately equivalent to

$$n = \frac{2 \bar{p} \bar{q} \cdot K}{(p_1 - p_2)^2}$$

to calculate power

$$Z_\beta = \frac{(p_1 - p_2) \cdot \sqrt{n}}{\sqrt{(p_1 q_1 + p_2 q_2)}} - Z_\alpha$$

case–control studies, given *OR* and $p_2$, then

$$p_1 = \frac{p_2 \cdot OR}{1 + p_2 (OR - 1)}$$

2. *Multiple controls per case*

Given *c* controls per case: $n$ = no. of cases or exposed subjects,

$cn$ = no. of controls.

$$n = \frac{(1 + 1/c) \cdot \bar{p} \bar{q} \cdot K}{(p_1 - p_2)^2}$$

$$Z_\beta = \frac{(p_1 - p_2) \cdot \sqrt{n}}{\sqrt{\{(1 + 1/c) \cdot \bar{p} \bar{q}\}}} - Z_\alpha$$

3. *1:1 matched studies*

$$M = \left[ \frac{Z_\alpha / 2 + Z_\beta \sqrt{\{H(1 - H)\}}}{H - 0.5} \right]^2 \bigg/ (p_2 q_1 + p_1 q_2)$$

where $H = OR/(1 + OR)$    $OR$ = odds ratio

and $M$ = number of matched pairs.

Notation

$n$ = number of subjects in each group

$p_1$ = probability of outcome in group 1   $q_1 = 1 - p_2$

$p_2$ = probability of outcome in group 2   $q_2 = 1 - p_2$

$\bar{p}$ = probability of outcome in whole study group   $\bar{q} = 1 - \bar{p}$

$K$ = constant dependent on significance level and power = $(Z_\alpha + Z_\beta)^2$

   (see Table 9)

$Z_\alpha$ = normal deviate corresponding to significance level (see Table 9)

$Z_\beta$ = normal deviate corresponding to power (see Table 9)

$c$ = number of controls per case
$M$ = number of matched pairs

## Table 8. Formulae for sample size determination: worked example

See Chapter 7, pp 256-263

## Table 9. Constants for use in sample size formulae

A. *Table relating normal deviates to power and to significance level*

| Power $(1 - \beta)$ (%) | Z-value (Normal deviate) | Significance level $(\alpha)$ | |
|---|---|---|---|
| | | One-sided | Two-sided |
| 99.5 | 2.58 | 0.005 | 0.01 |
| 99 | 2.33 | 0.01 | 0.02 |
| 98 | 1.96 | 0.025 | 0.05 |
| 95 | 1.64 | 0.05 | 0.1 |
| 90 | 1.28 | 0.1 | 0.2 |
| 80 | 0.84 | 0.2 | 0.4 |
| 70 | 0.52 | 0.3 | 0.6 |
| 50 | 0.0 | 0.5 | |

B. *Values of $K = (Z_\alpha + Z_\beta)^2$, for commonly used values of $\alpha$ and $\beta$*

| | | Power | | | | | |
|---|---|---|---|---|---|---|---|
| | | 50% | 80% | 90% | 95% | | |
| Sigificance level: | | | | | | Sigificance level: | |
| Two-sided | 0.1 | 2.7 | 6.2 | 8.6 | 10.8 | 0.05 | One-sided |
| Value | 0.05 | 3.8 | 7.9 | 10.5 | 13.0 | 0.025 | Value |
| | 0.02 | 5.4 | 10.0 | 13.0 | 15.8 | 0.01 | |
| | 0.01 | 6.6 | 11.7 | 14.9 | 17.8 | 0.005 | |

Normal deviates corresponding to frequently used values for significance levels $(Z_\alpha)$ and for power $(Z_\beta)$; and table of $K$ where $K = (Z_\alpha + Z_\beta)^2$. The value of $Z_\beta$ is the normal deviate corresponding to the one-sided test for (1–power)

## Table 10. Calculation of kappa to compare two sets of observations: formulae

1. *Format of table.* Shown for three categories.

$p_{ij}$ = proportions of total subjects in cell $i, j$ of the table

|  |  | Second survey $j = 1$ | 2 | 3 | Sum over $j$ |
|---|---|---|---|---|---|
| First | $i = 1$ | $P_{11}$ | $P_{12}$ | $P_{13}$ | $P_{1\cdot}$ |
| survey | 2 | $P_{21}$ | $P_{22}$ | $P_{23}$ | $P_{2\cdot}$ |
|  | 3 | $P_{31}$ | $P_{32}$ | $P_{33}$ | $P_{3\cdot}$ |
|  | Sum over $i$ | $P_{\cdot 1}$ | $P_{\cdot 2}$ | $P_{\cdot 3}$ | $P_{\cdot\cdot} = 1.0$ |

Note: $p_{\cdot 1}$ means summation of $p_{ij}$ over all $i$ values where $j = 1$; $p_{\cdot 1}$ means summation of $p_{ij}$ over all $j$ values where $i = 1$.

2. *Calculation of kappa, $\kappa$*

   Observed agreement $= O = \sum_{i} p_{ii}$  i.e. summation of cells showing agreement (on the diagonal of the table).

   Expected agreement

   by chance $= E = \sum_{ij} p_{i\cdot} p_{\cdot i}$  i.e. summation of products of marginal totals.

   Kappa, $\kappa$
   = (observed agreement − expected agreement)/ (1 − expected agreement)
   = $(O - E)/(1 - E)$

3. *Standard error of kappa, $SE(\kappa)$*
   $n$ = total number of subjects.
   Let $u_i = p_{i\cdot} \cdot p_{\cdot i}(p_{i\cdot} + p_{\cdot i})$  $u_i$ uses only the marginal totals.
   then

   $$SE(k) = \frac{\sqrt{E + E^2 - \sum_{i} u_i}}{(1 - E)\sqrt{n}}$$

   Test of significance of kappa compared with null value of 0 is given by $z = \kappa/SE(\kappa)$, but this is not very useful.

TABLE 10. CALCULATION OF KAPPA | 537

## Table 10. Calculation of kappa to compare two sets of observations: worked example

Data from Westerdahl *et al.* [14]; see also Ex. 5.6, p. 139.

1. *Question: Have you ever been sunburned causing erythema and pain for a few days? If yes, how many times after the age of 19 years?*

*Data: numbers of subjects*

|  |  | Second survey: |  |  |  |
|---|---|---|---|---|---|
|  |  | >5 times | 1–5 times | never | Total |
| First survey | >5 times | 57 | 37 | 4 | 98 |
|  | 1–5 times | 30 | 312 | 36 | 378 |
|  | never | 3 | 40 | 74 | 117 |
|  | Total | 90 | 389 | 114 | 593 |

*Proportions of total subjects*

|  |  | Second survey: |  |  |  |
|---|---|---|---|---|---|
|  |  | >5 times | 1 -5 times | never | Total |
| First survey | >5 times | 0.096 | 0.062 | 0.007 | 0.165 |
|  | 1–5 times | 0.051 | 0.526 | 0.061 | 0.637 |
|  | never | 0.005 | 0.067 | 0.125 | 0.197 |
|  | Total | 0.152 | 0.656 | 0.192 | 1.000 |

2. *Calculation of kappa*

Observed agreement $= (0.096 + 0.527 + 0.125) = 0.747$

Expected agreement by chance
$$= (0.165 \times 0.152 + 0.637 \times 0.656 + 0.197 \times 0.192) = 0.481$$

Kappa, $\kappa$
$$= (\text{observed agreement} - \text{expected agreement})/ (1 - \text{expected agreement})$$
$$= (0.747 - 0.481)/(1 - 0.481) = 0.512$$

3. *Standard error of kappa*

Number of subjects, $n = 593$

$U_1 = 0.00795$     from $0.165 \times 0.152 \times (0.165 + 0.152)$

$U_2 = 0.54084$

$U_3 = 0.01478$

hence $\sum_i u_i = 0.56357$

$$SE = \frac{\sqrt{0.481 + 0.481^2 - 0.564}}{(1 - 0.481)\sqrt{593}} = 0.031$$

Test of significance $Z = \dfrac{0.512}{0.031} = 16.8$    $p < 0.001$  (Appendix Table 15).

## Table 10. formulae, continued

4. *Confidence limits for kappa*
   Using the $Z$-values given in Table 9
   two-sided limits $= K \pm Z_{\alpha/2} \cdot SE(\kappa)$
   Other formulae are available to test the significance of a difference in
   kappa from a pre-specified value, and for weighted kappa.

5. *Relationship of kappa to odds ratio* (approximate)
   Let $OR_0 =$ observed odds ratio and $OR_T =$ true odds ratio
   then $OR_T = (\kappa + OR_0 - 1)/\kappa$
   and $OR_0 = \kappa (OR_T - 1) + 1$

   Sources:   2,        Cohen [15]
              3, 4      Fleiss *et al.* [16, 17]
              5         Thompson and Walter [18]

For weighted kappa and further development see Fleiss *et al.* [17]
For discussion of applications to study results see Armstrong *et al.* [19]

TABLE 10. CALCULATION OF KAPPA | 539

## Table 10. worked example, continued

4. *Confidence limits*

    95% two-sided confidence limits $= 0.512 \pm 1.96 \times 0.031 = 0.45, 0.57$

5. *Relationship of kappa to odds ratio*

    Suppose a study using this measure yields an odds ratio (observed) of 1.80, then estimated true odds ratio $= (0.512 + 1.80 - 1)/0.512 = 2.56$

## Table 11. Adjustment of results of a case–control study using values of sensitivity and specificity: formulae

1. *Observed results of case–control study: proportions of cases and controls exposed:*

|  | Cases | Controls |
|---|---|---|
| Exposed | $e_1$ | $e_0$ |
| Unexposed | $1 - e_1$ | $1 - e_0$ |
| Total | 1 | 1 |

Observed odds ratio $= e_1(1 - e_0)/e_0(1 - e_1)$

2. *Sensitivity and specificity values for exposure, for cases and for controls:*

|  |  | Cases | Controls |
|---|---|---|---|
| Sensitivity $=$ | $S =$ | $S_1$ | $S_0$ |
| Specificity $=$ | $F =$ | $F_1$ | $F_0$ |

3. *Hence estimated 'true' values:*

|  | Cases | Controls |
|---|---|---|
| Exposed | $e_1' = (e_1 - 1 + F_1)/(S_1 + F_1 - 1)$ | $e_0' = (e_0 - 1 + F_0)/(S_0 + F_0 - 1)$ |
| Unexposed | $1 - e_1'$ | $1 - e_0'$ |
| Total | 1 | 1 |

Estimated true odds ratio $= e_1' (1 - e_0')/e_0' (1 - e_1')$

TABLE 11. ADJUSTMENT OF MISCLASSIFICATION | 541

## Table 11. Adjustment of results of a case–control study using values of sensitivity and specificity: worked example

1. *Observed results of case–control study (hypothetical data)*

|  | Cases | Controls |
|---|---|---|
| Exposed | 200 | 100 |
| Unexposed | 300 | 400 |
| Total | 500 | 500 |

Observed odds ratio = $(200 \times 400)/ (300 \times 100) = 2.67$

*Results expressed as proportions exposed*

|  | Cases | Controls |
|---|---|---|
| Exposed | 0.40 | 0.20 |
| Unexposed | 0.60 | 0.80 |
| Total | 1 | 1 |

Observed odds ratio = $(0.40 \times 0.80)/(0.20 \times 0.60) = 2.67$

2. *Sensitivity and specificity of exposure assessment, in cases and in controls, from other sources*

|  |  | Cases | Controls |
|---|---|---|---|
| Sensitivity = | $S =$ | 0.90 | 0.85 |
| Specificity = | $F =$ | 0.80 | 0.83 |

For cases, 'true' proportion exposed = $(0.40 - 1 + 0.80)/(0.90 + 0.80 - 1) = 0.286$
and proportion unexposed = $1 - 0.286 = 0.714$

For controls, 'true' proportion exposed = $(0.20 - 1 + 0.83)/(0.85 + 0.03 - 1) = 0.044$
and proportion unexposed = $1 - 0.055 = 0.956$

Hence: estimated 'true' values for proportions exposed:

|  | Cases | Controls |
|---|---|---|
| Exposed | 0.286 | 0.044 |
| Unexposed | 0.714 | 0.956 |
| Total | 1 | 1 |

Estimated true odds ratio = $(0.286 \times 0.956)/(0.044 \times 0.714) = 8.67$

## Table 12. Meta-analysis: Mantel-Haenszel and Peto methods: formulae

1. *Format for each study is the same as given in Table 2*

|  | Success | Failure | Total |
|---|---|---|---|
| Treated | $a$ | $b$ | $N_1$ |
| Control | $c$ | $d$ | $N_0$ |
|  | $M_1$ | $M_0$ | $T$ |

For each study $i$,

observed number of successes on new treatment $= a_i$

expected number $\quad E_i = N_{1i}M_{1i}/T_i$

variance of $a_i$

$$V_i = \frac{N_{1i}N_{0i}M_{1i}M_{0i}}{T_i^2(T_i - 1)}$$

as in Appendix Table 2.

For meta-analysis of a number of studies, a format of one line per study is useful.

2. *Mantel–Haenszel method*

|  | Observed successes | Expected | Variance | $ad/T$ | $bc/T$ | Odds ratio |
|---|---|---|---|---|---|---|
| Each study | $a_i$ | $E_i$ | $V_i$ | $a_id_i/T_i$ | $b_ic_i/T_i$ | $a_id_i/b_ic_i$ |
| Summation over all studies | $\sum_i a_i$ | $\sum_i E_i$ | $\sum_i V_i$ | $\sum_i a_id_i/T_i$ | $\sum_i b_ic_i/T_i$ |  |

2A  Summary results: summary odds ratio $= \dfrac{\sum\limits_i a_id_i/T_i}{\sum\limits_i b_ic_i/T_i}$

2B  $\chi$ statistic $= \dfrac{\sum a_i - \sum E_i}{\sqrt{\sum V_i}}$

TABLE 12. META-ANALYSIS: MANTEL–HAENSZEL AND PETO METHODS | 543

## Table 12. Meta-analysis: Mantel–Haenszel and Peto methods: worked example

1. *Format of table*

   Data from three randomized trials
   assessing clomiphene in inducing ovulation [20]

| Study | Treated group: success | fail | Control group: success | fail | Total |
|---|---|---|---|---|---|
|  | $a$ | $b$ | $c$ | $d$ | $T$ |
| 1 | 20 | 4 | 8 | 14 | 46 |
| 2 | 16 | 6 | 5 | 14 | 41 |
| 3 | 35 | 30 | 7 | 58 | 130 |

2. *Mantel–Haenszel method*

| Study | $a$ = obs | $E$ | $V$ | $ad/T$ | $bc/T$ | $OR_i$ |
|---|---|---|---|---|---|---|
| 1 | 20 | 14.6087 | 2.7947 | 6.0870 | 0.6957 | 8.75 |
| 2 | 16 | 11.2683 | 2.6109 | 5.4634 | 0.7317 | 7.47 |
| 3 | 35 | 21.0000 | 7.1628 | 15.6154 | 1.6154 | 9.67 |
| Sum: | 71 | 46.8770 | 12.5684 | 27.1658 | 3.0427 |  |

2A Summary odds ratio:   $OR_s = \text{sum}(ad/T)/\text{sum}(bc/T) =$     8.93

2B Chi statistic   $\text{Chi} = (\text{sum } a - \text{sum } E)/\text{sum } \sqrt{V} =$   6.80

$\text{Chi sq} = \chi^2 =$   46.30

## Table 12. formulae, continued

### 2C *Confidence limits for summary odds ratio*

Precise limits given using the Robins *et al.* [1] formula for the variance of the ln summary odds ratio, given in Table 1, 5D

$$y\% \text{ limits for summary } OR = \exp\left[\ln OR_s \pm Z_y \cdot \sqrt{\text{var}}\right]$$

### 2D *Test for heterogeneity*

For each study calculate $Q_i = w_i(\ln OR_i - \ln OR_s)^2$
where $w_i$ = weight = 1/variance of ln $OR_i$, from Table 1.

$\ln OR_i = \ln OR$ for study $i$

$\ln OR_s = \ln$ summary $OR$

then $\sum_i Q_i$ is distributed as a $\chi^2$ statistic on $n-1$ degrees of freedom,

where $n$ = number of studies.

### 3. *Peto method*

| Each study | Observed successes $a_i$ | Expected $E_i$ | Variance $V_i$ | obs.-exp. $a_i - E_i$ | ln(odds ratio) $(a_i - E_i)/V_i$ | odds ratio $\exp(a_i - E_i)/V_i$ |
|---|---|---|---|---|---|---|
| Summation over all studies | $\sum_i a_i$ | $\sum_i E_i$ | $\sum_i V_i$ | $\sum_i (a_i - E_i)$ | | |

3A  summary ln odds ratio = $\dfrac{\sum_i (a_i - E_i)}{\sum_i V_i}$

summary odds ratio $= \exp\left[\dfrac{\sum_i (a_i - E_i)}{\sum_i V_i}\right]$

3B  summary $\chi$ (normal deviate) $= \dfrac{\sum_i (a_i - E_i)}{\sqrt{\sum_i V_i}}$

3C  *Confidence limits for summary odds ratio* $= \exp\left(\ln OR_s \pm Z_\alpha \Big/ \sqrt{\sum_i V_i}\right)$

where $Z_\alpha$ is the normal deviate for the significance level $\alpha$, from Table 9.

TABLE 12. META-ANALYSIS: MANTEL–HAENSZEL AND PETO METHODS | 545

## Table 12. worked example, continued

2C  *Confidence limits for* $OR_s$ $\ln OR_s = 2.1892$

variance of $\ln OR_s$ from Robins *et al.* [1] formula:   0.1173

95% confidence limits using this variance        4.56, 17.47

2D  Test of heterogeneity

| Study | ln OR | var ln OR | $w_i$ | $Q_i$ |
|---|---|---|---|---|
| 1 | 2.1691 | 0.4964 | 2.0144 | 0.0008 |
| 2 | 2.0104 | 0.5006 | 1.9976 | 0.0638 |
| 3 | 2.2687 | 0.2220 | 4.5044 | 0.0285 |
| Sum | | | | 0.0931 |

Sum $Q_i$ is a $\chi^2$ on two degrees of freedom: clearly non-significant

### Peto method

| Study | $a$ = obs | E | V | $a-E$ | ln $OR_i$ | $OR_i$ |
|---|---|---|---|---|---|---|
| 1 | 20 | 14.6087 | 2.7947 | 5.3913 | 1.9291 | 6.88 |
| 2 | 16 | 11.2683 | 2.6109 | 4.7317 | 1.8123 | 6.12 |
| 3 | 35 | 21.0000 | 7.1628 | 14.0000 | 1.9545 | 7.06 |
| Sum: | 71 | 46.8770 | 12.5684 | 24.1230 | | |

3A  Summary odds ratio

$\ln OR_s = \text{sum}(a-E)/\text{sum } V = 1.92$

$OR_s = \exp(\ln OR_s) = 6.82$

3B  Normal deviate

normal deviate $= \text{sum}(a-E)/\text{sum}\sqrt{V} = 6.80$

3C  *Confidence limits for summary odds ratio*

95% limits for $OR = 3.92, 11.85$

### Table 12. formulae, continued

3D  *Test of heterogeneity*

For each study $V_i$ and $a_i - E_i$ have been defined as in 3 above, and $(a_i - E_i)^2$ is also calculated. The heterogeneity statistic $Q$ is calculated as

$$Q = \sum_i \frac{(a_i - E_i)^2}{V_i} - \frac{\left(\sum_i (a_i - E_i)\right)^2}{\sum V_i}$$

$Q$ is distributed as a $\chi^2$ statistic on $n - 1$ degrees of freedom,
   where $n =$ number of studies.

As $\sum a_i - \sum E_i = \sum_i (a_i - E_i)$, the statistics produced by these two methods are
   the same. The odds ratio estimates are different.

Sources:   Mantel and Haenszel [2]
           Peto *et al.* [21]
           Petitti [22]

TABLE 12. META-ANALYSIS: MANTEL–HAENSZEL AND PETO METHODS | 561

## Table 12. worked example, continued

3D  *Test for heterogeneity*

| Study | $(a - E)^2/V$ |
|-------|---------------|
| 1     | 10.4004       |
| 2     | 8.5751        |
| 3     | 27.3636       |
| Sum:  | 46.3391       |

Heterogeneity $\chi^2 = 46.339 - [(24.12)^2/12.57] \doteq 0.04$

## Table 13. Meta-analysis: confidence limits method: formulae

### 1. Data required

The information required from each study is an appropriate measure of odds ratio, $OR^*$, and its variance, $V$, which can be calculated if the lower and upper confidence limits $OR_L$ and $OR_u$ are given, as

$$V = \left( \frac{\ln\,(OR_u/OR)}{Z} \right)^2 = \left( \frac{\ln\,(OR/OR_L)}{Z} \right)^2$$

where $Z$ corresponds to the significance level: e.g. for 95% two-sided confidence limits, $Z = 1.96$ (Table 9)

Then, for each study, the weight $w$ is $1/V$

| Each study | Odds ratio $OR_i$ | Variance $V_i$ | Weight $w_i = 1/V_i$ | wt. ln $OR$ $w_i \ln OR_i$ | Heterogeneity $Q_i = w_i(\ln OR_i - \ln OR_s)^2$ |
|---|---|---|---|---|---|
| Summation over all studies | | | $\sum_i w_i$ | $\sum_i (w_i \ln OR_i)$ | $\sum_i Q_i$ |

### 2. Calculation of summary odds ratio

$$\text{Summary ln } OR_s = \frac{\sum_i (w_i \ln OR_i)}{\sum_i w_i}$$

hence, $OR_s = \exp(\ln OR_s)$

### 3. Confidence limits for the summary odds ratio

$$\text{variance of ln } OR_s = V_s = \frac{1}{\sum_i w_i}$$

95% confidence limits for $\ln OR_s = \ln OR_s \pm 1.96\sqrt{V_s} = \ln OR_s \pm 1.96 \Big/ \sqrt{\sum_i w_i}$

95% confidence limits for $OR_s = \exp\left( \ln OR_s \pm 1.96 \Big/ \sqrt{\sum_i w_i} \right)$

### 4. Heterogeneity test

Heterogeneity statistic $= \sum_i Q_i = Q \quad I^2 = [Q-(n-1)]/Q$

which is a $\chi^2$ statistic on $n-1$ degrees of freedom, where $n =$ number of studies

Sources: Prentice and Thomas [23]
        Greenland [24]

*This method is applicable to relative risk also, and (without the log transformation) to risk difference.

TABLE 13. META ANALYSIS: CONFIDENCE LIMITS METHOD | 549

## Table 13. Meta analysis: confidence limits method: worked example

1. Meta analysis of seven case–control studies relating sunburn to melanoma.

| Study $i$ | Odds ratio $OR_i$ | 95% CL lower | 95% CL upper | Variance $v_i$ | Weight $w_i$ | $w_i \ln OR_i$ | heterogeneity $Q_i$ |
|---|---|---|---|---|---|---|---|
| 1 | 1.30 | 0.90 | 1.80 | 0.03 | 31.86 | 8.36 | 4.39 |
| 2 | 1.20 | 0.60 | 2.30 | 0.12 | 8.50 | 1.55 | 1.73 |
| 3 | 3.70 | 2.30 | 6.10 | 0.06 | 16.14 | 21.12 | 7.35 |
| 4 | 2.40 | 0.80 | 7.30 | 0.32 | 3.14 | 2.75 | 0.18 |
| 5 | 6.50 | 3.40 | 12.30 | 0.11 | 9.29 | 17.40 | 14.25 |
| 6 | 1.49 | 0.97 | 2.32 | 0.05 | 20.20 | 8.06 | 1.11 |
| 7 | 1.60 | 1.00 | 2.60 | 0.06 | 16.83 | 7.91 | 0.45 |
| Summation | | | | | 105.97 | 67.14 | 29.47 |

2. Summary $\ln OR_s = 67.14/105.97 = 0.63$   Summary $OR_s = \exp(0.63) = 1.88$

3. 95% CL for summary $OR_s = \exp(0.63 \pm 1.96/\sqrt{105.97}) = $ lower 1.56

   upper 2.28

4. Test for heterogeneity: sum $Q_i = 29.47$

   Sum $Q$ is a $\chi^2$ statistic on $n - 1 = $ six degrees of freedom; from Table 16 $P < 0.0001$, so consideration has to be given to the results which are discordant, as shown by their $Q_i$ results.

   $I^2 = (29.47 - 6)/29.47 = 0.80$

   $= 80\%$

## Table 14. Random effects model (DerSimonian–Laird) applied to confidence limits data

1. The random effects model of DerSimonian and Laird uses the same data as the fixed effects model shown in Table 13. For each study, the odds ratios $OR_i$, and their variances $v_i$ are as in Table 13.

   Weights $w_i = 1/v_i$ are calculated. The fixed effects summary odds ratio $OR_s$ is calculated as before, and the quantities $Q_i = w_i(\ln OR_i - \ln OR_s)^2$ and sum $Q_i = Q$

2,3. For the random effects model, revised weights $dw_i$ are used where

$$dw_i = \frac{1}{(D+w_i)}$$

$$D = \frac{(Q-n-1)\times \text{sum } w_i}{(\text{sum } w_i)^2 - \text{sum}(w_i^2)}$$

where $n$ is the number of studies.

$D$ cannot be negative. If $(n-1)$ is greater than $Q$, then $D = 0$.

If there is little heterogeneity, $Q$ will be small, so $D$ will be small, and the DerSimonian and Laird weights will be similar to the fixed effects weights.

4. The percentage distribution of weights is shown, showing how the D–L method gives a more even weight distribution than the fixed effects method.

*Source*: DerSimonian and Laird [25]

TABLE 14. RANDOM EFFECTS MODEL (DERSIMONIAN–LAIRD) | 551

## Table 14. Random effects model (DerSimonian–Laird) applied to confidence limits data

1. Data as in Table 13: seven studies relating sunburn to melanoma

| | Fixed effects model (as in Table 13) | | | | | | | | Random effects model | |
|---|---|---|---|---|---|---|---|---|---|---|
| Odds ratio and 95% limits | | | variance | weight | | | heterog. | | DL weight | |
| Study | OR | lower | upper | $v$ | $w$ | $w^2$ | $w \ln RR$ | Q | DL $w$ | DL $w \ln OR$ |
| 1 | 1.30 | 0.90 | 1.80 | 0.03 | 31.86 | 1015.34 | 8.36 | 4.39 | 3.55 | 0.93 |
| 2 | 1.20 | 0.60 | 2.30 | 0.12 | 8.50 | 72.28 | 1.55 | 1.73 | 2.72 | 0.50 |
| 3 | 3.70 | 2.30 | 6.10 | 0.06 | 16.14 | 260.56 | 21.12 | 7.35 | 3.20 | 4.19 |
| 4 | 2.40 | 0.80 | 7.30 | 0.32 | 3.14 | 9.88 | 2.75 | 0.18 | 1.76 | 1.54 |
| 5 | 6.50 | 3.40 | 12.30 | 0.11 | 9.29 | 86.37 | 17.40 | 14.25 | 2.80 | 5.23 |
| 6 | 1.49 | 0.97 | 2.32 | 0.05 | 20.20 | 408.15 | 8.06 | 1.11 | 3.34 | 1.33 |
| 7 | 1.60 | 1.00 | 2.60 | 0.06 | 16.83 | 283.12 | 7.91 | 0.45 | 3.23 | 1.52 |
| Summations | | | | | 105.97 | 2135.70 | 67.14 | 29.47 | 20.597 | 15.241 |

**2. Fixed effects model:**

**3. Random effects model:**

number of studies $(k)$     7

$Q = 29.47$

$D = ((29.47 - 6) \times 105.97) / (105.97^2 - 2135.70)$

    $= 0.2502$

*As in Table 13:*

| | | |
|---|---|---|
| Summary odds ratio | **1.88** | |
| ln $OR_s$ | | 0.634 |
| Variance of ln $OR_s$ = 1/(sum $w$) = | | 0.0094 |
| **95% C.I. For summary $OR$** | **1.56** | **2.28** |
| Heterogeneity test $Q$ = | 29.47 | |
| Degrees of freedom, $P$-value | 6 | 0.00005 |
| $I^2$ =   79.60% | | |

| | | |
|---|---|---|
| DL summary odds ratio | | **2.10** |
| ln $OR_s$ | | 0.740 |
| Variance of ln $OR_s$ = 1/(sum $w$) = | | 0.0486 |
| **95% C.I. for summary $OR$** | **1.36** | **3.23** |

**4. Weight distribution**

| Study | weight % Fixed | Random |
|---|---|---|
| 1 | 30.1 | 17.2 |
| 2 | 19.1 | 16.2 |
| 3 | 15.9 | 15.7 |
| 4 | 15.2 | 15.6 |
| 5 | 8.8 | 13.6 |
| 6 | 8.0 | 13.2 |
| 7 | 3.0 | 8.5 |
| Sum | 100.0 | 100.0 |

## Table 15. Table of probabilities (P-values) and corresponding values of $\chi^2$ on 1 d.f., standardized normal deviate 2-sided, and 1-sided

| P-values | $\chi^2$ 1 d.f. | Normal deviate 2-sided | Normal deviate 1-sided |
|---|---|---|---|
| 0.000001 | 23.9 | 4.89 | 4.75 |
| 0.00001 | 19.51 | 4.42 | 4.27 |
| 0.0001 | 15.14 | 3.89 | 3.72 |
| **0.001** | **10.83** | **3.29** | **3.09** |
| **0.01** | **6.63** | **2.58** | **2.33** |
| 0.02 | 5.41 | 2.33 | 2.05 |
| 0.03 | 4.71 | 2.17 | 1.88 |
| 0.04 | 4.22 | 2.05 | 1.75 |
| **0.05** | **3.84** | **1.96** | **1.64** |
| 0.06 | 3.54 | 1.88 | 1.55 |
| 0.07 | 3.28 | 1.81 | 1.48 |
| 0.08 | 3.06 | 1.75 | 1.41 |
| 0.09 | 2.87 | 1.70 | 1.34 |
| **0.10** | **2.71** | **1.64** | **1.28** |
| 0.11 | 2.55 | 1.60 | 1.23 |
| 0.12 | 2.42 | 1.55 | 1.18 |
| 0.13 | 2.29 | 1.51 | 1.13 |
| 0.14 | 2.18 | 1.48 | 1.08 |
| 0.15 | 2.07 | 1.44 | 1.04 |
| 0.16 | 1.97 | 1.41 | 0.99 |
| 0.17 | 1.88 | 1.37 | 0.95 |
| 0.18 | 1.80 | 1.34 | 0.92 |
| 0.19 | 1.72 | 1.31 | 0.88 |
| **0.20** | **1.64** | **1.28** | **0.84** |
| 0.25 | 1.32 | 1.15 | 0.68 |
| 0.3 | 1.07 | 1.04 | 0.52 |
| 0.35 | 0.87 | 0.93 | 0.39 |
| 0.4 | 0.71 | 0.84 | 0.25 |
| 0.45 | 0.57 | 0.76 | 0.13 |
| 0.5 | 0.45 | 0.67 | 0.0 |
| 0.6 | 0.27 | 0.52 | |
| 0.7 | 0.15 | 0.39 | |
| 0.8 | 0.06 | 0.25 | |
| 0.9 | 0.02 | 0.13 | |

TABLE 15 TABLE OF PROBABILITIES (*P*-VALUES) AND CORRESPONDING VALUES | 553

## Table 15. Table of probabilities (*P*-values) and corresponding values of $\chi^2$ on one degree freedom, standardized normal deviate two-sided, and standardized normal deviate, one-sided

*The values tabulated*

1. The chi-square $\chi^2$ statistic on one degree of freedom. For any other number of degrees of freedom, use Table 16

   The table gives the probability of the given $\chi^2$ or a larger value under the null hypothesis.

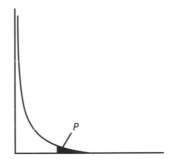

Although this is a one tail probability on a $\chi^2$ distribution, because the $\chi^2$ distribution is given by a normal deviate squared, this gives a two-sided test; assessing a variable $x^2$ using a $\chi^2$ distribution is equivalent to assessing $x$ using a normal distribution and a two-sided test.

2. The standardized normal deviate (often called *Z* or chi) using a two-sided test.

   The probability given is that of the given value $\pm Z$ or a more extreme value of either sign, under the null hypothesis.

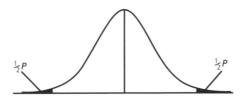

TABLE 15 TABLE OF PROBABILITIES (*P*-VALUES) AND CORRESPONDING VALUES | 555

3.  The standardized normal deviate (often called $Z$ or chi), using a one-sided test.
    The probability given is that of the given value $Z$ or a more extreme value of the same sign.

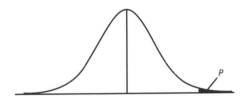

*Relationships between these*
1.  For a given value of $P$, the corresponding $\chi^2_{(1)}$ value is equal to the two-sided standardized normal deviate squared.
    e.g. for $P = 0.05$    $\chi^2 = 3.84$    $Z = 1.96 = \sqrt{3.84}$
2.  For a given normal deviate, the two-sided probability is twice the one-sided.
    e.g. for $Z = 1.96$, two-sided probability $= 0.05$, one-sided $= 0.025$

*How to use the tables*
1.  Be sure you know which statistic you wish to use!

2.  To find the value of a statistic corresponding to a given $P$-value: look down the table to find the $P$-value or the nearest to it; read off the corresponding statistic.
    Examples: What $\chi^2_{(1)}$ value corresponds to $P = 0.05$? Result: 3.84
    What one-sided deviate corresponds to $P = 0.01$? Result: 2.33

3.  To find the $P$-value corresponding to a given statistic:
    find the correct column;
    look down the table to find the given value or the nearst to it;
    read off the corresponding $P$-value.
    Examples: What $P$-value corresponds to $\chi^2_{(1)} = 7.4$? Result between 0.001 and 0.01; can be written $0.001 < P < 0.01$
    What $P$-value corresponds to a one-sided test giving a deviate of 1.04?
    Result: 0.15

TABLE 16. FUNCTIONS IN MICROSOFT EXCEL SPREADSHEETS | 571

Table 16. Functions in Microsoft Excel spreadsheets to convert between test statistics and probability (P) values

| To get from: | to: | function | Example | | Result | |
|---|---|---|---|---|---|---|
| Z statistic | P value, 2 sided | =2*(1-normsdist(z)) | Z stat | 1.96 | P value | 0.049996 |
| | | | Z stat | 3 | P value | 0.002700 |
| | | | Z stat | 4.89 | P value | 0.000001 |
| Z statistic | P value, 1 sided | =(1-normsdist(z)) | Z stat | 1.96 | P value | 0.024998 |
| | | | Z stat | 1.64 | P value | 0.050503 |
| | | | Z stat | 4.75 | P value | 0.000001 |
| P value, 2 sided | Z statistic | =abs(normsinv(P/2)) | P value | 0.05 | Z stat | 1.96 |
| | | | P value | 0.001 | Z stat | 3.29 |
| | | | P value | 0.1 | Z stat | 1.64 |
| P value, 1 sided | Z statistic | =abs(normsinv(P)) | P value | 0.05 | Z stat | 1.64 |
| | | | P value | 0.1 | Z stat | 1.28 |
| | | | P value | 0.01 | Z stat | 2.33 |
| Chi squared stat, df | P value | =chidist(chi, df) | Chi stat, df | 3.84, 1 | P value | 0.050044 |
| | | | Chi stat, df | 10.3, 3 | P value | 0.016181 |
| | | | Chi stat, df | 38.932, 21 | P value | 0.010000 |
| P value, df | Chi sq | =chiinv(P, df) | P value, df | 0.01, 1 | Chi sq | 6.63 |
| | | | P value, df | 0.2, 1 | Chi sq | 1.64 |
| | | | P value, df | 0.05, 30 | Chi sq | 43.77 |
| t test result, df | P value | =tdist(test, df, tails) | T test, df, tails | 4, 1, 1 | P value | 0.077979 |
| | | | T test, df, tails | 4, 1, 2 | P value | 0.155958 |
| | | | T test, df, tails | 1.96, 160, 2 | P value | 0.051733 |

## References for Appendix

1. Robins JM, Breslow NE, Greenland S. Estimation of the Mantel–Haenszel variance consistent with both sparse-data and large-strata limiting models. *Biometrics* 1986; **42**: 311–323.

2. Mantel N, Haenszel W. Statistical aspects of the analysis of data from retrospective studies of disease. *J Natl Cancer Inst* 1959; **22**: 719–748.

3. Wolff B. On estimating the relationship between blood group and disease. *Ann Hum Genet* 1955; **19**: 251–253.

4. Rothman KJ, Greenland S. *Modern epidemiology* Second ed. Philadelphia: Lippincott - Raven; 1998.

5. Shapiro S, Slone D, Hartz SC, et al. Anticonvulsants and parental epilepsy in the development of birth defects. *Lancet* 1976; **i**: 272–275

6. Breslow NE, Day NE. *Statistical methods in cancer research. Volume 1: The analysis of case-control studies.* Lyon: IARC Scientific Publication No 32; 1980.

7. Armitage P, Berry G, Matthews JNS. *Statistical methods in medical research.* 4 ed. Oxford: Blackwell Scientific; 2002.

8. Saral R, Burns WH, Laskin OL, Santos GW, Lietman PS. Acyclovir prophylaxis of herpes-simplex-virus infections: a randomized, double-blind, controlled trial in bone-marrow-transplant recipients. *N. Engl. J Med* 1981; **305**, 63–67.

9. McNemar Q. Note on the sampling of the difference between corrected proportions or percentages. *Psychometrika* 1947; **12**: 153–157.

10. Collette HJA, Day NE, Rombach JJ, de Waard F. Evaluation of screening for breast cancer in a non-randomised study (the DOM project) by means of a case-control study. *Lancet* 1984; **1**: 1224–1226.

11. Elwood JM. Maternal and environmental factors affecting twin births in Canadian cities. *Br J Obstet Gynaecol* 1978; **85**: 351–358.

12. Armitage P. Test for linear trend in proportions and frequencies. *Biometrics* 1955; **11**: 375–386.

13. Mantel N. Chi-square tests with one degree of freedom; extensions of the Mantel-Haenszel procedure. *Am Stat Assoc J* 1963; **58**: 690–700.

14. Westerdahl J, Anderson H, Olsson H, Ingvar C. Reproducibility of a self-administered questionnaire for assessment of melanoma risk. *Int J Epidemiol* 1996; **25**(2): 245–251.

15. Cohen J. A coefficient of agreement for nominal scales. *Educ. Psychol. Meas.* 1960; **20**: 27–46.

16. Fleiss JL, Cohen J, Everitt BS. Large sample standard errors of kappa and weighted kappa. *Psychol Bull* 1969; **72**:323–327.

17. Fleiss JL, Levin B, Paik MC. *Statistical methods for rates and proportions.* 3 ed. New York: John Wiley & Sons; 2003.

18. Thompson WD, Walter SD. Variance and dissent. A reappraisal of the kappa coefficient. *J Clin Epidemiol* 1988; **41**: 949–958.

19. Armstrong BK, White E, Saracci R. *Principles of Exposure Measurement in Epidemiology.* Oxford: Oxford University Press; 1992.

20. Hughes E, Collins, J., Vandekerckhove, P. Clomiphene citrate vs. placebo for ovaluation induction in oligo-amenorrhoeic women. *Cochrane Database of Systematic Reviews* 1995; **2** (CD-ROM). (This review has since been updated)

21. **Peto R, Pike MC, Armitage P, Breslow NE, Cox DR, Howard SV et al.** Design and analysis of randomized clinical trials requiring prolonged observation of each patient. II. analysis and examples. *Br J Cancer* 1977; **35**(1):1–39.

22. **Petitti DB.** *Meta-analysis, decision analysis, and cost-effectiveness analysis. Methods for quantitative synthesis in medicine* Second ed. New York: Oxford University Press; 2000.

23. **Prentice RL, Thomas DB.** On the epidemiology of oral contraceptives and disease. In: Klein G, Weinhouse S, editors. *Advances in Cancer Research Volume 49.* 49 ed. Orlando: Academic Press; 1987. 285–401.

24. **Greenland S.** Quantitative methods in the review of epidemiologic literature. *Epidemiol Rev* 1987; **9**:1–30.

25. **DerSimonian R, Laird N.** Meta-analysis in clinical trials. *Control Clin Trials* 1986; **7:** 177–188.

# Appendix

# References

1. Robins JM, Breslow NE, Greenland S. Estimation of the Mantel–Haenszel variance consistent with both sparse-data and large-strata limiting models. *Biometrics* 1986; **42**: 311–323.

2. Mantel N, Haenszel W. Statistical aspects of the analysis of data from retrospective studies of disease. *J Natl Cancer Inst* 1959; **22**: 719–748.

3. Wolff B. On estimating the relationship between blood group and disease. *Ann Hum Genet* 1955; **19**: 251–253.

4. Rothman KJ, Greenland S. *Modern Epidemiology* (2nd edn). Philadelphia, PA: Lippincott–Raven, 1998.

5. Shapiro S, Slone D, Hartz, SC. Anticonvulsants nad parental epilepsy in the development of birth defects. *Lancet* 1976; **i**: 272–275

6. Breslow NE, Day NE. *Statistical Methods in Cancer Research.* Vol. 1: *The Analysis of Case–Control Studies.* Lyon: IARC Scientific Publication No. 32, 1980.

7. Armitage P, Berry G, Matthews JNS. *Statistical Methods in Medical Research* (4th edn). Oxford: Blackwell Scientific, 2002.

8. Saral R, Burns WH, Laskin OL, Santos GW, Lietman PS. Acyclovir prophylaxis of herpes-simplex-virus infections: a randomized, double-blind, controlled trial in bone-marrow-transplant recipients. *N Engl J Med* 1981; **305**: 63–67.

9. McNemar Q. Note on the sampling of the difference between corrected proportions or percentages. *Psychometrika* 1947; **12**: 153–157.

10. Collette HJA, Day NE, Rombach JJ, de Waard F. Evaluation of screening for breast cancer in a non-randomised study (the DOM project) by means of a case–control study. *Lancet* 1984; **i**: 1224–1226.

11. Elwood JM. Maternal and environmental factors affecting twin births in Canadian cities. *Br J Obstet Gynaecol* 1978; **85**: 351–358.

12. Armitage P. Test for linear trend in proportions and frequencies. *Biometrics* 1955, **11**: 375–386.

13. Mantel N. Chi-square tests with one degree of freedom; extensions of the Mantel–Haenszel procedure. *Am Stat Assoc J* 1963; **58**: 690–700.

14. Westerdahl J, Anderson H, Olsson H, Ingvar C. Reproducibility of a self-administered questionnaire for assessment of melanoma risk. *Int J Epidemiol* 1996; **25**: 245–251.

15. Cohen J. A coefficient of agreement for nominal scales. *Educ Psychol Meas* 1960; **20**: 37–46.

16. Fleiss JL, Cohen J, Everitt BS. Large sample standard errors of kappa and weighted kappa. *Psychol Bull* 1969; **72**: 323–327.

17. Fleiss JL, Levin B, Paik MC. *Statistical Methods for Rates and Proportions* (3rd edn). New York: John Wiley, 2003.

18. Thompson WD, Walter SD. Variance and dissent. A reappraisal of the kappa coefficient. *J Clin Epidemiol* 1988; **41**: 949–958.

19. Armstrong BK, White E, Saracci R. *Principles of Exposure Measurement in Epidemiology.* Oxford: Oxford University Press, 1992.

20. Hughes E, Collins J, Vanderkerckhove P. Clomiphene citrate vs. placebo for ovulation induction in oligo-amenorrhoeic women. *Cochrane Database Syst Rev* 1995; **2** (CD-ROM)

21. Peto R, Pike MC, Armitage P, *et al.* Design and analysis of randomized clinical trials requiring prolonged observation of each patient. II: Analysis and examples. *Br J Cancer* 1977; **35**: 1–39.

22. Petitti DB. *Meta-Analysis, Decision Analysis, and Cost-Effectiveness Analysis: Methods for Quantitative Synthesis in Medicine* Second ed. New York: Oxford University Press, 2000.

23. Prentice RL, Thomas DB. On the epidemiology of oral contraceptives and disease. *Adv Cancer Res* 1987; **49**: 285–401.

24. Greenland S. Quantitative methods in the review of epidemiologic literature. *Epidemiol Rev* 1987; **9**: 1–30.

25. DerSimonian R, Laird N. Meta-analysis in clinical trials. *Control Clin Trials* 1986; **7**: 177–188.

26. Charlton A. Children's coughs related to parental smoking. *BMJ* 1984; **288**: 1647–1649.

# Index

The most important entries are in **bold.**